LOCAL AUTHORITIES AND THE SOCIAL DETERMINANTS OF HEALTH

Edited by
Adrian Bonner

Foreword by Rhodri Williams QC

GW00496779

P

First published in Great Britain in 2020 by

Policy Press, an imprint of
Bristol University Press
University of Bristol
1-9 Old Park Hill
Bristol
BS2 8BB
UK
t: +44 (0)117 954 5940
e: bup-info@bristol.ac.uk

Details of international sales and distribution partners are available at
policy.bristoluniversitypress.co.uk

British Library Cataloguing in Publication Data
A catalogue record for this book is available from the British Library

ISBN 978-1-4473-5623-3 hardcover
ISBN 978-1-4473-5624-0 paperback
ISBN 978-1-4473-5625-7 ePdf
ISBN 978-1-4473-5626-4 ePub

Cover design: Andrew Corbett
Front cover image: Let's Imagine (www.letsimagine.co.uk)

Bristol University Press and Policy Press use environmentally responsible
print partners.

Printed in Great Britain by CMP, Poole

To Gill, Adam, Kirsten, Gemma, Jake, Hope,
Thea, Cassian, Freya, Zachary

Contents

Contents

List of figures, tables and boxes

Figures

Tables

Boxes

Notes on contributors

Editor

Adrian Bonner currently focuses his research on the impact of economic austerity policies on health, social care and housing strategies, reflected in the publication *Social Determinants of Health: An Interdisciplinary Approach to Social Inequality and Wellbeing* (Policy Press, 2018). A key theme emerging from this current collaborative work is the recognition of the need for partnerships between the public, private and third sectors in addressing the range complex issues ('wicked issues') related to the social determinants of health. *Local Authorities and Social Determinants of Health*, the second book in the social determinants series, has provided a platform for the development of the Centre for Partnering (CfP), co-founded by Adrian and other contributors in this book, a network of universities working with the public, private and third sectors.

Adrian's early research was concerned with neurobiological aspects of alcohol, as reflected in publications and teaching activities in the 1990s at the Universities of Surrey and Kent. At this time, he became Chairman of the Congress of the European Society for Biomedical Research into Alcohol (Bonner, 2005). *Social Exclusion and the Way Out: An Individual and Community Response to Human Social Dysfunction* (Bonner, 2006) provided the basis for research into *The Seeds of Exclusion* (Bonner et al, 2008), a major report that continues to influence Salvation Army strategic planning. These activities were undertaken while he was a Reader in the Centre for Health Service Studies, University of Kent, and Director of the Addictive Behaviour Group, which facilitated the development of undergraduate and postgraduate teaching and research activities.

From 2010 to 2012, he was seconded from the University of Kent to become the Director of the Institute of Alcohol Studies. This involved participating in the UK government's Responsibility Deal and membership of the European Alcohol Health Forum, an advisory group supporting the work of the European Commission. These insights into UK and European policy development have influenced his current activities, which include interdisciplinary research into health inequalities and membership of HealthWatch and the Joint Mental Health and Wellbeing Clinical Commissioning Group in the

London Borough of Sutton. He is an honorary Professor in the Faculty of Social Sciences, University of Stirling.

Contributors

Isobel Anderson is Chair in Housing Studies and Research Director for the Faculty of Social Sciences at the University of Stirling, Scotland, where she has worked since 1994. She has research, teaching and supervision interests in housing policy and governance; inequality and social exclusion; homelessness; health and wellbeing; and international comparisons. She has held research grants from a range of funding agencies and published widely for scholarly, policy and practice audiences. Isobel was a founder of the European Network for Housing Research working group on Welfare Policy, Homelessness and Social Exclusion, which she jointly coordinated from 2003 to 2013; and in 2015 she joined the network's coordination team for the working group on Housing in Developing Countries. She is also a member of the Women's Homelessness in Europe Network, is on the International Advisory Committee of the *European Journal of Homelessness* and is a board member of Homeless Action Scotland.

Kate Arden is Director of Public Health, Wigan Council. Kate attended Manchester High School and read Medicine at Manchester University. She was awarded the Royal College of General Practitioners Professor Patrick Byrne Prize for General Practice. Kate has an MSc in Epidemiology and Health and Membership of the Faculty of Public Health. She was awarded Fellowship of the Faculty of Public Health 2006. Kate has an Honorary Professorship at Salford University, where she is a co-researcher on the National Institute for Health Research-funded evaluation of Greater Manchester's innovative Communities in Charge of Alcohol programme. Kate is also a Visiting Professor at Chester University. She is Lead Director of Public Health for the Greater Manchester Combined Authority for Health Protection and Emergency Planning & Response, in addition to her substantive post as Director of Public Health for Wigan, where she is also Chief Emergency Planning Officer and the council's Chief Commissioner for Leisure Services. She is currently lead Director of Public Health for the Greater Manchester Health and Social Care Partnership for alcohol and substance misuse harm reduction and health protection transformation, including the development of a multi-agency antimicrobial resistance programme for the conurbation and has led the Greater Manchester health protection sector-led improvement work on which she was asked to attend and give evidence to the House of Commons Health Select Committee as part of their inquiry into public health functions in England, post-2013. Kate co-chairs the Greater Local Health Resilience Partnership and is a member of both the Greater Manchester Resilience Forum and the Greater Manchester High Rise Taskforce set up by Mayor Burnham in response to the Grenfell fire. Since March 2016, Kate has been a trustee of the Royal Society of Public Health, and she was one of the external experts consulted on the Scottish Government's national public health review.

Dave Ayre is the Property Networks Manager for the Chartered Institute of Public Finance and Accountancy (CIPFA) and advises on asset management, partnering and wider property issues throughout the United Kingdom (UK). He is a qualified public service manager with extensive experience in the development, procurement and implementation of innovative public/private partnerships. He has considerable local government experience and has also worked as a consultant to public and private sector organisations delivering public services. He has contributed at a national level to the development of successive government performance management regimes for planning, property and construction through the Planning Officers Society, the Local Government Construction Taskforce and Constructing Excellence, and written guidance on collaboration between public sector organisations. In his contribution, Dave draws on his own experience and sets it against the wider social and political trends governing the relationships between public and private sectors.

Nigel Ball is the Executive Director of the Government Outcomes Lab (GO Lab), which is based in Oxford University's Blavatnik School of Government. Nigel leads the work of engaging government commissioners and decision-makers with evidence about how to effectively commission services for populations with complex social needs. Prior to joining the GO Lab, Nigel was part of the founding team of West London Zone for Children and Young People, where he set up a Collective Impact Bond that leveraged multiple public and private sources of funding to be paid when a partnership of mainly local charities supported at-risk children to achieve better outcomes. Nigel's previous roles include Head of Innovation at Teach First, the leading education charity, and supporting social entrepreneurship in East Africa. He is a qualified teacher, having learnt his craft in a secondary school in Eccles, Manchester. He holds a first-class BA in English and Linguistics from the University of York.

Michael Bennett is a Co-Founder of the Centre for Partnering and the Director of Public Intelligence. Previously, he was a Director of the Society of Local Authority Chief Executives, where he held a number of senior policy roles.

Adam Bonner has an academic background in Human Resource Management at the University of Kent. He has worked professionally and voluntarily with regional and national youth organisations in the UK for 20 years. This work involved creating new community-funded and volunteering programmes. In 2007, he became regional and then national community development manager for the Shaftesbury Society, developing community initiatives for young people and focusing on those in deprived communities. Following the merger of the Shaftesbury Society with John Grooms to create the newly branded Livability 2007, he became Director for Community and Communications and then in 2013 became Executive Director of Public Engagement. In 2018, he became Director of the Youth United Foundation, an umbrella organisation working with 11 uniformed groups, including Scouts and Guides, to engage with young people on the margins of society. In 2019, he was the founder and director of a community interest company, Sutton Community Dance.

Harry Burns graduated in medicine from Glasgow University in 1974. He trained in surgery and became a consultant surgeon in the University Department of Surgery at the Royal Infirmary in Glasgow. Working with patients in the east end of Glasgow gave him an insight into the complex interrelationships between social and economic status and illness. He completed an MA in Public Health in 1990 and shortly afterwards was appointed Medical Director of The Royal Infirmary. In 1994, he became Director of Public Health for Greater Glasgow Health Board and he continued research into the social determinants of health. In 2005, he became Chief Medical Officer for Scotland. His responsibilities included public health policy, health protection and, for a time, sport. He was knighted in 2011, and in April 2014 became Professor of Global Public Health at Strathclyde University, where he continues to research how societies create wellness.

Tony Chasteauneuf has an MA in Voluntary Administration from London South Bank University and an Honours degree from Durham University. He has been involved in the development and strategic management of homelessness services, community development projects, community services, not-for-profit management and the faith sector in the UK and Australia. Currently, he is the Regional Specialist for Community Services (Yorkshire and the North East of England), The Salvation Army.

Keith Clements is a researcher and policy expert focussing on children's health and social care services in England. Over the course of his career he has led and contributed to the development of a number of high-impact reports exploring the effects of inequalities on children and young people. This includes leading research on behalf of the All Party Parliamentary Group for Children on children's social care and on behalf of the National Children's Bureau on the impact of health inequalities in the early years. His work has also focussed on joint working between public sector and voluntary organisations to meet the needs of vulnerable children. Keith is currently Senior Researcher at the National Children's Bureau. He has previously worked for the Council for Disabled Children and Ambitious About Autism.

Anna Coleman is Senior Research Fellow in the Health Organisation, Policy and Economics research group at the University of Manchester. She is a skilled policy researcher, having extensive experience over many years researching into and publishing on health and care policy, partnership working and commissioning. She investigated the implementation of health scrutiny for her PhD (2003–6) and has most recently been looking at new models of care, integration and place-based planning in health and care – Vanguards, integrated care systems and Greater Manchester health and social care devolution. Previously, Anna worked in policy and research within local government and is recognised beyond the university as an expert in the increasingly important intersection between health policy and local government, having been invited to speak at an international conference on municipalities and health, provided written evidence to Health Select Committees and given personal advice to a member of the House of Lords and to external organisations.

Mark Cook is partner at Anthony Collins Solicitors, having advised on procurement and public–private partnerships for 30 years. He is the lawyer who has most contributed to the inclusion of community benefits at the core of public contracts in the UK. He contributed to the drafting of the Public Services (Social Value) Act 2012 and the content of the Procurement Reform (Scotland) Act 2014. He also contributed to the Can Do Toolkits in Wales. He is company secretary to catalytic do-tank Collaborate, and he is deeply committed to creating alternatives to the commissioner– contractor dynamic.

Penny Cook is Professor of Public Health and leads a research group, Equity, Health and Wellbeing at the University of Salford. She has attracted £4 million in research funding in her career to date, investigating health impacts of alcohol and tobacco as well as research into sedentary behaviour, physical activity and the health and wellbeing benefits of green space. Current projects include investigating an asset-based community development intervention, whereby members of a community can support each other with alcohol advice (funded by the National Institute for Health Research). Penny also researches on foetal alcohol spectrum disorders (FASD). She is currently developing a parenting intervention for families affected by FASD (funded by the Medical Research Council) and is leading the first UK study into their prevalence. Penny is a co-investigator on the National Environment Research Council-funded Green Infrastructure and the Health and Wellbeing Influences on an Ageing Population project. She also teaches on the MSc in Public Health.

Keith Cunliffe is the Deputy Leader of Wigan Council and has had the Portfolio for Health and Adult Social Care since 2008. He is Joint Chair of the Wigan Health and Wellbeing Board. Keith is a member peer at the Local Government Association, providing peer review, mentoring and workshops to a number of local authorities. He is also the national Vice-Chair of the Industrial Communities Alliance.

Jeanelle de Gruchy is President of the Association of Directors of Public Health and Director of Population Health, Tameside Metropolitan Borough Council. Formerly, Jeanelle was Director for Public Health for Haringey, and public health lead on health inequalities and public mental health, becoming director for Haringey Clinical Commissioning Group (CCG) in 2010.

Paul Dennett was elected Salford City Mayor in May 2016. Before then, Paul served as a local councillor in the Langworthy ward of the city, and held the workforce and equalities portfolio on the city council's cabinet. Being born in Warrington into a working-class family had a significant impact on Paul's politics and life-long appreciation for the public sector, health care, education and the emergency services. He worked in customer services at a BT call centre and, after completing his degree, lectured in Business at

Manchester Metropolitan Business School. Paul is currently also the Greater Manchester Combined Authority portfolio lead for housing, planning and homelessness.

Ruth Dombey has been the Leader of the London Borough of Sutton and has chaired its Health and Wellbeing Board since 2012. She is a trained facilitator for the Local Government Association, specialising in courses for councillors and general practitioners who chair health and wellbeing boards. She is also one of the Vice-Chairs of London Councils and Deputy Leader of the Liberal Democrat group on the Local Government Association.

Catherine Farrell is based in Cardiff Business School and her research interests are in the areas of public management and governance. She has published widely on school governance and the role of public boards in public service improvement. She is currently researching different models of public board governance including the stakeholder, elected, appointed and skills-based approaches in a range of different services, including the fire and rescue service. She has undertaken an evidence review of aspects of the Well-Being of Future Generations Act and public services. Her work has been published in journals including *Public Administration*, *Policy and Politics*, *Local Government Studies* and *Human Relations*.

Chris Fox is Professor of Evaluation and Policy Analysis at Manchester Metropolitan University where he is also Director of the Policy Evaluation and Research Unit and co-lead of Metropolis – an academic-led think tank. Chris is involved in a wide range of evaluation and research projects in a number of policy areas, including criminal justice, social investment and welfare reform. He is particularly interested in the role of co-design in public sector reform.

Max French is a lecturer in Systems Leadership at Newcastle Business School, Northumbria University, and a Visiting Fellow at the Open Lab, Newcastle University. His research focusses on two areas of practice. Firstly, he studies the implications of complexity and complexity-informed practice for public administration and non-profit management, centring on the development of new methods, models and approaches. Secondly, he researches the use of action-oriented approaches to social research as a means to improve research relevance.

Gillian Gibson is Director of Public Health, Sunderland. She has lived in Sunderland for most of her life and worked in the National Health Service (NHS) from 1984 until 2013, when responsibility for public health transferred to local government. She is a registered public health specialist and has been a consultant in public health in Sunderland since 2011, taking responsibility for the integration of public health services. She became Acting Director of Public Health in April 2015.

Tim Gilling is a Director at the Centre for Public Scrutiny (CfPS), the leading UK governance and scrutiny organisation. He delivers national programmes in England for major clients such as the Department of Health and Social Care, NHS England, Public Health England and the Care Quality Commission. Tim also has experience of local government and health issues in Scotland and Wales. He works with councils and health bodies around integration and service reconfiguration and strengthening relationships between health bodies and council scrutiny. He recently published a guide for council scrutiny committees to ask about social value policy and outcomes. As well as his public policy, local government and healthcare experience, Tim also works with the private sector, currently in construction and energy. He also brings practical experience of governance in the education and charitable sectors. He is a member of the UK Administrative Justice Council and a Fellow of the Royal Society of Arts.

Peter Hain has led a colourful life. The child of South African parents who were jailed, banned and forced into exile during the freedom struggle, in 1969 and 1970 he led anti-apartheid campaigns to stop all-white South African sports tours. MP for Neath from 1991 to 2015 and a Privy Councillor, Peter served in the UK Government for 12 years, seven of these in the Cabinet. He negotiated the 2007 settlement to end the conflict in Northern Ireland and was a Foreign Minister with successive responsibilities for Africa, the Middle East and Europe. He has chaired the United Nations Security Council and negotiated international treaties. He was also Secretary of State for Work and Pensions, Secretary of State for Wales, Leader of the House of Commons and Energy Minister. His concise and readable biography *Mandela His Essential Life* was published in 2018, his memoirs *Outside In* in 2012 and his co-authored *Pitch Battles: Protest, Prejudice and Play* in May 2020. He has written or edited 21 books, and has also appeared regularly on television and radio and written for most UK newspapers.

Melissa Hawkins is currently a researcher at Newcastle University Business School, and is conducting action research into developing complexity-informed practice in public and third-sector organisations. Research interests have been influenced by time spent as a classroom teacher, and they are focused upon how complexity theory can be used to critically analyse current performance management practices, and how action research can be utilised as a methodology for innovating in complex conditions.

David J. Hunter is Professor of Health Policy and Management, Institute of Health and Society, Newcastle University. David graduated in political science from Edinburgh University. His academic career spans over 40 years, during which he has researched complex health systems, with a focus on how health policy is formed and implemented. Between 1999 and July 2017, David was Director of the Centre for Public Policy and Health at Durham University. The centre was designated a World Health Organization Collaborating Centre in Complex Health Systems Research, Knowledge and Action in 2014. In August 2017, he transferred to the Institute of Health & Society, Newcastle University, and became an Emeritus Professor in August 2018. Recent former positions include being a non-executive director of the National Institute of Health and Care Excellence (2008–16); an Appointed Governor of South Tees Hospitals NHS Foundation Trust (2009–17); and a special advisor to the UK Parliamentary Health Committee. He is an honorary member of the UK Faculty of Public Health and Fellow of the Royal College of Physicians (Edinburgh).

Edward Kunonga is currently a consultant in public health working for Tees, Esk and Wear Valleys Mental Health NHS Foundation Trust and County Durham and Darlington Acute NHS Foundation Trust. Edward spent nine years as the Director of Public Health and Public Protection for Middlesbrough Council, and during the last three years of that tenure he was the joint director of public health across Middlesbrough and Redcar and Cleveland Borough Councils (the first joint public health service in the North-East). As part of this arrangement, Edward was instrumental in the development of the joint health and wellbeing board across these two local authorities, chief officer for emergency preparedness and response for the council and took a regional lead role for public mental health. Edward has an MSc in Epidemiology from the London School of Hygiene and Tropical Medicine, an MBA from Leicester University and a Diploma in Epidemiology and Public Health from the Faculty of Public Health of the Royal College of Physicians UK. He also has a diploma in Lifestyle Medicine and is a certified lifestyle medicine practitioner. He was awarded Fellowship of the Faculty of Public Health 2011. Edward has Honorary Professorship at Teesside University and contributes to a wide range of teaching and research activities.

Jennifer Law is an expert on local government, particularly in relation to public service improvement, performance measurement and strategy. She has published widely in these areas and has also provided advice and consultancy to organisations including Public Health Wales, Welsh Government, CIPFA, as well as a number of local authorities and other public bodies. Her most recent work has been for Public Health Wales and has focused on the enablers and barriers of the Well-being of Future Generations Act and on the equality implications of the Act.

Toby Lowe is a senior lecturer in Newcastle Business School at Northumbria University, working on partnerships to achieve social change. This work includes research and collaborative publications in the funding of complex ecologies. Previously, he was Chief Executive of Helix Arts, and he works with Collaborate to support funders and help senior commissioners respond to complexity.

Jim McManus is Vice-President, Association of Directors of Public Health and Director of Public Health, Hertfordshire County Council, is a chartered Psychologist, Chartered Scientist and public health specialist.

Gayle Munro is Head of Research and Evidence at the National Children's Bureau, London. Gayle's doctoral work (Geography, University College London) explored the transnational experiences of migrants from the former Yugoslavia to Britain. Gayle has worked in the voluntary sector for more than 20 years and has held research and teaching positions at The Salvation Army (London), the Organisation for Security and Cooperation in Europe (Bosnia & Herzegovina), the European Centre for Minority Issues (Germany), Lemos & Crane (London) and Sichuan University (China).

Alison Navarro has 30 years' experience of working with local communities, the voluntary and community sector, partnership bodies and public sector agencies. Her first role was a Community Development Officer within the City Challenge Regeneration

Programmes in Liverpool and then later as a Programme Manager for an inner city Single Regeneration Budget Programme in Liverpool. As a Partnership Manager, Alison supported the development of local strategic partnerships and community strategies. In the early 2000s, she set up her own training and consultancy firm where she worked with a range of people and organisations, all of her work being linked to her passions for social justice. In later years, Alison has been involved in the Infrastructure movement, and she spent some time at Community Links Bromley before becoming the chief executive officer at Community Action Sutton in 2016.

Chris O'Leary is a public policy specialist and Deputy Director of the Policy Evaluation and Research Unit at Manchester Metropolitan University. He has written and commented on issues around commissioning and procurement, particularly on the barriers faced by local charities and small businesses. His empirical research focuses on social innovation, particularly where different parts of social provision interact. Much of his published research is around housing/homelessness and its interaction with health and social care, and the criminal justice system

Dean Pallant is Secretary for Communications (The Salvation Army UK and Republic of Ireland), previously Director of The Salvation Army's International Social Justice Commission-based in New York City. His doctoral studies at King's College London resulted in the publication of his first book, *Keeping Faith in Faith-Based Organisations*, in 2012. Dean was a founding member and director of the Joint Learning Initiative on Faith and Local Communities.

Catherine Parker is a consultant in public health and has lived and worked in the North-East all her life. Her career in health started in 2003 as part of the NHS graduate management programme, where a passion for public health was quickly established. Catherine has held a variety of roles in health and public health commissioning and strategic management working at local and regional to national level on health improvement and inequalities. She is a registered public health specialist since and Consultant since 2018.

Glenda Roberts currently works for Avante Care and Support as Head of Care Homes – Kent, assisting with reviewing and directing all aspects of the organisation's work in a portfolio of care homes. Prior to her current position, she was Deputy Director of Older People's

Service for The Salvation Army. She was Master's educated at the University of Stirling, with a specific interest in dementia studies, and has been a qualified Registered Adult Nurse since 2002, with 18 years of experience supporting young adults with complex needs and older adults in health and social care settings in both the third sector and private sector.

Jacquie Russell is the Assistant Director Policy and Performance at Salford City Council, a post she has held since 2012. In this role, Jacquie has worked with colleagues across the city council and Salford CCG to successfully create integrated funding, governance and joint working arrangements for health and care in the city, Jacquie has also led work to bring together the city's Tackling Poverty and Inequality Strategy. Before working in Salford, Jacquie held posts in Manchester City Council, Government Office for the North West and the Home Office. Before then, she held various policy positions in the Australian civil service.

Jolanta Shields has recently submitted her PhD in the School of Social Sciences at the University of Manchester. Her research, funded by the Economic and Social Research Council (ESRC) and a Manchester President's Doctoral Scholar Award, concerns the role of new providers of health care services, Community Interest Companies, in the NHS. During her PhD, the ESRC funded an internship at CfPS where Jolanta published *Governance of Sustainability and Transformation Plans*. She was a researcher for the report 'A Shared Responsibility: Tackling Inequalities in Health Across Greater Manchester', commissioned by the Oglesby Trust. Prior to academia, Jolanta had a successful career in local government working for the Third Sector and Policy Team at Manchester City Council.

Richard Simmons is a senior lecturer in Public and Social Policy and Co-Director of the Mutuality Research Programme at the University of Stirling. Over the last decade or so, he has led an extensive programme of research on voice and cooperation in public policy. This includes four studies funded by the ESRC/Arts and Humanities Research Council, a Single Regeneration Budget-funded study and work for the NHS, Scottish Executive, National Consumer Council, Carnegie Trust, the Organisation for Economic Co-operation and Development, World Bank, Co-operatives UK, Nesta and the Care Inspectorate. He is currently working on a European Union (EU) Horizon 2020 project, working with local municipal governments and schools to improve the quality of primary school meals through better procurement. He writes widely on these issues for academic, policy and practitioner audiences. His book, *The Consumer in Public Services* is published by the Policy Press. As well as a series of journal articles in high-quality international journals such as *Social Policy and Administration, Policy and Politics, Annals of Public and Co-operative Economics* and *Public Policy and Administration*, Richard has written a number of policy-oriented publications and professional journal articles for a practitioner audience. His research interests are broadly in the field of user voice, the governance, delivery and innovation of public services and the role of mutuality and cooperation in public policy. The Mutuality Research Programme has acquired an international reputation as a centre of excellence for research, knowledge exchange and consultancy on these issues.

Richard Smith has enjoyed various senior management positions in both public and private sectors. He has developed a variety of commercial skills within the defence sector and legal skills, qualifying as a barrister in 1978. In the second phase of his career, he founded Public Sector Plc, a private sector organisation utilising a new and innovative legal framework based on a cultural relationship between partners forming in advance of formal legal commitments. His work has been based on the principles of 'insourcing', which was the notion of the market strengthening the public sector not replacing it. His work in the public/private partnering field formed part of the Public Sector Plc Government Pilot Partnership Network established to consider Best Value and its introduction. This opportunity came about at the same time as he presented evidence to a House of Commons Select Committee. Currently he is in discussions with a number of universities to establish the CfP to undertake research programmes in this partnering field and to consider the positive impact it can have on delivering socio-economic benefits to local communities, particularly in the field of health. This work builds upon his experience of setting up the Local Government Council Consortium Group, which was a group of 22 councils that delivered a 'Commission' Report containing 11 recommendations on unlocking additional value from local authority property estates. Richard is an Honorary Professor at the University of Stirling and Chairman of CfP.

Steve Thomas has over 30 years of experience working within local government. In 2004, he became Chief Executive of the Welsh Local Government Association, the representative body of the 22 Welsh councils. Here he also co-developed with Public Health Wales the Cymru Well Wales partnerships aimed at tackling key determinants of ill health. Having retired from this role, Steve now lectures in the Faculty of Business and Society at the University of South Wales within the fields of strategy, leadership and organisational change.

Tony Thornton is Regional Manager, Homelessness Services Unit (HSU) North-East Region, The Salvation Army. Educated and living in Darlington, County Durham, he has worked for The Salvation Army since 1993: he was a centre manager for over eight years, working with vulnerable homeless adults and managing a staff team of 21. He was awarded an MBE in 2008 for services to Homelessness. He then joined The Salvation Army Housing Association (SAHA), which, working as an Independent Quality Inspectorate, inspected all SAHA and Salvation Army services. He remained with SAHA for three years before joining The Salvation Army again as the Assistant Regional Manager HSU North East, and he is now the Regional Manager – having had in total five years' experience of regional management, at the same time gaining a Master of Science in Housing Studies in 2017 from Stirling University.

Lord Graham Tope CBE was a councillor in the London Borough of Sutton for 40 years until 2014 and leader of that council for 13 years. He was a member of the London Assembly from 2000 to 2008 and leader of the five-member Liberal Democrat Group for six of those years. He was a UK delegate to the EU Committee of the Regions (the voice of regional and local government in the EU decision-making process) for 20 years, leading its European Liberal Group for part of that time. Graham was Liberal MP for Sutton & Cheam from 1972 to 1974 and was made a life peer in 1994. He has been Liberal Democrat Education spokesperson in the Lords and was co-chair of the Lib Dem Communities & Local Government Parliamentary Committee throughout the five years of the Coalition government. He is Co-President of London Councils.

Acknowledgements

I wish to extend my thanks to those who have contributed to insights and contacts with front-line services and national and local management of community resources, both in the publication of this volume and in the first volume of this series, *Social Determinants of Health: An Interdisciplinary Approach to Social Inequality and Wellbeing* (Policy Press, 2018).

I would particularly like to acknowledge the continued support of the following:

Professor Alison Bowes, Dean of the Faculty of Social Sciences, and other colleagues at the University of Stirling who continue to provide an academic base that is well grounded in research for the public good.

Commissioner Anthony Cotterill, Lt-Col. Drew McCombe, and Lt-Col. (Dr) Dean Pallant senior leaders of The Salvation Army, and Nick Redmore, Director of the Research and Development Unit, have supported this exploration of the changing socio-economic environment in which this world-wide organisation continues to support people at the margins of the community.

I am indebted to Professor Richard Smith for his considerable experience and insight into the legal profession and its role in changing the culture of procurement and commissioning. This book has provided an opportunity to engage with Richard and colleagues in establishing the Centre for Partnering.

I do not take for granted the support of my wife, Gill, and her insight into children and families and their experience of the educational system, as well as her continued discussion and proofreading of this and other publications.

Finally, I must thank Laura Vickers-Randell, Amelia Watts Jones, Elizabeth Stone and the editorial team at Policy Press for their helpful and professional support in preparing this publication.

Foreword

Rhodri Williams QC

The General Election on 12 December 2019 resulted in a Conservative government that, with a majority of 80, was mandated to 'Get Brexit Done'. The socio-economic background to the Referendum result, in 2016, to leave the European Union (EU), has its origins in the 19th century. The industrial revolution contributed to Britain becoming a wealthy colonial power. The dark side to this economic growth included slavery, exploitation of working people and poor health for those who stoked the fires of the 'dark satanic mills'. The extremes of wealth and social deprivation had political consequences, resulting in the emergence of trade unions and origins of the welfare state. The political drivers resulting in the United Kingdom (UK) leaving the EU in 2020 include a significant response from people living in traditional labour-supporting communities, particularly in South Wales and the northern parts of England. People voting to leave the EU have experienced the outcomes of authority budgets undermining welfare support, pressures on the National Health Service (NHS) and social care and concerns about threats, real or imagined, to employment owing to the free movement of people within the EU. Feelings of being left out of the economic growth of the UK, the increasing gaps between socially deprived and those better off, and the lack of personal actualisation is noted by Burns in Part I, Chapter 1, as a key determinant of the 'deaths of despair' and decreasing life expectancy.

The growing concern about the links between social conditions and the state of public health led to the emergence of modern local government in the UK. In recent years, a greater understanding that wellbeing of people is an important determinant of the economic prosperity is demonstrated by the 'wellbeing' budget being introduced by the New Zealand Government, reported in *The Guardian*, 30 May 2019.

In 1945, Clement Attlee's Labour government was elected at a time of severe post-war austerity. It marked the start of a new social-democratic consensus that was to develop over 30 years under successive governments. The election of Margaret Thatcher's Conservative government in 1979 up-ended this post-war consensus. The free market think tanks of the Adam Smith Institute, the Institute for Economic Affairs and the Centre for Policy Studies influenced the government to embark on a programme of wholesale privatisation. The Local Government Acts of 1988 and 1992 introduced and extended compulsory competitive tendering (CCT). Services such as waste collection, construction, grounds maintenance and catering were some of the first to be affected. This was later to be extended to white collar architectural and civil engineering design services towards the end of the John Major Conservative government. Although an enthusiastic proponent of CCT, the Major government was keen to portray a less ideological approach to public services than its predecessor.

The relationship of public and private sectors in the UK and the commissioning, procurement and development of public private partnerships has been driven by the prevailing political and economic environment. In 1992, the Major government introduced the Private Finance Initiative (PFI) and branded it as a new form of public–private partnership. The New Labour government of Tony Blair embarked on an ambitious programme of new hospitals, schools and highways infrastructure funded by PFI. While the Major government signed 21 PFI deals, by the end of Blair's term as prime minister in 2007, 850 had been signed.

The health and wellbeing of people is linked with the economic status of the country. This book presents the social determinants of health rainbow model (Dahlgren and Whitehead, 1991) perspective on local authorities and their changing approaches to procurement and commissioning. While this model of health and wellbeing, promoted by the World Health Organization, has influenced the development of health systems globally, only recently has local government begun to adopt this approach in integrated planning. Centralisation, delegation, devolution and privatisation have been adopted by successive governments in addressing growing demands across the health and social care system. Chapters from a number of local authorities (LAs) in Part II of this book indicate a cultural change in recognition that social determinants and 'health in place' should underpin responses to joint needs assessments. The chapters in Part II provide an insight into the impact of austerity on local authority budgets and individual LAs' responses to protect the wellbeing of their communities. This response is influenced by geo-sociopolitical circumstances, such as local opportunities for employment (particularly in the North-East, Chapter 7), the extent of devolution (for example, so-called 'devo max' in the North-West, Chapters 5, 8) and the culture of commissioning.

The Localism Act and the Care Act, conceived by the Coalition government (2010–15) have brought a major cultural shift in thinking and planning. These were well-intentioned legislative changes but LAs, with decreasing funding from Central government, have greater responsibilities for their communities undermined by austerity budgeting. In searching for innovative approaches to dealing with the rise in the diseases of modern society, such as obesity and Type 2 diabetes, this wider view of health and wellbeing has promoted prevention and the embedding of public health strategies in all policies. LAs are seen to be uniquely positioned to facilitate this transformation, as they are close to local communities and have an understanding and responsibility for issues such as environment.

Observations that life expectancy in the current century is stalling and health inequalities are rising, are concerning and have political implications with the gap in life expectancy between the richest and poorest areas of England and Wales widening over the past decade. Harry Burns, in Chapter 1, suggests that public policies fail as a result of attempts in the 1980s to make public services 'more business like'. New Public Management approaches, adopted by the NHS, have focused on customer service, financial control, value for money and increasing efficiency. 'Senior managers drive change by setting targets and indicators and performance monitoring. The wellbeing of the community, being difficult to conceptualise, rarely features in strategic plans or managers' objectives' (Burns, Chapter 1).

In Part III, the changing responses of LAs are reviewed. Public services are commissioned and delivered, often on the basis of a hard-lined demarcation between the responsibilities of council and contractor, when in fact if wellbeing is to be truly embraced, as suggested by Mark Cook, introducing Part III, a much more nuanced dynamic has to exist. This dynamic needs to take account of culture and competence on all sides: 'The connection between Best Value and wellbeing is one that is not well understood in central and local government.' The Wigan Deal (Part II, Chapter 8) is an example of a consultative approach in which cultural changes in public attitude and behaviour complement financial gains and cost savings in the council budget. As with the examples from other local authorities, place-based policies and working with local communities appear to provide a socio economic and political context to developing and supporting healthy communities.

CCT provided an opportunity to take over and run public services, but culture and competence would often be inappropriate to achieve outcomes necessary to address the needs. The inadequacy of the market came to be fully recognised with the externalisation process introduced in 1994 to 1995. It has become very apparent that if future partnering is to be effective then there must be more emphasis on social, economic and community wellbeing issues being more effectively combined with the commercial and profit motive.

To do this, there must be more time to have joint dialogue within a flexible legal framework. If there can be more use of benchmarking for comparison of proposals and fewer automatic assumptions that tendering will always deliver best results, then this could be advantageous.

Richard Smith, a barrister by training, has considerable experience working within the public and private sectors in the local government, demonstrates in Chapter 10 that to overcome the different cultures and environments, time is required to jointly design project opportunities. This need not preclude competition and, if organised properly, enhances the outcomes financially and qualitatively for both partners.

EU law, particularly the EU treaty and the Procurement Directive 2014/24/EU, currently underpins the broad terms under which public procurement and competitive tendering operate in the UK; see Chapter 9. The rules have been transposed into national law as the Public Contracts Regulations 2015 by the UK's governments, establishing how public authorities, including health and social care commissioners, purchase goods, works and services.

Existing domestic legislation, such as the Health and Social Care Act 2012 and the NHS (Procurement, Patient Choice and Competition) Regulations 2013 in England, currently enshrines effectively the same rules as EU law. These laws, for example, prohibit NHS England or clinical commissioning groups (CCGs) from favouring a single provider and gave powers to the regulator Monitor, and its successor NHS Improvement, to enforce competition rules on NHS trusts.

The collapse of giant outsourcer Carillion in January 2018 was one of the highest-profile failures of the traditional outsourcing model. Carillion was a major strategic supplier to the UK public sector, its work ranging from building roads and hospitals to providing school meals and defence accommodation. It collapsed in January 2018 with some 420 public sector contracts. The Local Government Association estimated that 30 councils and 220 schools were directly affected. It had around 43,000 employees, including 19,000 in the UK. Many more people were employed in its extensive supply chains. Thousands of people lost their jobs. Carillion left a pension liability of around £2.6 billion.

The complex nature of public service requires public servants to be properly equipped with new, 'complexity-informed tools', as described by Toby Lowe, Max French and Melissa Hawkins in

Part III, Chapter 13. The task of creating positive social outcomes (such as improved wellbeing, increased employment or reduced crime) in complex environments as seen, in this chapter through the lens of public sector performance measurement and management (PSPMM), and how this has evolved towards increased complexity by moving from an output (activity) to an outcome (results) focus. Outcome commissioning is being used by an increasing number of local authorities, as noted in Part II, Chapter 6.

The original local government aims, as a first-line defence thrown up by the community against poverty, sickness, ignorance, isolation, mental derangement and social maladjustment, are severely challenged by severe cutbacks, which are causing them to target reductions in discretionary services in order to provide relative protection for statutory and more acute services. Improvements in public health during recent years resulted from heavy investment in alleviating adverse social conditions for children. The last ten years have seen a rapid withdrawal from this and other community assets, such as funding for youth clubs by local authorities: see Part IV, Chapters 15 and 16.

Michael Bennett, in Part V, Chapter 18, writes that although sustainability is cast as fulfilling legal obligations, rather than creating outcomes acceptable or desirable to society, there is ongoing rationing, with scarce resources being focused on a narrower group of people with highest care needs at the expense of prevention and wider social benefits. This is counter-intuitive to the social model of health, where there is an 'interconnectedness and interdependence of socio-economic, cultural, environmental, living and working conditions, social and community networks, and lifestyle choices that contribute to a person's health and well-being' (Bonner, 2018: xxi).

If we think about the future of partnering and overcoming the considerable culture differences that exist between public, private and voluntary sectors, then we must address the need to forge stronger relationships before entering into contractual commitment. A procurement regime that does not provide sufficient opportunity to build trust and transparency between potential partners at the outset risks a stiff inflexible relationship driven by contractual specification and tendering assumptions obtained during an expensive exercise in bidding for contracts.

The future opportunity that a post-Brexit environment offers is a chance to rewrite rules and regulations, not superimpose more changes and amendments on the existing regime. Let us put relationships first and contracts second!

Note

Rhodri Williams QC is a barrister specialising in EU law, local government law, public and administrative law. He deals with cases involving local and regional government, including advising the Welsh Government and other government departments and local authorities. He has represented the UK Government on several occasions before the Court of Justice of the EU in Luxembourg.

References

Bonner, A. (ed) (2018) *Social Determinants of Health: An Interdisciplinary Approach to Social Inequality and Wellbeing*, Bristol: Policy Press.
New Zealand Government (2020) 'New Zealand "wellbeing" budget promises billions to care for most vulnerable',
The Guardian, 30 May 2019. Available from: https://www.theguardian.com/world/2019/may/30/new-zealand-wellbeing-budget-jacinda-ardern-unveils-billions-to-care-for-most-vulnerable [Accessed 12 May 2020].

Summary

This book addresses the key issues facing local authorities as they provide services and support their local populations.

Although the municipal corporations in the 19th century had responsibility for the community, populations were stratified, with those in the lower levels not well supported. The generation of wealth and the influence of socialist and liberal policies in the 20th century led to a cultural change in which respect and help for individuals was addressed by the setting up of the welfare state and the National Health Service.

With continued cultural and political change, expectations of support for the individual from the state have risen. We are now faced with the question as to who is responsible for the health and wellbeing of individuals and their communities. The simple answer could lie in the appropriate and fair allocation of resources by the locally elected members of councils that commission services. However, our changing understanding of the social determinants of health, regional differences in wealth and opportunities, and the defence of human rights should promote a fundamental rethinking of local approaches to health and wellbeing.

This book explores the challenges and responses of local authorities to the changing sociopolitical landscape by means of five sections addressing: Health, social care and community wellbeing; The role of local authorities in promoting health and wellbeing in the community; Local authority commissioning; The third sector; and Socio-economic political perspectives.

This interdisciplinary approach is being captured by a number of universities in discussion, collaborating in this publication, to promote relationship-building and the establishment of a Centre for Partnering (CfP); see Part IV, Chapter 10. This is a new initiative that is considering partnership and the future delivery of public services. Among the aims of the CfP are consideration of the various issues raised in this book, particularly as they relate to place-based services, and how collaborative economies could assist in the establishment of future sustainable economic models. This book raises 'wicked issues' within the context of the social determinants of health. The aim of the CfP, through universities working together, and collaborating with local authorities and the third sector, will be to consider how best to translate the issues and experiences encountered by the authors into positive and practical outcomes.

Introduction:
Key sociopolitical changes affecting the health and wellbeing of people

Adrian Bonner

Following on from *Social Determinants of Health: An Interdisciplinary Perspective on Social Inequality and Wellbeing* (Bonner, 2018b), this volume provides a unique insight into the relationship between health and housing, regional disparities and responses across England, Wales and Scotland in the provision of health and social care and local authority commissioning. While references to the health care system will be found in the book, its primary focus is on health as defined in the Constitution of the World Health Organization (WHO), which was adopted by the WHO in 1946 and has not been amended since 1948: 'Health is a state of complete physical, mental and social well-being and not merely the absence of disease and infirmity' (Anon, 1946).

The cultural changes leading to the development of the welfare state and contemporary system transformations are reviewed using examples of innovative approaches which involve shared responsibilities between statutory, third sector, community organisations and the private sector.

Cameron's Big Society (Anon, 2015a) was launched two weeks after the formation of the Coalition government following the general election of 6 May 2010. The key aims of the policy were, to increase 'community empowerment' by decentralisation with more power devolved to local councils and neighbourhoods; to promote 'social action' by encouraging people to play a more active role in communities; and 'opening up public services' by enabling charities, cooperatives social enterprises, and also private companies to compete in the delivery of public services.

> Because we believe that a stronger society will solve our problems more effectively than big government has or ever will, we want the state to as act an instrument for helping to create a strong society … Our alternative to big government is the Big Society. (Cameron, 2009)

Cameron's Big Society can be traced back to Tony Blair's Third Way, which aimed to unlock potential within society, promoting social capital to provide added value to the state and financial markets. Gordon Brown promised to 'empower communities and citizens and ensure that power is more fairly distributed across the whole of society'. A number of strategies have been launched and relaunched by the main political parties. However, a three-year review, by Civil Exchange (Anon, 2015b) concluded that 'social action' had not increased, communities have not been empowered and the Big Society has not reached those most in need. In 2019, volunteering within the third sector is thriving, as noted in Part IV; but it was a fallacy of the Third Way and the Big Society that gaps in resources due to downsizing of the welfare state could be filled by volunteers. Austerity policies, resulting from the global economic recession of 2008, and some would say political ideology, have resulted in family budgets being significantly squeezed, and social mobility has decreased. Welfare reform and shortages in the housing market, financial uncertainty due to the protracted negotiations relating to the United Kingdom (UK) leaving the European Union (EU), all provide challenges to local authorities, whose elected members are faced with increasing problems owing to diminishing funds from central government. Many local councils have cut and reduced services, impacting on health and wellbeing; this has the paradoxical effect of increasing acute health costs in the long term. Community services such as bus services, clubs for young people and safety nets such as children's centres impact on health directly, as mobility, social interaction and family support are affected. Indirect effects result from the loss of self-esteem and other psychological factors, as highlighted in the Marmot Review (Marmot, 2010).

Recent policy developments have to a large extent been based on amplifying social capital (human relationships and networks), in addition to human capital (skills and knowledge of individuals, and workforce shaping). However, a pivotal resource in developing communities is wealth and its distribution. The control of financial resources is central to past and current support for people and their communities. There have been major changes in the control of financial capital from the 19th to the 21st centuries.

Municipalisation and social reform

The Municipal Corporations Act (1835) led to the establishment of elected town councils. Welfare provision was at the heart of these councils, with 'municipal socialism' inspiring work for the common good, significantly influenced by social reformers including Joseph Rowntree (1836–1925), Lord Shaftesbury (1811–51), Charles Booth

(1840–1916), William Booth (1829–1912) and others (Bonner, 2006). The actions of these social reformers and philanthropists laid the foundations of the third sector; see Part IV. The Beacon Project, from the Centre for Philanthropy at the University of Kent (Breeze, 2019), provides helpful insights into the historical and contemporary importance of philanthropy, and was based around ongoing work into third sector activity.

Local council activity led to the building of houses and hospitals, the creation of parks, museums, libraries and swimming pools, and welfare provision. Municipalisation included the purchase of gas, electricity, water and tramway systems, as it seemed logical that a local authority should ensure the availability of essential services for its residents. The benefits of affordable prices for these services, their safety and the reinvesting of income into further improvements was evident: 'by 1901, one reformer looked forward to the time when joy will be considered as much a necessity in a city as anything else. In that time citizens, well convinced that all the prime necessities of life must be municipalised' (Anon, 2015b). In 1930, a Member of Parliament observed that 'a young person today lives in a municipal house, and he washes himself in municipal water. He rides a municipal tram or omnibus, and I have no doubt that before long he will be riding in a municipal aeroplane. He walks on a municipal road; he is educated in a municipal school. He reads in a municipal library and he has his sport on a municipal recreation ground. When he is ill he is doctored by a municipal hospital and when he dies he is buried in a municipal cemetery...' (Anon, 2015b). The management of water supplies, sewage systems, air quality, and the physical and social environment are key contributors to public health, as reviewed in Chapter 2.

The origins of local authorities

In the mid- to late 20th century, municipalisation gave way to centralised government, which subverted the autonomy of local authorities. Council-owned water, electricity, water assets were nationalised in 1945. Municipal hospitals were nationalised within the National Health Service (NHS) and gradually local authority powers were reduced, in the control of local assets, to agencies of the centralised welfare state. By 2019, the UK is the most centralised country in the Western world, with 91 pence in every pound controlled and allocated by the Westminster Parliament (Crewe, 2016). The importance of local authorities in promoting health in the community is highlighted by Michael Bennett in Chapter 18.

Historical and political perspectives on the public concern and understanding of the UK health care system were demonstrated at the UK General Election in 2015, when funding for the (NHS) was one of the key issues highlighted by the main political parties. In opinion polls, the electorate's main concerns were related to the shrinking size of the welfare state, the UK budget deficit and protecting the NHS. In attempts to attract voters, each of the major parties used their manifestos to outbid each other by promises to increase NHS budgets. In July 2018, the NHS celebrated its 70th birthday, provoking a focus for the critical issues that currently account for the crisis in this service with the largest number of employees in the UK (also see Bonner, 2018a). In August, Theresa May announced £200 million per week to support the NHS. Although there are questions as to how this money will be found, it provides the basis for a ten-year plan. HealthWatch England is beginning NHS100, an ongoing survey of public attitudes into the perceived needs of the population within the context of technological and medical advances, the changing roles, relationships and responsibilities of individuals and the providers of health and social care. Although people will be living longer, and hopefully will be engaged in meaningful activities in retirement, the diseases of old age could be mitigated by greater individual new technological approaches to monitoring personal health, increased understanding of human development, health and wellbeing, and successful ageing. However, the health care system as reflected in the NHS and growing private organisations providing services to physical and mental health contribute to 20 per cent or less of the personal support of health and wellbeing. Good health and achieving a flourishing and fulfilling life require more, involving the interdependence of the domains outlined in Dahlgren and Whitehead's rainbow model of the social determinants of health (Dahlgren and Whitehead, 1991).

Health and wellbeing in 2020

Currently, social care is provided and funded by local authorities and private funders. The main objective of social care is to help people to live well and happily, and live as long as they can. This person-centred approach is in contrast to the systems that have been developed to support the health care needs of people. Local social services support a wide range of needs including autism, conduct disorder, mental health issues, children, family, working age adults and care for the fragile elderly, dementia and bereavement support. These complex behavioural issues are less amenable to technological monitoring and support than the clinical dimensions of health. Difficulties in the integration of health and social care systems (see Part I, Chapters 2 and 3) relate to physical, mental and emotional issues that challenge individual, family and community health. Cultural and professional differences between the NHS and social care, traditionally managed by local authorities, are some of the key challenges in the integration of the NHS and social care.

With the ongoing decline in revenue support grant for local authorities (50 per cent reduction within the last five years, leading to 100 per cent reduction by 2020), from central government, the most likely source of funding is from increases in council tax. Elected members and officers running local authorities have a difficult task in balancing the needs of diverse communities within a politically contested environment. Most people are unaware of how social care is funded. This, in part, is owing to the complexity of the service provision and the lack of high-quality information, as is the case for the NHS. There is a need for people to have standardised information and advice (for example regarding care providers and care homes; see Part III, Chapter 12), so that they can make informed decisions about their own and their families care-support needs. There are inequalities regarding the comparative funding of physical versus social care, as demonstrated by the funding from the NHS for cancer care in contrast to the requirement to provide personalised funding of, for example Alzheimer's disease. There is a general misunderstanding of what is and is not provided by the state. The politics of social care was evident when Gordon Brown announced changes to inheritance tax (Death Tax) and Theresa May's capping of costs to 75 per cent of actual care costs (the Dementia Tax). Addressing these politically sensitive issues has not seen any significant changes from the implementation of the ten reports on social care produced during the last ten years. Currently, a Green Paper on social care is being developed, and this will address social care across the lifespan. The successful outcomes of the resulting White Paper will depend on cross-party agreement, relevant approaches to the wide range of social needs, as noted above, and appropriate funding being available. The probability that this will resolve problems with increasing social needs is low, in view of the problems of implementing the Care Act 2014, as reviewed by Paul Burstow (Burstow, 2018). Appropriate funding of social care is important, but the actual needs of people, for example loneliness, depression, problematic substance misuse, obesity and lifestyle disorders, are somewhat more complex than treatments provided for physical health needs. In many respects, these 'wicked issues' (Rittel and Webber, 1973) are not too dissimilar from those challenges faced by people and communities prior to the establishment of the welfare state.

Health and wellbeing across the life course

In 2020, poverty still remains a key driver of poor health and wellbeing. The relationship between poverty, child abuse and neglect (Bywaters et al, 2016), is associated with domestic violence (Fahmy et al, 2016), human trafficking and modern slavery (Bulman, 2018) and other 'wicked issues'.

An important contribution to the Social Determinants of Health conceptual framework is provided by the work of Michael Marmot and the University College London Institute of Health Equity. One of the nine key messages of the landmark Marmot Review (Marmot, 2010) is that reducing health inequalities requires policy objectives to:

- give every child the best start;
- enable all children, young people and adults to maximize their capabilities and have control over their lives;
- create fair employment and good work for all;
- ensure healthy standard[s] of living for all;
- create and develop healthy sustainable places and communities;
- strengthen the role and impact of ill health prevention.

The current deterioration in standards of living in the UK is apparent from the Human Rights Watch Report (Anon, 2019a) released on 20 May 2019. This accuses the UK government of breaching its international duty of care by 'cruel and harmful policies' that are exacerbating child poverty in Hull, Cambridgeshire and Oxford. The report, commenting on 'a troubling development in the world's fifth largest economy', identifies tens of thousands of families who do not have enough to eat, with parents and schools resorting to food banks to feed their children. Food banks, managed by the Trussell Trust and a range of independent organizations (see Chapter 17), are a common feature of community support for people struggling to survive precarious social situations, impacted in many cases by welfare reform, delayed benefit payments, sanctions and unreliable disability assessments. A recent report in the *British Journal of Nutrition and Dietetics*, into food provided by Trussell Trust and other independent food banks in Oxfordshire, indicates that although food banks are providing a regular source of basic food for an increasing number of families, such provision has poor nutritional value (Fallaize et al, 2020).

The United Nations Rapporteur, Philip Alston, has previously drawn attention to the political context of poverty in children and families in the UK (Anon, 2019b), and attributes these adverse conditions to a UK government that is preoccupied with leaving the EU. The final report was published on Wednesday 23 May 2019. In this final version of his report, Alston accused UK ministers of 'immiseration of a significant part of the British Population', and warned of the worsening prospects of vulnerable people if Brexit proceeds: it 'was a tragic distraction from the social and economic policies shaping a Britain that it's hard to believe any political parties really want'. Alston's comments that ministers had designed a digitised version of 19th-century workhouses, as depicted by Charles Dickens, was rejected by Amber Rudd, the Work and Pensions Secretary, saying that the report was politically motivated. However, the UK government does not have a good track record in dealing with this 'wicked Issue' (see introduction to Part IV). In response to the riots in August 2011, The Troubled Families programme was announced in June 2013 (HMG, 2019), and rolled out from 2015. This was aimed at 'turn[ing] around' 120,000 households, but appears to have run into difficulties. According to the BBC (BBC, 2019), the 'damning' report into this programme was suppressed, and in any case, according to a senior civil servant, was 'window dressing'. Of 56 local authorities, there was a 'lack of obvious effect … across a range of outcomes … within the time frame [18 months] … of the report'. This policy was implemented during the progression of the Children and Families Act 2014 (Kerr, 2018).

The demographic projections of an ageing population present considerable challenges for national and local government. Four independent reviews, and a number of Green and White Papers of the funding of social care, including a Royal Commission and the Dilnot Commission (Dilnot, 2010), have not resolved this demographic crisis. The problems of an ageing population and housing is the focus of Chapter 18. Paradoxically, lower house prices in the North-East have resulted in movement there of an increasing number of people after retirement, and this is also the case for other areas with lower-cost housing. This gives councils with the added liability of councils for increased social care costs (see Chapter 7).

There are both political and health-based connotations for 'taking [back] control'. However, although personal control is an important bio-psycho driver, a sense of coherence, identified by Antonovsky, supported by extensive evidence from Lindström and Eriksson (2010), is central to our sense of identity. This approach, which involves 'head, hands and heart' is being adopted by policymakers and commissioners of services, as noted in Part IV, Chapter 16. 'Deaths of despair', reviewed by Harry Burns (Part I, Chapter 1), are a sad indictment of our society, and too often are the result of negative sociopolitical attitudes, the flames of which are fanned by social deprivation and social and health inequalities.

In order to achieve the best outcomes for individuals and their communities, local authority leaders should consider the interconnectedness of communities, social networks, resilience and psycho-social health based on an 'asset-based' approach to health and social care (Lindström and Eriksson, 2010). A combination of individual, family and environmental factors can create risk and increase the probability of adverse life events. These can be mitigated by protective factors, an accumulation of which increases the chances of positive effects and resiliency dependent on the level of risk factors.

The paradox of the paralysis of the UK parliament, due to Brexit, is that it is predicted that a significant proportion of 52 per cent of the UK population who voted to leave the EU in the 2015 referendum are those most likely to be adversely affected by the continuing austerity budgets and anticipated downturn in the UK if the UK leaves the EU 'without a deal'.

Developing assets in people and the community

Building on our knowledge of developmental processes across the lifecourse, particularly family and community influences (Lindström and Eriksson, 2010), clearly the more assets that are present within a person's life, the more likely they are to have positive outcomes and the less likely they are to engage in poor lifestyle choices. This use of developmental assets (Rippon and Hopkins, 2015) promotes a holistic, joined-up approach to healthy development by highlighting areas that can be improved in order to thrive. The developmental assets framework provides the possibility of identifying children and young people at risk, and identifies specific areas of support required. The factors identified within Action for Children Research (Anon, 2009) have preventative potential and economic benefit from providing nurturing environment and service provision around specific pathways. Both viewpoints reinforce the value of positive psychology, and the resilience-building effects of positive activities and involvement within communities.

A thriving community results from an individual reaching their potential, underpinned by positive childhood and personal resilience nurtured within a community led by informed elected members working within local, regional and central government. The Care Act 2014 is a political response to promote wellbeing and make wellness a common purpose of health and social care (Chapter 15). Promotion of this community-organising principle recognises that relationships are critical to a good life. Relationships are also important in the response of local authorities in the provision of services and support for people and their community (see Part III, Chapters 11, 12, and Part IV, Chapter 15).

From a Social Determinants of Health perspective, the interdependence of an individual's assets and their socio-economic environment is 'glue' that promotes health and a healthy community. Community assets are, in the main, managed by local authorities. This book presents a number of challenges to each one of us as we influence local policy by the election of local councils, which are responsible for the selection and activities of council officers.

Maintaining social connections, looking to the strengths and resources of statutory services and promoting partnerships are all central to enabling healthy communities to thrive. However, fiscal restraints in implementing the Care Act 2014, welfare reforms, economic uncertainty with the UK leaving the EU and current perturbations in the UK political system all point to the need for a critical review of community anchors and the evolving role of local authorities.

COVID-19

Following the reporting of a cluster of cases of pneumonia by the Wuhan Municipal Health Commission in China on 31 December 2019, the COVID-19 crisis has brought unprecedented challenges to every family, neighbourhood, local authority and government department in the UK, not to mention a devastating impact on the world economy.

The news on 4 January 2020 of the first recorded case of COVID-19 outside China, in Thailand, was the start of a chain of transmission across the world, with the first cases in the UK being confirmed on 31 January 2020. By 5 March 2020, the first UK death was confirmed, and on the same day England's Chief Medical Officer, Chris Whitty, announced that the UK was moving to the second stage of dealing with COVID-19 from 'containment' to the 'delay' phase. On 9 March 2020, the FTSE 100 plunged by more than 8 per cent, its largest intraday fall since 2008, amid worries over the spread of COVID-19.

Deeply concerned by the alarming levels of spread and severity, and by the alarming levels of inaction, the World Health Organization made the assessment that COVID-19 should be characterised as a pandemic on 11 March 2020. The next day the FTSE 100 plunged again by over 10 per cent, its biggest drop since 1987, with other markets around the world being similarly affected by the ongoing economic turmoil. The UK government response came in a series of announcements; from advice to work from home if possible and to avoid visiting public places on 16 March, to closing schools from 20 March along with the closure of pubs, restaurants, theatres, leisure centres and other similar locations, and eventually, on 23 March, the Prime Minister, Boris Johnson, announced a UK-wide partial lockdown that was to come into force on 26 March. On 16 April 2020 a three-week extension to the nationwide lockdown measures was announced as the number of confirmed COVID-19 cases in the UK rose to more than 100,000 (see Appendix for a synopsis of the COVID-19 timeline).

On 22 April, the government announced that the outbreak was at its peak but that the UK would have to live with some social distancing measures for at least the rest of the year. By 5 May 2020, the number of recorded deaths from COVID-19 in the UK had risen to 29,427, giving the country the highest number of COVID-19 related deaths in Europe and second only in the world to the USA.

This book, providing a range of different perspectives into 'wicked issues', will I hope stimulate conversations, relationships and partnerships for the public good.

References

Anon (1946) Constitution of the World Health Organization. Available from: https://www.who.int/governance/eb/who_constitution_en.pdf [Accessed 8 April 2020].

Anon (2009) 'Action for children' research, 2009'. Available from: https://www.actionforchildren.org.uk/resources-and-publications/reports/neglect-research-evidence-to-inform-practice-2009/ [Accessed 8 April 2020].

Anon (2015a) 'The big society audit'. Press release, 20 January. Available from: https://www.civilexchange.org.uk/wp-content/uploads/2015/01/Whose-Society_The-Final-Big-Society-Audit_final.pdf [Accessed 12 May 2020].

Anon (2015b) 'Civil exchange'. Press release, 20 January. Available from: http://www.civilexchange.org.uk/press-release-20-january-2015 [Accessed 8 April 2020].

Anon (2019a) 'Human rights watch report: the UK'. Available from: https://www.hrw.org/world-report/2019/country-chapters/united-kingdom [Accessed 8 April 2020].

Anon (2019b). 'Report of the special rapporteur on extreme poverty'. Available from: https://www.bbc.co.uk/news/uk-48354692 [Accessed 8 April 2020].

BBC (2019) BBC report on the troubled families programme. Available from: https://www.bbc.co.uk/news/uk-politics-37686888 [Accessed 8 April 2020].

Bonner, A.B. (2006) *Social Exclusion and the Way Out: An Individual and Community Response to Human Social Dysfunction*, Chichester: John Wiley & Sons.

Bonner, A.B. (2018a) 'The individual growing into society', in A.B. Bonner (ed) *Social Determinants of Health: An Interdisciplinary Perspective on Social Inequality and Wellbeing*, Bristol: Policy Press, pp 3–15.

Bonner, A.B. (ed) (2018b) *Social Determinants of Health: An Interdisciplinary Perspective on Social inequality and Wellbeing*, Bristol: Policy Press.

Breeze, B. (2019) The Beacon Project, from the Centre for Philanthropy at the University of Kent. Available from: https://research.kent.ac.uk/philanthropy. [Accessed 8 April 2020].

Bulman, M. (2018) 'Hundreds of modern slavery victims pushed into poverty after escaping abuse, report finds'. Available from: https://www.independent.co.uk/news/uk/home-news/modern-slavery-victims-trafficking-poverty-food-abuse-hestia-home-office-a8588591.html [Accessed 8 April 2020].

Burstow, P. (2018) 'The Care Act, 2014', in A.B. Bonner (ed) *Social Determinants of Health: An Interdisciplinary Perspective on Social Inequality and Wellbeing*, Bristol: Policy Press, pp 311–24.

Bywaters, P., Bunting, L., Davidson, G., Hanratty, J., Mason, W., McCartan, C. and Steils, N. (2016) 'The relationship between poverty, child abuse and neglect: an evidence review'. JRF. Available from: https://www.jrf.org.uk/report/relationship-between-poverty-child-abuse-and-neglect-evidence-review [Accessed 8 April 2020].

Cameron, D. (2009) 'The Big Society'. Conservative Party speech, 10 November. https://conservative-speeches.sayit.mysociety.org/speech/601246.

Crewe, T. (2016) 'The strange death of municipal England', *London Review of Books* (15 December), 38(24). Available from: https://www.lrb.co.uk/the-paper/v38/n24/tom-crewe/the-strange-death-of-municipal-england [Accessed 8 April 2020].

Dahlgren, G. and Whitehead, M. (1991) *Policies and Strategies to Promote Social Equity in Health*. Stockholm: Institute for Futures Studies.

Dilnot, A. (2010) 'Commission on funding of care and support'. Available from: https://webarchive.nationalarchives.gov.uk/20130221121534/http://www.dilnotcommission.dh.gov.uk/our-report/ [Accessed 8 April 2020].

Fahmy, E., Williamson, E. and Pantazis, C. (2016) 'Evidence and policy review: domestic violence'. JRF/University of Bristol. Available from: https://research-information.bristol.ac.uk/files/128551400/JRF_DV_POVERTY_REPORT_FINAL_COPY_.pdf [Accessed 8 April 2020].

Fallaize, R., Newlove, J., White, A. and Lovegrove, J.A. (2020) 'Nutrition adequacy and content of food bank parcels in Oxfordshire, UK: a comparative analysis of independent and organisational provision', *Journal of Human Nutrition and Dietetics*. 11 February. Available from https://onlinelibrary.wiley.com/doi/full/10.1111/jhn.12740.

HMG (UK Government) (2019) 'National evaluation of the Troubled Families Programme 2015 to 2020: findings'. Available from: https://www.gov.uk/government/publications/national-evaluation-of-the-troubled-families-programme-2015-to-2020-findings [Accessed 8 April 2020].

Kerr, K. (2018) 'Addressing inequalities in education', in A.B. Bonner (ed) *Social Determinants of Health: An Interdisciplinary Perspective on Social Inequality and Wellbeing*, Bristol: Policy Press, pp 17–27.

Lindström, B. and Eriksson, M. (2010) 'The Hitchhikers guide to salutogenesis: salutogenesis pathways to health promotion', Helsinki: Folkhälsan Research Centre, Health Promotion Research Programme and IUHPE Global Working Group on Salutogenesis.

Marmot, M. (2010) 'Fair society, healthy lives', The Marmot Review, Institute of Health Equity. Available from: http://www.instituteofhealthequity.org/resources-reports/fair-society-healthy-lives-the-marmot-review [Accessed 8 April 2020].

Rippon, S. and Hopkins, T. (2015) 'Heads, hands and heart: asset-based approaches in health care. A review of the conceptual evidence and case studies of asset-based approaches in health, care and wellbeing', The Health Foundation. Available from: https://www.health.org.uk/sites/default/files/HeadHandsAndHeartAssetBasedApproachesInHealthCare.pdf [Accessed 8 April 2020].

Rittel, H.J. and Webber, M.M. (1973) 'Dilemmas in a general theory of planning', *Policy Sciences*, 4(2): 155–69. Available from: https://www.researchgate.net/publication/225230512_Dilemmas_In_a_General_Theory_of_Planning [Accessed 8 April 2020].

PART I

Health, social care and community wellbeing

Introduction

Adrian Bonner

In Chapter 1, Harry Burns sets the context of this book by drawing our attention to the decline in life expectancy in the United States (US), United Kingdom (UK) and other European countries since 2014. This demographic phenomenon appears to be related to underlying social and economic factors, leading to 'deaths of despair'. Social isolation and poor labour market opportunities negatively impact on physical and mental health. There are particular concerns regarding increasing levels of premature deaths in younger age groups. In many cases, deaths are due to drug overdoses, suicide, alcohol-related problems and 'external causes', such as violence and accidents. The author of Chapter 1, as former Chief Medical Office for Scotland, has a unique view of diseases linked to contemporary lifestyles (often referred to as 'non-communicable diseases'), which are significantly linked to social, cultural and psychological environments. These social determinants are, to a large extent, influenced by local and national politics. Following the devolution of statutory powers to Scotland (see Chapter 20) and Wales (see Chapter 21), there are quite distinct health and social care policies emerging across UK regions. Burns provides a critique of the hierarchy of needs, proposed by Maslow in the 1940s, highlighting the pivotal nature of self-actualisation and the spiritual concept of cultural propensity, the capacity of which depends on early life experiences of nurturing and attachment, setting the scene for later lifestyle choices and resilience. In contrast to the hard structures developed through health, social and local authority policy implementation, reviewed throughout this book, the soft structural approach, as promoted in Part IV, provides a 'salutogenic' perspective through which health, wellbeing and self-actualisation can be promoted. With reference to the Improvement Collaborative, developed in Scotland, and the 100 Million Healthier Lives Project, convened in Boston, US, this chapter provides the possibility of positively changing the outcomes of complex systems in health and social care.

Chapter 2, representing the perspectives of the Association of the Directors of Public Health, largely focuses on England, with some comparisons from the rest of the UK. It plots the changing positioning of public health, moving between the National Health Service (NHS) and local government.

The strategic movement, across both developed and developing countries, from concentrating health resources on communicable disease to a focus on non–communicable disease, is a response to modern epidemics of obesity, alcohol-related diseases and the politics of health care. However, communicable diseases can still have major health, social and economic impacts, as demonstrated by the potential pandemic caused by the rapid global of COVID-19 (Coronavirus); see Chapters 2, 3 and 4.

Clearly, austerity budgets have an effect on the health of particular segments of the population, with those people at the lower end of the social gradient being most affected by both quality of the environment and availability of health and social care.

Public Health was incorporated into the NHS in 1974, and then, influenced by the Marmot Review (2010), it was returned to local authorities in 2013. Building on the 'science' of public health, public health professionals have been challenged to develop skills in the 'art' of public health that are required to influence policy change and systems leadership within their wider remit in local authorities.

A review of organisational changes in the delivery of health and social care is presented in Chapter 3. These significant system changes provide a backdrop to current challenges in moving towards an integrated system of health and social care, as presented in Chapter 3. Here challenges, related to NHS services being free at the point of use and their integration with means-tested social care, are discussed. Working in Greater Manchester, the authors show how one of the first UK regions in which health budgets have been devolved to the local authority has allowed the development of governance arrangements and agreed strategic plans across the health and social care sector, to promote relationship building. These developments have been underpinned by politically driven reorganisation, expanded in Chapter 5. The Greater Manchester Partnership has increased the possibility of dealing with the complexity of 'wicked issues' (related to individual and community needs), supported by a Transformational

Fund. The wider determinants of health perspective, as proposed by Dahlgren and Whitehead's 'rainbow' model, have been useful in developing holistic responses; these include considerations of transport, housing and unemployment, among other determinants.

In Chapter 4, David Hunter emphasises the need for partnership working, which has been a long-standing objective of health and social policy. For many years, the NHS and local authorities have been attempting to deal with 'wicked issues'. Issues such as homelessness, disaffection of young people and the ageing society that have complex multiple causes require joined-up approaches by the statutory and third sectors at national and local levels. In 2012, at the time when Public Health responsibilities were transferred from the NHS to local authorities (see Chapter 2), health and wellbeing boards (HWBs) were established in England. The author of Chapter 4 has been involved in reviewing the development of HWBs during recent years. He suggests that, although partnerships have never been out of vogue in the UK, the need for them has never been greater. With few exceptions, HWBs punch below their weight and are not the powerful system leaders that were hoped for. Evidence of their value and impact is negligible, with poor performance indicators and the difficulties in overcoming deep-seated departmentalism and a silo approach, prevalent in government and public services, leaving 'wicked issues' as deep-seated as ever. 'After nearly a decade of austerity, which has contributed to a sharp rise in health inequalities and entrenched the North–South divide, and with the potential fallout from Brexit with as yet unknown but almost certainly negative consequences, the need for powerful HWBs that can bring about real change to improve the lot of ravished communities has never been greater.'

Chapter 1 provides a stark insight into some of the 'wicked issues' confronted by the statutory sectors. The complexities of providing an integrated health and social care system are immense. This complexity is particularly problematic owing to regional sociopolitical differences between UK regions. Political changes, such as devolution of responsibilities to Scotland and Wales and metropolitan areas in England, provide a method of disaggregating geo-specific issues. The system changes within the NHS and between the NHS and local authorities could benefit from greater effectiveness of HWBs. However, to date, there is little evidence of their impact in dealing with complex person-centred needs, especially for those at the margins of communities.

What emerges from this section of the book is the need to consider the importance and effectiveness of partnerships. To address major resource issues and health inequalities across the UK, there is clearly a need to increase prevention and community-based approaches that take account of both hard and soft determinants of health, for instance by reference to 'salutogenesis' (see Chapter 1), working with the third sector (see Part IV) and focusing on the causative drivers of 'wicked issues', as discussed in Chapter 4.

Aligned with the aims of the book, this section emphasises the need to critically examine the role of public, private and third sector partnerships. The success of such partnerships will depend on the relationships between the various sectors, pivotal to which is the development of trust and understanding between those who manage and implement this central element of the welfare state.

A key determinant underpinning the provision of formal and non-formal support for people in the UK is the state of the economy. The end of austerity and future of the UK with the European Union (EU) and the US is currently unknown. Following the general election in December 2019, the majority Conservative Government has legislated for the UK to leave the EU by the end of 2020. The extent to which privatisation of the health service is used by the UK government in trade negotiations with the US will clearly impact on the hard structures supporting the health and wellbeing of people across the UK.

Deaths of despair – causes and possible cures

Harry Burns

Introduction

Increasing life expectancy is an accepted indicator of human progress in a country. Except in times of war, high income countries have experienced many decades of steady growth in life expectancy. Such growth is largely associated with improving social and economic conditions as well as advances in health care. The long-term trend in life expectancy suggests that the determinants of health and wellbeing were improving. However, there are increasing reports that recent years have seen a slowing in life expectancy growth in many countries. Some countries, including the United States (US), the United Kingdom (UK) and several other European countries, are reporting an actual decline in life expectancy over the past few years since 2014 (Ho, 2018).

This chapter considers the possible causes of this sudden change in the pattern of growth in life expectancy. It is likely that a change in the pattern of the social determinants of health underlies this abrupt deterioration. Simply, the authors consider the possibility that social change has produced a decline in the wellbeing of populations in high income countries. They examine how wellbeing is defined and how it is created, and the methods by which societies can improve wellbeing in their citizens are considered.

What has caused the decline in life expectancy?

Some studies have attributed this relative decline in life expectancy to increasing mortality among the elderly from heart disease, Alzheimer's and respiratory disease. Some have suggested that this increase in deaths might be associated with serious influenza outbreaks (Ho, 2018; Kwong et al, 2018). However, increases in premature deaths in the US and the UK have also been seen in younger age groups.

The causes in younger people have been identified as drug overdoses, suicide, alcohol-related problems and external factors, such as violence and accidents. This pattern of mortality strongly suggests that underlying social and economic issues are responsible for this worrying trend (Leyland et al, 2007; Case and Deaton, 2015). Economic insecurity has been suggested as an important influence on what has been described by Case and Deaton (2015) as an increase in 'deaths of despair'.

They used this term to describe the emergence in the US of a marked increase in the all-cause mortality of middle-aged, white, non-Hispanic men and women between 1999 and 2013. This increase was primarily due to deaths from drugs, alcohol and suicide. The authors suggested that these mortality increases are a reflection of the distress that mid-life blue collar workers in the US are experiencing owing to increasing social isolation, poor labour market opportunities and, consequently, poorer physical and mental health.

This picture is very similar to the situation seen earlier in areas of the UK that also experienced collapse of industry and loss of social cohesion as communities sank into poverty. The effect has been closely studied in West Central Scotland, which saw catastrophic loss of traditional industries such as steel and shipbuilding in the decades following the Second World War (Hanlon et al, 2007; Walsh et al, 2017). Slow improvement in life expectancy in Scotland has been accompanied by a relative widening in mortality across socio-economic classes (Popham and Boyle, 2010). Extensive analysis suggests that the problem in Scotland has been caused by increasing mortality among poor, young and middle-aged Scots due to drugs, alcohol, suicide and violence. The pattern seen in Scotland's post-industrial areas mirrors the 'deaths of despair' described in the US.

Increasing poverty, which accompanied the loss of high-quality jobs in the second half of the 20th century, and a series of town planning policies based on social selection caused significant social dislocation and economic upheaval. In effect, Scotland experienced the social effects of austerity many decades before anywhere else.

Reversing the decline in life expectancy seen across several countries will not be achieved by more health care. Increasing mortality from drugs, alcohol, suicide and violence is symptomatic of deeper societal problems. These issues, which seem to affect predominantly poor post-industrial areas, will not be cured by hospitals and doctors. The problem faced by these areas is not too much illness; the problem is a lack of wellness.

Wellbeing – what is it?

The World Health Organization defines health as a 'state of complete physical, mental and social wellbeing, not merely that absence of illness or infirmity'. It is a definition that is often quoted but it is not entirely helpful. It tells us that to be healthy you need to experience wellbeing, but what is wellbeing? It is difficult to find a concise definition.

Wellbeing is subjective. If people feel their lives are going well, they will report a sense of wellbeing. If they feel safe and secure in their living conditions and feel in control of their lives, they will feel well. If they have a sense that their lives have purpose and meaning and, as a result, they have a desire to engage with the world and its problems, they are likely to feel well (Antonovsky, 1979).

Furthermore, creating wellbeing is not a simple matter. Wellbeing across a society emerges from a complex adaptive system in which many influences interact. Wellbeing is not something that can be created by a single, simple intervention (Cloninger et al, 2012). Yet public policy often relies on such solutions when it turns to legislation to control access to cigarettes or alcohol or sugar-containing beverages. Such solutions may have some effect, but their contribution to broader wellbeing in society is often difficult to quantify.

Conditions that support wellbeing include living in safe and congenial communities. There is evidence, for example, that living close to green space is associated with better health (Ward Thompson and Silveirinha de Oliveira, 2016). Security of housing tenure, access to education and opportunities, and adequate income from that satisfying employment are important determinants of wellbeing, as are the relationships that come from living in a supportive community. All these aspects of society contribute to the wellbeing of citizens.

How is wellbeing created?

There are many theories about how wellbeing in individuals emerges. One of the most influential theories used by public health practitioners to explain the relationship between external influences and positive outcomes is Abraham Maslow's hierarchy of human needs (Figure 1.1) (Maslow, 1943). Maslow was an American psychologist who proposed a theory of health and wellbeing that was based on the idea of serial fulfilment of basic human needs. He suggested that humans perceived needs as a hierarchy and, if they were fulfilled in order of need, humans would attain a state of 'self-actualisation'. Self-actualised people are considered to be those who are fulfilled and doing all they are capable of.

Figure 1.1: Maslow's hierarchy of human needs

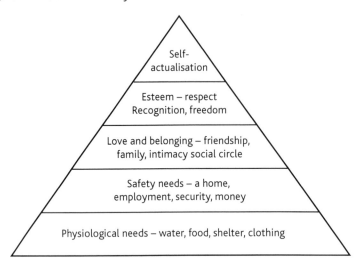

Self-
actualisation

Esteem – respect
Recognition, freedom

Love and belonging – friendship,
family, intimacy social circle

Safety needs – a home,
employment, security, money

Physiological needs – water, food, shelter, clothing

Source: Maslow, 1943

The term refers to the person's desire for self-fulfilment. Maslow proposed it as the capacity of individuals to achieve all that they have the potential to be. Famously, Maslow showed these needs as a triangle or pyramid with self-actualisation at its apex, and so suggested that it could only be achieved after other needs had been met.

This theory has had significant influence on public health thought and practice. If self-actualisation is regarded as the state of peak wellbeing, the idea is encouraged that self-actualisation cannot occur without attention to issues lower down the hierarchy. If individuals lack wellbeing, Maslow's theory is used to support the argument that poverty, social exclusion and needs must be identified and dealt with before people can function at a level consistent with their full capacities.

However, there is considerable evidence that suggests Maslow was wrong in suggesting this order of events.

In 1938, Maslow visited a Blackfoot Indian reservation in Canada (Blackstock, 2011). There, he learned how the Native Americans sought to preserve a strong, traditional culture. They drew for him a different hierarchy that had as its *base* the need for self-actualisation (Figure 1.2).

If, they argued, young people grew up to feel positive about their lives and in control of their destinies, they could contribute effectively to community actualisation. If, as a consequence, communities were functioning to their full capacity, their traditional cultures would be preserved. Cultural perpetuity was their aspiration. Self-actualisation

Figure 1.2: The hierarchy of needs as suggested to Maslow by the Blackfoot Indians

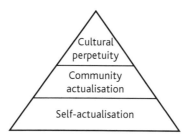

Source: Blackstock, 2011

for the indigenous people was the foundation of the way in which they preserved their culture, not the end result. This view of self-actualisation seems more plausible. In prehistoric times, it is unlikely that prehistoric *Homo sapiens* would solve all the problems of survival before learning to cooperate and live successful lives in community with others.

Why did Maslow move self-actualisation to the top of his hierarchy? It is difficult to say. It may be that he felt uncomfortable with the more spiritual concept of cultural perpetuity and respect for ancestors described by the Native Americans. He may have wanted to assert the importance of individual decision-making and development, as was being advocated by economists of the time. However, since then, a greater understanding of neuroscience and the biology of stress has given us insight into how and when personality develops. This work suggests that the development of the capacity for self-actualisation depends on the experience of nurture and attachment during very early childhood (McEwen, 2008; Hill et al, 2018).

Unlike Maslow's theory of self-actualisation, which suggests that individuals attain the ability to feel in control of their lives after a series of other conditions have been satisfied, science tells us that self-actualization is an attribute that develops from birth, and is experienced in parallel with and influences all the other stages outlined by Maslow. In order to progress to a fulfilled life, it seems we must learn self-actualisation in early life if we are to progress. Self-actualisation is a means to an end, not, as Maslow suggested, an end in itself. Understanding these processes, therefore, has significance for public policy as it tries to improve wellbeing.

Salutogenesis and the science behind wellbeing

Over the years, salutogenesis has become an established concept in public health and health promotion. The key elements of the salutogenic model are the focus on supporting the individual's problem-solving capacity and, secondly, developing the capacity to use physical and social resources available to solve the problems encountered.

It was the American sociologist Aaron Antonovsky who introduced the term 'salutogenesis' in 1979. Antonovsky's idea was that we should view the health of an individual as being a point on a continuum from complete ill health (dis-ease) to complete health (ease). His insight was that we should focus on building people's resources and capacity to create health rather than adopt a medical focus on ill health and disease. This concept was based on work he carried out in the 1960s, studying the health of menopausal women in Israel. He found that women who had been exposed to severe stress in early life had poorer health in later life. However, one-third of women who had been exposed to the same severe stress, in this case the Holocaust, had normal health. It seemed to him that those who were healthy had found resources to cope with external stressors, and he set out to understand how this capacity might be created.

Antonovsky evolved the concept that the key factor underpinning wellbeing and the capacity to manage external stressors was the extent to which the individual had developed in early life a *sense of coherence* (Antonovsky, 1993). He defined this as:

> [A] global orientation that expresses the extent to which one has a pervasive, enduring, though dynamic, feeling of confidence that:
> 1. the stimuli derived from one's internal and external environment are structured, predictable and explainable
> 2. The resources are available to one to meet the demands posed by these stimuli
> 3. These demands are challenges, worthy of investment and engagement.

To experience wellbeing, Antonovsky suggested, individuals must feel the world around them as understandable, manageable and meaningful, otherwise they will experience a state of chronic stress. The idea that stress levels are higher in those individuals who do not feel in control over their lives has allowed Antonovsky's ideas to be tested.

The biological consequences of adversity in childhood

The relationship between social and economic circumstances and evidence of altered metabolic processes has been studied in a number of settings. Children who have experienced neglect and subsequent adoption have higher stress hormone levels than children who have no such history (Kertes et al, 2008). Children born into families at the lower end of the socio-economic spectrum are more likely to have poorer cognitive function and lower educational attainment than children from more affluent families (Hackman et al, 2010).

Brain imaging studies have shown that children who experience neglect or abuse or whose parents have serious mental illness have a pattern of brain development that makes them more emotionally labile and less likely to be able to control impulsive behaviour (McEwen, 2008; Hackman et al, 2010) They become more anxious, aggressive, fearful and more likely to react to stressful situations with poorly thought-out responses.. The more adversity children encounter, the more likely they are to grow up with addiction issues, fail in obtaining employment, engage in partner violence and acquire criminal convictions.

In 1972, researchers in New Zealand began a study of the health and wellbeing of 1,000 babies born in Dunedin that year (Poulton et al, 2015). Forty-seven years later, most of those people are still being studied. Risk factors for poor wellbeing in later life have been identified: low family socio-economic status, low parental education, time in a single-parent family, having multiple caregivers or residential changes, experiencing domestic violence, physical abuse and sexual abuse were all associated with a higher risk of aggression, hyperactivity, conduct disorder, anxiety, antisocial behaviour, mental health problems and lower self-esteem. These children endured longer periods of youth unemployment, and 20 per cent of the group studied accounted for 80 per cent of the criminal behaviour observed.

A study of adverse experiences in childhood carried out in the US also showed a strong association between poor early childhood experiences and risk of violent behaviour as an adult (Felitti et al, 1998). Closer to home, a study carried out in England reported that adults experiencing serious levels of neglect were 14 times more likely than those children not experiencing abuse and neglect to have been a victim of violence, 15 times more likely to have committed a violent crime in the last year and 20 times more likely to go to prison during their lives (Bellis et al, 2014). A study carried out in Wales suggested that 14 per cent of the population had a level of exposure to adverse experiences that would result in them carrying these risks. In addition, the study quantified the longer-term risk of chronic disease in people affected by childhood adversity (Bellis et al, 2016).

It is clear that the ability to feel in control of one's life is largely determined by the circumstances in which people are born and raised. Failure to experience consistent, nurturing parenting impairs children's ability to see the world as structured, predictable and explainable. They are less likely to acquire the skills and insights that allow them to meet the challenges they face in an acceptable way. In short, they do not acquire a sense of a coherent world with which to engage. If we are to tackle the causes of inequity in outcome, we need to create a society that helps young people to feel in control of their lives.

How can societies create health and wellbeing?

Most countries know how much they spend on health care and treating disease. Few countries will know how much they spend on creating wellbeing in their citizens. This is understandable given the subjective nature of the term. For example, spending money creating green space or installing public art might make some people feel well while others are, at best, neutral in their feelings.

There have been some attempts to measure the economic implications of failure to create the capacity for wellbeing in children. In particular, studying the impact of adverse childhood experiences on adult wellbeing has been used to calculate the lifetime economic impact of failure to provide support to families and children. In studying the economic burden of child maltreatment in the United States, Fang et al (2012) estimated the aggregated lifetime cost of child maltreatment in 2008 by multiplying per-victim lifetime cost estimates by the estimated number of new child maltreatment cases in 2008. They estimated total lifetime economic burden resulting from new cases of fatal and non-fatal child maltreatment in the US in 2008 was approximately $124 billion. This cost is approximately equivalent to the cost of chronic disease such as stroke and Type 2 diabetes (Fang et al, 2012). However, more recent estimates of the annual cost of adverse childhood experiences suggest the impact is much greater. Bellis and colleagues (2019) suggest that the annual cost attributable to chaotic childhoods is equivalent to $581 billion in Europe and $748 billion in the US (Bellis et al, 2019).

Without clearly appreciating the impact of their failure to tackle the circumstances that result in a lack of wellbeing in large sections of the population, policymakers will just keep on doing what they have always done – expecting different results. Einstein, it is reported, thought this was a definition of insanity.

Why does public policy fail?

In the 1980s, attempts were made in the UK to make public services 'more businesslike'. Known as New Public Management (NPM), the system focuses on customer service, financial control, value for money and increasing efficiency. Senior managers drive change by setting targets and using indicators and performance monitoring. The wellbeing of the community, being difficult to conceptualise, rarely features in strategic plans or managers' objectives.

Public services tend to focus on people's problems, needs and deficiencies. We design services to fill gaps and fix people's problems for them. Studying many projects that have transformed the lives of people living with socio-economic deprivation suggests that helping people develop a sense of self-efficacy and control are important drivers of wellbeing. Public services do things to people rather than with them. As a result, citizens become passive recipients of services.

The projects that are successful in transforming the lives of people living with socio-economic deprivation are those that help people develop a sense of control over their lives. Public services often undermine the already low sense of self-efficacy and self-esteem of people living in difficult circumstances. Whatever we do to improve wellbeing will involve helping people to take control over their lives.

A method for improvement

Wellbeing emerges from the complex interaction of many factors. It is not something that can be created by a single intervention. The linear thinking encouraged by NPM is unable to take account of the complexity from which wellbeing emerges. Setting targets without understanding the actions required to achieve those targets is certain to alienate front-line workers, who are probably the best informed about the complexity of the problems facing them.

Scotland recently began to tackle complex problems in health using concepts of improvement science. This is an approach that emphasises testing in the field the ideas for change that emerge from practitioners. The results of many tests of the impact of change are quickly spread in order to generate learning about the changes that produce the desired improvements. It brings together the empirical knowledge of people who have to deliver the change and provides them with tools to implement the desired improvements.

Projects begin by specifying a clear and stretching aim for improvement and a measurement plan, and then the practitioners begin small tests of those changes they think will lead to improvement over a short period of time. As these small tests are refined and successfully implemented, the learning is shared and improvements are scaled up across the system. Implementing this approach requires us to answer four questions.

- What do we want to change?
- By how much do we want to change it?
- By when do we want to achieve the change?
- What method will we use to make the change?

This was the approach used in Scotland to improve outcomes in Scottish hospitals. The Scottish Patient Safety Programme has produced a highly significant reduction in harm to patients and, notably, a 37 per cent reduction in post-operative deaths, largely associated with the regional improvement collaboratives. It is also being used to improve outcomes for children in the Children and Young People Improvement Collaborative. The system was first used in industrial process improvement by W. Edwards Deming. It was then applied to health care in the US by the Institute for Healthcare Improvement in Boston, when it developed its 100 Million Healthier Lives campaign, noted below.

The method is one in which front-line staff identify several interventions that have a small but positive effect on desired outcomes. Taken in isolation, each intervention might only produce a small effect that might not be seen as significant if tested by conventional statistical methods. If, however, we identify 30 small changes that each produce a 1–2 per cent improvement and apply them consistently, we might see a 30–50 per cent improvement. It was this method of concentrating on 'marginal gains' that brought success to UK cycling teams in international events (Pentecost et al, 2017).

Applying improvement methods to wellbeing

An improvement programme aimed at improving wellbeing across a whole society is a formidable prospect. In any such programme, it would be critical to ensure it was designed by citizens working closely with front-line staff from the agencies most closely involved in supporting communities. This work should not be designed by academics and experts advising ministers, who then issue policy papers that they expect front-line staff to implement. It is difficult for people to be committed to a programme that they have had no involvement in designing. To be effective, the programme design must involve the people being supported and those who support them.

In essence, an improvement collaborative has four stages. First, set a stretching aim for the project. Secondly, agree a set of drivers that will help achieve the stretch aim. Thirdly, identify actions that will implement change in the drivers. Finally, agree the metrics that should be used to assess the degree of improvement.

The most ambitious wellbeing improvement programme currently under way is the 100 Million Healthier Lives campaign. The following description comes from the website that supports the campaign and those involved in it.[1]

This international programme is convened by the Institute for Healthcare Improvement in Boston, US. It brings together community organisations, educational establishments, governments, funders and a variety of organisations that contribute to health and wellbeing. It works to a broad definition of health and wellbeing that acknowledges health is not solely the absence of disease but involves the addition of 'confidence, skills, knowledge and connection'. It goes on to say that health is a 'means to an end – which is a joyful, meaningful life'. This definition is broad and its parameters are difficult to measure. However, it is perfectly accurate and reasonable to suggest that the aim of the project is to enhance the chance that people are able to live a 'joyful, meaningful life'. The only problem is how to do it.

Having set a stretching and worthwhile aim – that 100 million people should be more able to live a healthier life by 2020 – the next question to answer was 'what do you want to change?'.

To shape the list of 'whats', the conveners gathered recommendations from groups of experts working across all the agencies that might contribute to health

Address equity gaps – required for all participants.

1. Help all kids have a great start in life with all the skills they and their families need to flourish from cradle to career.
2. Support veterans and refugees to thrive.
3. Reclaim the health, wellbeing and dignity of indigenous communities.
4. Address the social and behavioural determinants of health across health care, community and social services, with a special focus on vulnerable populations.
5. Make mental health everybody's job, across the continuum of health care, community, public health and social services.
6. Improve access to primary health care for all.

7. Create the best possible wellbeing in the elder years and at the end of life.
8. Engage everyone in improving their own health.

This list involves several high-level aims. The third question is 'how are we going to make the change happen?'. The 'how' list was drawn up based on the extensive consultation.

1. Shift culture and mindset
   - Use storytelling as a strategy to create a change in culture.
   - Develop a culture of partnership.
   - Develop a culture of wellbeing.
   - Develop leaders at every level who are empowered to carry out the vision.
2. Develop workforce strategies – engage students and youth as leaders in the transformation.
3. Integrate peer-to-peer support systems into every relevant initiative.
4. Integrate improvement and change methods at the community level.
5. Use the top chronic diseases in each community and core risk factors to build a continuum of health across home, community, public health and health care.
6. Develop and adopt financing strategies that align funding at the community level.
7. Integrate data across silos (health care, community, public health and social services).
8. Engage employers and businesses to improve workforce health and wellbeing.
9. Transform health care to be good at health and good at care

Each community will develop its own ideas as to how these drivers of improvement can be delivered locally. They test the effectiveness of these ideas and share the results across the network. Shared learning allows identification of many effective interventions that can drive improvement.

The final part of the improvement journey is to establish a measurement framework that allows improvements in health and wellbeing achieved by the tests of change to be identified and recorded. The societal drivers of wellbeing are complex, and it is difficult in any complex system to identify which intervention was responsible for a particular change in outcome. However, measuring improvements in wellbeing is essential in encouraging the many stakeholder agencies involved in promoting improvement to maintain their efforts.

The 100 Million Healthier Lives website gives a comprehensive description of the measurement framework being used in the project. Measurement of healthy life expectancy and assessment of how inequalities in health are narrowing are key measures. Other aspects of improvement are also important. Psychological and emotional development of children and assessment of healthy behaviour changes are also included.

The improvement collaborative approach is a proven method for changing the outcome of a complex system in health and care. The 100 Million Healthier Lives project is an immensely ambitious use of the technique. It is to be hoped that it will produce learning that can be used to transform lives across social and ethnic divides, and make the people of the world kinder and more supportive of those living difficult lives.

Conclusion

Improvements in life expectancy in high income countries have slowed considerably. It is argued in this chapter that this deterioration in health is due to increasing problems with social determinants of wellbeing. The processes by which wellbeing can be enhanced are described and seen to focus very much on the way families with children are supported. Many suggestions have been made for policies that can improve wellbeing, but the most effective seem to be those using improvement science methods. These involve front-line staff working closely with citizens to design, test and implement successful change.

Note
[1]   https://www.100mlives.org

References
Antonovsky, A. (1979) *Health, Stress and Coping*, San Francisco: Jossey-Bass.

Antonovsky, A. (1993) 'The structure and properties of the sense of coherence scale', *Social Science and Medicine*, 6: 725–33.

Bellis, M.A., Ashton, K., Hughes, K., Ford, K., Bishop, J. and Paranjothy, S. (2016) 'Adverse childhood experiences (ACEs) in Wales and their impact on health in the adult population: Mariana Dyakova', *European Journal of Public Health*, 26(1): ckw167.009. Available at https://doi.org/10.1093/eurpub/ckw167.009 [Accessed 8 April 2020].

Bellis, M.A., Hughes, K., Ford, K., Rodriguez, G.R., Sethi, D. and Passmore, J. (2019) 'Life course health consequences and associate annual costs of adverse childhood experience across Europe and North America: a systematic review and meta-analysis', *Lancet Public Health*. Available from: https://doi.org/10.1016/S2468-2667(19)30145-8 [Accessed 8 April 2020].

Bellis, M.A., Lowey, H., Leckenby, N., Hughes, K. and Harrison, D. (2014) 'Adverse childhood experiences: retrospective study to determine their impact on adult health behaviours and health outcomes in a UK population', *Journal of Public Health*, 36(1) (March): 81–91.

Blackstock, C. (2011) 'The emergence of the breath of life', *Journal of Social Work Values and Ethics*, 8(1).

Case, A. and Deaton, A. (2015) 'Rising morbidity and mortality in midlife among white non-Hispanic Americans in the 21st century', *Proceedings of the National Academy of Sciences of the USA*, 112(49): 15078–83.

Cloninger, C.R., Salloum, I.M. and Mezzich, J.E. (2012) 'The dynamic origins of positive health and wellbeing', *International Journal of Person-Centered Medicine*, 2(2): 179–87.

Fang, X., Brown, D.S., Florence, C.S. and Mercy, J.A. (2012) 'The economic burden of child maltreatment in the United States and implications for prevention', *Child Abuse & Neglect*, 36(2): 156–65.

Felitti, V.J., Anda, R.F., Nordenberg, D., Williamson, D.F., Spitz, A.M., Edwards, V., Koss, M.P. and Marks, J.S. (1998) 'Relationship of childhood abuse and household dysfunction to many of the leading causes of death in adults: the adverse childhood experiences (ACE) Study', *American Journal of Preventive Medicine* (May), 14(4): 245–58.

Hackman, D.A., Farah, M.J. and Meaney, M.J. (2010) 'Socioeconomic status and the brain: mechanistic insights from human and animal research', *Nature Reviews Neuroscience*, 11(9): 651–9.

Hanlon T.E., Carswell, S. and Rose, M. (2007) 'Research on the caretaking of children of incarcerated parents: findings and their service delivery implications', *Child and Youth Services Review*, 29(3): 348–62. Available from https://doi.org/10.1016/j.childyouth.2006.09.001 [Accessed 28 July 2020].

Hill, P.A., Turiano, N. and Burrow, A.L. (2018) 'Early life adversity as a predictor of sense of purpose during adulthood', *International Journal of Behavioral Development*, 42(1): 143–7.

Ho, J.Y. (2018) 'Recent trends in life expectancy across high income countries: retrospective observational study', *British Medical Journal*, 362. Available from: https://doi.org/10.1136/bmj.k2562 [Accessed 8 April 2020].

Kertes, D.A., Gunnar, M.R., Madsen, N.J. and Long, J.D. (2008) 'Early deprivation and home basal cortisol levels: a study of internationally adopted children', *Development and Psychopathology*, 20(2): 473–91. Available from: https://doi.org/10.1017/S0954579408000230 [Accessed 18 May 2020].

Kwong, J.C. et al (2018) 'Acute myocardial infarction after laboratory-confirmed influenza infection', *New England Journal of Medicine*, 378(4): 345–53.

Leyland, A.H., Dundas, R., McLoone, P. and Boddy, F.A. (2007) 'Cause-specific inequalities in mortality in Scotland: two decades of change; a population-based study', *BMC Public Health*, 7: 172.

Maslow, A.H. (1943) 'A theory of human motivation', *Psychological Review*, 50(4): 370–96.

McEwen, B.S. (2008) 'Understanding the potency of stressful early life experiences on brain and body function Metabolism' (October), 57(Suppl. 2): S11–S15.

Pentecost, C., Richards, D. and Frost, F. (2017) 'Amalgamation of marginal gains (AMG) as a potential system to deliver high-quality fundamental nursing care: a qualitative analysis of interviews from high-performance AMG sports and healthcare practitioners'. Available from: https://doi.org/10.1111/jocn.14186 [Accessed 8 April 2020].

Popham, F. and Boyle, P. (2010) 'Assessing socio-economic inequalities in mortality and other health outcomes at the Scottish national level', Scottish Collaboration for Public Health Research and Policy. Available at: https://calls.ac.uk/output-entry/assessing-socio-economic-inequalities-in-mortality-and-other-health-outcomes-at-the-scottish-national-level/ [Accessed 13 May 2020].

Poulton, R., Moffitt, T.E. and Silva, P.A. (2015) 'The Dunedin multidisciplinary health and development study: overview of the first 40 years, with an eye to the future', *Social Psychiatry and Psychiatric Epidemiology*, 50(5): 679–93.

Walsh, D., McCartney, G., Collins, C., Taulbut, M. and Batty, G.D. (2017) 'History, politics and vulnerability: explaining excess mortality in Scotland and Glasgow'. Available from: https://www.publichealthjrnl.com/article/S0033-3506(17)30203-2/abstract)_ [Accessed 8 April 2020].

Ward Thompson, C. and Silveirinha de Oliveira, E.M. (2016) 'Evidence on health benefits of urban green spaces', in A. Egorov, P. Mudu, M. Braubach and M. Martuzzi (eds) *Urban Green Spaces and Health: A Review of Evidence*, pp 3–20, Copenhagen: World Health Organization Regional Office for Europe.

The role of English local authorities in addressing the social determinants of health: a public health perspective

Jeanelle de Gruchy and Jim McManus

Introduction

While the term 'social determinants' would have been alien to local government in England at the time of the Public Health Act 1848, the concepts and actions would have been well understood and core to its activities. Parks, decent housing, education, libraries and more have been the staple work of local authorities for many decades. This chapter explores the social determinants of health through the lens of directors of public health in local government – and considers the challenges and opportunities today, and in the years ahead.

The focus is largely on England because of different legislative and constitutional contexts in the four nations of the United Kingdom (UK). At the time of writing, life expectancy is stalling (ONS, 2018) and health inequalities are worsening; with the gap in life expectancy between the richest and poorest areas of England and Wales widening over the past decade (ONS, 2019).

The conditions that create good health are more social than personal (Marmot, 2010). While genetics, individual behaviour and medical services, such as the UK's National Health Service (NHS), contribute to our health outcomes, the dominance given to these factors is more rooted in cultural and ideological prejudices than evidence. These drivers are over-represented when it comes to public health policy and investment decisions.

Health care contributes a significant but small proportion of the public's overall health – and in the UK, the NHS is free at the point of need for all. It is the unequal social, economic and environmental circumstances throughout a person's life course that contribute to enduring and widening inequalities in health. But current government policy on the NHS and prevention seems to privilege both clinical measures and NHS funding over social determinants (House of Commons Health Committee, 2016; Fell and McManus, 2020). This reliance on clinical prevention over addressing social determinants hampers the effective addressing of health inequalities (Milne, 2018.)

This dual imbalance, worsening health inequalities and a move to clinical measures rather than funding action on social determinants, has been made worse by years of austerity and sustained cuts to local authority, voluntary and community sector-provided services and interventions – including youth clubs, children's centres, social care provision and much more besides. Yet despite experiencing considerable funding cuts, local government continues to play a critical role in shaping the social determinants of health.

Public health in local government

Since the Victorian era, local government has led public health improvement in the UK. Councils themselves emerged, in part, because of the health needs of communities during industrialisation. Overcrowding and the spread in the 19th century of communicable diseases required local health boards to develop sewerage systems, provide clean water and undertake slum clearance projects. Legislation covering topics as diverse as parks, education, social housing initiatives and public washhouses (Public Health Act, 1936) were driven by the aspiration to improve the health of the population.

In 1974, the NHS took over most public health functions with the exception of environmental health – which remained within the remit of local government. From their new NHS base, the directors of public health – the independent advocates for the health of the population – had fewer levers to influence the social determinants of health.

Despite this, the work of local authorities on the social determinants of health continued. Figure 2.1 (LGA, 2010) illustrates the role of local authority services and functions in population health. The ability of these services to be effective is, inevitably, related to the level of funding available. Austerity over the last decade has, according to many analysts, hampered this (Gray and Barford, 2018; Institute for Fiscal Studies, 2019.)

And it was within the challenging context of austerity that public health moved from the NHS to local government in England in 2013, with a remit to champion public health across the whole of the local authority's business and constructively engage the NHS and other

Figure 2.1: The role of local authorities in social determinants of health

The social determinants of health and well-being

Global Ecosystem
Natural Environment
Built Environment
Activities
Local Economy
Community
Lifestyle
People

age, sex
hereditary factors

How local government can make a difference

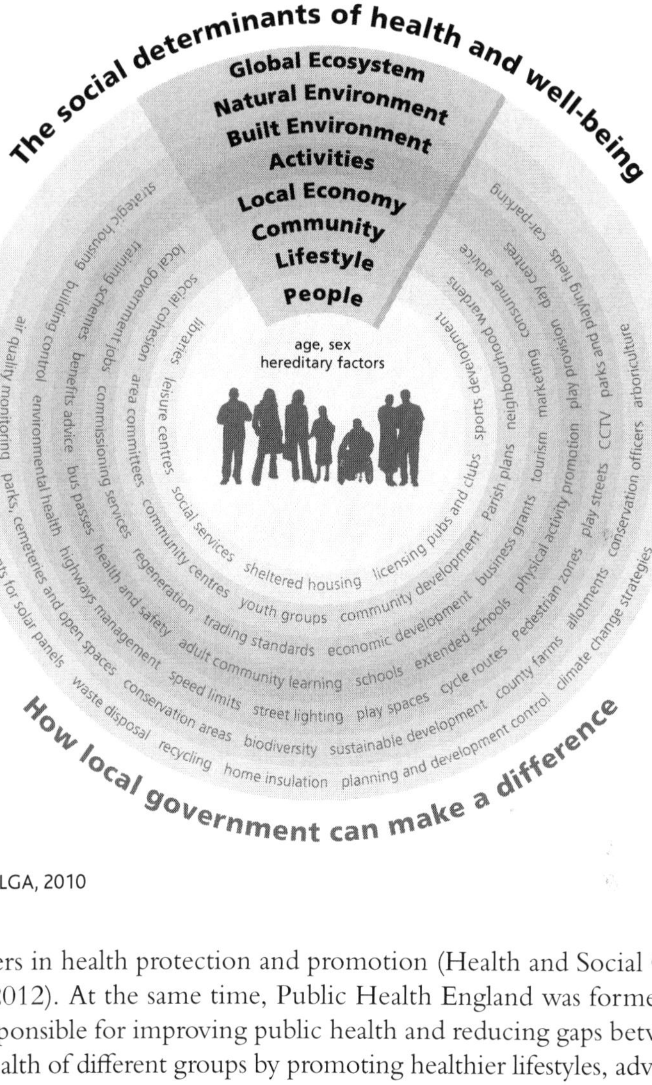

Source: LGA, 2010

partners in health protection and promotion (Health and Social Care Act, 2012). At the same time, Public Health England was formed to be responsible for improving public health and reducing gaps between the health of different groups by promoting healthier lifestyles, advising government and – crucially in the context of social determinants – supporting action by local government, the NHS and the public.

A recent review (King's Fund, 2020) concluded that the transfer was the right thing to do, but austerity was unhelpful and harmful. Public health teams were well embedded in local government and are well placed to work on social determinants. The deep cuts (up to 50 per cent of local government budgets), despite being unwelcome, generated innovation in commissioning, delivery and a focus on prevention. While specialist public health functions remain more NHS-centred in Wales and

Scotland, both nations have introduced policy frameworks that recognise the importance of local government in addressing health inequalities. This has not happened in England, despite the obvious capability of local government and the renewed impetus that the transfer of public health back into local government has brought to prevention efforts.

Meeting 21st-century public health challenges

The Marmot Review (2010) set the direction for improving health and reducing health inequalities in England and continues to shape public health services. It is estimated that over 70 per cent of local authorities are explicitly using Marmot principles to guide the way they carry out their public health responsibilities (LGA, 2017).

The principles are:

- give every child the best start in life;
- enable all children, young people and adults to maximise their capabilities and have control over their lives;
- create fair employment and good work for all;
- ensure a healthy standard of living for all;
- create and develop healthy sustainable places and communities;
- strengthen the role and impact of ill–health prevention.

A decade after this report, people in deprived areas continue to live shorter lives, as well as spending more of those years in poor health. The gap in healthy life expectancy is about 19 years for both males and females, and those living in the most deprived areas spend nearly a third of their lives in poor health, compared with only about a sixth for those in the least deprived areas (Raleigh, 2018).

Public health teams, now firmly at home in English local government, are a vital component of the local place leadership team – developing vital links across the council, the NHS and other local partners – with children's and adults' services, community safety, housing, planning and economic development all around the table. Within local government, public health is much more able to work collaboratively with communities to create healthy places for all and be part of local systems to address the social determinants of health.

Delivering place-based population health approaches

Given the wide range of determinants of health, most major achievements in public health happen when stakeholders across sectors develop common purposes and work together on shared goals. Key partners for councils include the NHS, the wider public sector, voluntary and community sectors, and businesses.

The directors of public health play a key leadership role in developing the local systems needed to tackle the complex issues impacting on health. Here we explore three aspects:

- the framing of public health;
- making the financial case;
- whole systems approaches.

The framing of public health

While the directors of public health have always claimed expertise in the 'science' of public health – which was well respected while within the NHS – the move to local government challenged them professionally to develop a stronger mastery of the 'art' of public health – influencing, policy change and systems leadership. The King's Fund (2020) assessment is that this has been largely successful. Working in a more explicitly political environment has stimulated careful consideration of how to frame public health efforts and tailor messages to different audiences. How we choose to frame things is critical, as the language we use, how we explain things and what we do not say influences how people make sense of and engage with issues. Some words and phrases illustrate the importance of paying attention to this: 'health', 'lifestyle', 'prevention', 'health in all policies' and 'a public health approach to…'.

The Health Foundation and the FrameWorks Institute have together been leading an exciting programme of work to reframe the conversation on the social determinants of health (Health Foundation and FrameWorks Institute, 2019). They have looked in detail at how the public understands the word 'health'. They note that:

> despite extensive evidence of the impact of social determinants on people's health, public discourse and policy action is limited in acknowledging the role that societal factors such as housing, education, welfare and work play in shaping people's long-term health.

Their research concludes that the dominant way people conceptualise health is through models of individual choice and health care – and the purported solution is 'raising awareness' so people make different choices. It is not surprising therefore that policymakers home in on individually focused interventions, primarily framed as changing 'lifestyle choices' and providing treatment through NHS services.

The use of 'lifestyle' has its origins in business marketing, a word capturing how to create desire and promote consumption. This is done by using very sophisticated techniques targeting segments of society – groups of people, not individuals – with products and services, from alcohol to gambling to Easter eggs. The term 'commercial determinants of health' is often used to describe the impact economic activity can have on our health and wellbeing. 'Lifestyle' both puts the emphasis on the individual, framing health-harming behaviour as an individual choice, and it takes the focus away from the socio-economic determinants of health and the health inequalities experienced by certain groups of people. 'Lifestyle' still problematically dominates national and local conversations about improving public health. And despite the evidence, we continue to situate answers with individuals and the need for them to alter their 'lifestyle choices'.

'Prevention' is another term that has gained remarkable traction over the last decade. While there is general agreement nationally and locally that this is what is needed, there is less agreement about what is meant by the term – and the 'fully engaged' scenario that Derek Wanless argued for (Wanless, 2002) remains little understood, let alone realised. The directors of public health have been influencing and shaping how people understand and use preventative approaches, trying to shift from the dominant focus on tertiary or secondary prevention to primary prevention and from a focus on the individual and one-to-one services, to communities and population health. Recognising that a systems-wide approach will deliver greater population-level improvements, they work to develop collectively owned, multidisciplinary, coherent models and narratives that enable strong local leadership on prevention agendas.

Advocating for 'health in all policies' has become increasingly popular. This phrase is often used by directors of public health to denote their new role of influencing their colleagues across a council to understand and develop the health-promoting potential of their functions and services and create a 'public health council'. In that sense, the transformational potential of public health being in local government would be realised by having healthy policies embedded in all aspects of what a council and its partners do.

The phrase 'health in all policies' remains a rather technical one, having arguably failed to gain general use beyond public health professionals. However, different framing is emerging, such as 'population health' or 'wellbeing of future generations': both show signs of being much more successful in energising and galvanising many more people to the cause.

Finally, public health contributes a set of skills to help systems address the complex challenges we face. Recently, the term 'a public health approach' has been used to understand and develop responses to knife violence, air quality and gambling. This language is particularly helpful for directors of public health and their teams as it provides an opportunity once again to bring their skills – and the science – to 21st-century public health challenges. How we talk about public health – with its focus on systemic approaches and determinants, rather than individual lifestyles or clinical interventions and the contribution of local government to this – is crucial, especially in the context of the current UK government, which, alongside sections of the media, remains overly dependent on individualist narratives.

Making the financial case

The framing of prevention is critical to ensuring sustainable funding flows at both national and local levels. Given the current financial climate, the case for investment in prevention must be as robust as possible. This applies both to maintaining current funding and the oft-stated and little-achieved collective ambition of shifting resources to prevention while maintaining treatment services. The ambition of whole-system integrated approaches can also founder when the payer organisation is not the financial beneficiary of improved outcomes.

Locally, in practice, these issues can only be resolved by strong partnerships with high levels of trust and a willingness to share both budgets and pool risks. Directors of public health need to develop a strong narrative and case for investment to advocate for prevention in planning and budgeting processes.

The future of public health funding must necessarily be seen in the context of NHS funding. Much could be achieved through judicious pooling of health and social care budgets, which could help to clearly identify the return on investment for everyone from prevention investments. Whether the national political will to deliver this is in place remains to be seen.

The public health grant supports public health teams – and the skills and experience within them – as well as funding the key frontline services for which directors of public health have responsibility. Rather than increasing this funding – and thus signalling real commitment behind the rhetoric on public health and prevention – there have been considerable reductions, with concomitant major impact on local services, such as sexual health, drug and alcohol services, stop smoking support, health visiting and school nursing. These cuts disadvantage particular population groups with high needs – and therefore increase inequalities. It also epitomises the current short-term approach to public health and ignores the much larger long-term costs associated with not investing in public health. It fails to appreciate the great dividends to be paid, both to the economy and society, through investing in improved public health.

At the same time, the Public Health Grant has made public health spending more transparent than was ever the case in the NHS, but the significant focus on the role of this ring-fenced grant has in some respects focused attention too narrowly on mandated service commissioning functions of the directors of public health and downplayed their potential system leadership role – which is crucial in addressing the social determinants of health. Directors of public health should influence across systems and public sector budgets. However, the cuts undermine their ability and capacity to have this very influence.

At the time of writing in May 2020, the future of English local government funding is in discussion, and with it the future of public health funding. The government's aim is to introduce 75 per cent business rate retention. It is very important that the system is designed in such a way that this does not mean disinvestment in prevention, does not widen health inequalities and enables directors of public health to continue to lead improvements in the health of their local populations. As the King's Fund (2020) states, 'changes to local government financing (for example, a proposed increase in local retention of business rates) must not unintentionally put public health spending at risk'. An increasing coalition of voices agrees that English public health needs better and more sustainable funding. The mechanism by which this is delivered and distributed is an open question.

After years of cuts, there is a growing movement of non-governmental organisations, policy commentators, think tanks and professional bodies calling for a commitment to restoring £1 billion of real-terms per head cuts to the public health grant (Finch et al, 2018; Buck, 2019; House of Commons Health Committee, 2016) as part of a long-term funding package, similar to that given to the NHS to implement the Long Term Plan.

Whole systems approaches

The last five years have seen a rapid rise in consideration of systems approaches to population health (Bagnall et al, 2019), and alongside this a rise in approaches to the leadership styles and behaviours needed to be effective (Bolden et al, 2019). Whole systems approaches are becoming increasingly widespread, including on topics such as healthy weight (Public Health England, 2019), with the appreciation that focusing on individual choices alone will not reduce levels of obesity – only whole system working will achieve the scale of change required. The following describes the latest definition of this way of working.

> A local whole systems approach responds to complexity through an ongoing, dynamic and flexible way of working. It enables local stakeholders, including communities, to come together, share an understanding of the reality of the challenge, consider how the local system is operating and where there are the greatest opportunities for change. Stakeholders agree actions and decide as a network how to work together in an integrated way to bring about sustainable, long-term systems change. (LGA, 2019a)

A whole systems approach to obesity has several key benefits (LGA, 2019a):

- effect of collective actions is greater than the sum of the individual actions – identifies, implements and aligns actions that have wider impact across the local system;
- reflects the local leadership role of local authorities – enables reach and penetration into local places, working with and through an extensive range of stakeholders, including communities;
- aligns with a 'Health in All Policies' approach – recognises the range and complexity of causes of obesity, supporting a system-wide approach to understand and address health inequalities;
- maximises all the assets in the local area, including community assets – recognising and identifying local assets can help build on the strengths of communities;
- supports a community-centred approach to tackling health inequalities – involving local communities, especially disadvantaged groups, can better reflect the local realities, help improve health and wellbeing and reduce health inequalities;
- develops transferable workforce skills and capacity – relevant and applicable for other complex issues;
- recognises the potential of all partners to contribute – NHS organisations, local authority departments and the education,

business and voluntary sectors all have a significant role to play in improving the population's health.

For directors of public health on the ground, this means utilising their expertise not just on weight management services but on public health influence over licensing (to halt the proliferation of takeaways) and planning (to put active travel such as walking and cycling at the heart of regeneration plans). It means always thinking about how whole systems approaches can reduce health inequalities. For instance, evidence shows that there are elevated levels of obesity in communities with high concentrations of fast food outlets (Zenk et al, 2009) and further evidence that such concentrations are highest in areas of greatest deprivation (LGA, 2015).

Funding for social infrastructure and a clear understanding of the health-promoting role of places and communities both remain neglected. Good, healthy lives need a strong social fabric, involving attractive places that allow us to connect to each other, advice and support when we encounter difficulties and activities that create relationships, purpose and resilience. A healthy society is not one that waits for people to become ill, but one that sees how health is shaped by social, cultural, political, economic, commercial and environmental factors, and acts on these.

Transforming services

Public health in local government delivers key frontline services or significantly influences other services to address the social determinants of health. These services can roughly be divided into four categories: the best start in life, living and ageing well, a good place to live and support in difficult times. These interventions can only work if properly funded and backed up by good national policy and sufficient levels of funding.

Austerity has been a major driver of change in the way we deliver these services. In part, it has driven necessary transformation and efficiencies within public services; but mostly it has driven unnecessary demands on many services and arguably is now costing the government more than it is saving – as well as leading to all sorts of distortions within the public sector. Many of the services that transferred with directors of public health from the NHS to local government brought with them long-standing challenges – from the underfunding of school nursing and fragmentation in health visiting, including poor links with general practitioners – to overly medicalised and expensive sexual health services, or drug services focused on clinical treatment and not recovery.

Public health in local government has brought new energy and rigour to the commissioning of the services for which directors of public health have responsibility, often transforming who delivers them, where and how, making integration and partnership-working real – and, in the context of rising demand and huge cuts, largely delivering good outcomes. Redesign in many areas has focused on integration – integration with other public services, such as criminal justice, adult services, children and young people's services, and integration across the wider health economy. It has also looked to commission the community and voluntary sectors and to increase social value through its contracts.

Many local authorities have taken decisions that the NHS could not or would not make. Several reports indicate that local government has been successful in delivering services under difficult circumstances and has prioritised increasingly scarce resources effectively. For instance, analysis of the Public Health Outcomes Framework – which tracks 112 health indicators – shows that in the last six years 80 per cent of those indicators have been level or improving (LGA, 2019b). This strong performance is unsustainable in the context of falling budgets.

Directors of public health in England are providing leadership and expertise to meet 21st-century public health and financial challenges and deliver strong place-based, population health approaches – as well as leading the transformation of those services they are responsible for commissioning – substance misuse, sexual health and 0–19 services.

The modernisation of sexual and reproductive health services offers good examples of how this shift is taking shape on the ground. In Norfolk, for instance, the county council commissioned an integrated sexual health service. In response to a rising number of attendances at their sexual health clinics, the council was looking for other ways to support people. The development of an online platform enables people who are concerned about their sexual health to request a sexually transmitted infection kit to be sent to their home, self-test, return via post and receive the results to their mobile phone within days. With better triaging, the right tests can be sent to the right people at the right time; while moving forward, the service is looking to reduce the costs of over-testing (LGA, 2019b).

A new national Sexual and Reproductive Health Strategy is long overdue: building on the integrated care pathways being developed in different parts of the country and reducing health inequalities should be essential components. Similar principles must be applied across all public health services.

National leadership for wellbeing

Local authorities are not islands; they cannot tackle the social determinants alone – a range of policy and investment decisions must be made in Whitehall to support town halls. Nationally, recent policy announcements relating to prevention, such as the publication of a Green Paper (Cabinet Office, 2019) on the subject, have stimulated conversations within, and between, the different departments that should hold a shared responsibility for addressing the social determinants of health.

Delivering change means putting a greater emphasis on improving housing, air quality, education, income and food; it means supporting people into good work and creating healthy workplaces – all factors which overwhelmingly shape our health and wellbeing: and drive down inequalities in how long we live in good health. Whether we call it wellbeing or happiness or something else, the commitment to a common narrative across government that makes our health and wellbeing of equal importance to our economic success is the next big milestone.

The idea of wellbeing as an organising principle of society has become increasingly prominent. Politicians and policymakers have also been attracted by the concept of a national measurement of success that is more concerned with happiness than a narrow focus on our economic output. The UK government has pledged to launch a new health index (Cabinet Office, 2019) to help Whitehall track the health of the nation. This could provide the driver for every department to make policy and spending decisions that improve wellbeing – essentially a gross domestic product-type indicator for health.

In 2018, Scotland, Iceland and New Zealand established the network of Wellbeing Economy Governments, which seeks to promote the sharing of expertise and transferable policy practices among governments that have a shared ambition of delivering wellbeing through their economic approach. New Zealand has become the first country in the world to produce a 'wellbeing budget' – a commitment to prioritise population wellbeing as the main mission of the government (Wellbeing Budget, 2019). A similar philosophy was adopted in Wales in 2015 through the Well-being of Future Generations Act, which requires public bodies to think about the long-term impact of their policies on both people and places (Welsh Government, 2015).

This is a bold new development in the story of public health, an approach that puts the highest value on quality of life when it comes to national policy and investment decisions. The Association of Directors of Public Health has long championed taking a whole system and a long-term view about how we create, enable and sustain the health and wellbeing of everyone in society.

Local government has not often seized the passion of public health research as much as it could have, and we believe, in concluding, that there remains much to be learned in comparative research about how local government has been engaged in addressing health inequalities across the four nations of the UK, especially in the context of devolution (Greer, 2016). This is a research agenda that could yield significant fruit.

Conclusion

Ten years since the publication of the Marmot Review, for the first time in more than 100 years life expectancy has failed to increase across the country, and for the poorest 10 per cent of women it has declined (Marmot et al, 2020). Health and wellbeing problems remain complex – shaped by international and national political, economic and social trends – and require approaches that work across these systems. Tackling poverty, serious violence, domestic abuse, air quality, childhood obesity or unhealthy ageing means thinking about the environments we call home. We need places that help us to live and thrive – good schools, good homes, good jobs, good open spaces and good social and civic infrastructure for connecting people and enabling relationships.

As we look to the future, we see a welcome and renewed ambition to improve healthy life expectancy so that, by 2035, we will be enjoying at least five extra years of healthy, independent life, while closing the gap between the richest and poorest. If public health – and local government – funding continues to be cut, this noble goal will not be met, with the costs – in pounds and loss of human potential – being borne by the NHS, the economy and individuals. For too long, the role of local authorities and their actions on wider determinants have been understated and undervalued. That will not deter local authorities from acting, but this view continues to impoverish English health policy. The dual imbalance of austerity and privileging clinical approaches continues to hamper progress on inequalities, and makes neither moral nor economic sense.

References

Bagnall, A., Radley, D., Jones, R., Gately, P., Nobles, J., Van Dijk, M., Blackshaw, J., Montel, S. and Sahota, P. (2019) 'Whole systems approaches to obesity and other complex public health challenges: a systematic review', *BMC Public Health*, 19(1): article 8.

Bolden, R., Gulati, A. and Edwards, G. (2019) 'Mobilizing change in public services: insights from a systems leadership development intervention', *International Journal of Public Administration*, 43(1): 26–36.

Buck, D. (2019) 'Public health spending: where prevention rhetoric meets reality'. Available from: https://www.kingsfund.org.uk/blog/2019/07/public-health-spending-blog [Accessed 29 July 2019].

Cabinet Office (2019) 'Advancing our health: prevention in the 2020s'. London: Cabinet Office. Available from: https://www.gov.uk/government/consultations/advancing-our-health-prevention-in-the-2020s [Accessed 14 August 2019].

Fell, G. and McManus, J. (2020) 'Public health within local government, six years on', *British Medical Journal*, 368, m572. Available from: https://doi.org/10.1136/bmj.m572 [Accessed 8 April 2020].

Finch, D., Bibby, J. and Elwell-Sutton, T. (2018) 'Taking our health for granted: plugging the public health grant funding gap'. Available from: https://www.health.org.uk/publications/taking-our-health-for-granted [Accessed 29 July 2019].

Gray, M. and Barford, A. (2018) 'The depths of the cuts: the uneven geography of local government austerity', *Cambridge Journal of Regions, Economy and Society*, 11(3): 541–63. Available from: https://doi.org/10.1093/cjres/rsy019 [Accessed 15 August 2019].

Greer, S.L. (2016) 'Devolution and health in the UK: policy and its lessons since 1998', *British Medical Bulletin*, 118(1): 16–24.

Health and Social Care Act (2012) UK Public General Acts. Available from: http://www.legislation.gov.uk/ukpga/2012/7/contents/enacted [Accessed 12 August 2019].

Health Foundation and FrameWorks Institute (2019) 'Briefing: reframing the conversation on the social determinants of health'. Available from: https://www.health.org.uk/sites/default/files/upload/publications/2019/Reframing-the-conversation-on-social-determinants.pdf [Accessed 15 August 2019].

House of Commons Health Committee (2016) 'Public health post-2013 inquiry'. Available at: https://www.parliament.uk/business/committees/committees-a-z/commons-select/health-committee/inquiries/parliament-2015/public-health-post-2013-inquiry-15-16/ [Accessed 11 August 2019].

Institute for Fiscal Studies (2019) 'English local government funding: trends and challenges in 2019 and beyond'. London: IFS. Available from: https://www.ifs.org.uk/publications/14563 [Accessed 31 January 2020].

King's Fund (2020) 'Looking ahead to 2020', blog post, 1 January. Available from: https://www.kingsfund.org.uk/blog/2020/01/looking-ahead-2020 [Accessed 28 July 2020].

LGA (Local Government Association) (2010) 'The social determinants of health and the role of local government'. Available from: https://www.local.gov.uk/sites/default/files/documents/foreward-and-introduction-c1c.pdf [Accessed 11 August 2019].

LGA (Local Government Association) (2015) 'Tipping the scale'. Available from: https://www.local.gov.uk/sites/default/files/documents/L15-427%20Tipping%20the%20scales%20WEB.pdf [Accessed 21 August 2019].

LGA (Local Government Association) (2017) 'Prevention: how do you know that your council is doing all it can to deliver on prevention?' Available from: https://www.local.gov.uk/sites/default/files/documents/22.10%20-%20Must%20Know%20for%20Elected%20members%20on%20Prevention_05.pdf [Accessed 11 August 2019].

LGA (Local Government Association) (2019a) 'LGA/ADPH annual public health conference and exhibition 2019', March. Available from: https://www.local.gov.uk/lgaadph-annual-public-health-conference-and-exhibition-2019-21-march-2019 [Accessed 29 July 2020].

LGA (Local Government Association) (2019b) 'LGA case studies – Norfolk County Council: easing demand on clinics'. Available from: https://www.local.gov.uk/norfolk-county-council-easing-demand-clinics [Accessed 10 August 2019].

Marmot, M. (2010) 'Fair Society, Healthy Lives', The Marmot Review, Institute of Health Equity. Available from: http://www.instituteofhealthequity.org/resources-reports/fair-society-healthy-lives-the-marmot-review [Accessed 8 April 2020].

Marmot, M. et al (2020) 'Health Equity in England: The Marmot Review in England'. Available from: http://www.instituteofhealthequity.org/resources-reports/marmot-review-10-years-on/marmot-review-10-years-on-full-report.pdf [Accessed 8 April 2020].

Milne, E. (2018) 'The transfer of public health to local authorities suggests alternatives are possible – the *BMJ*'. Available from: https://blogs.bmj.com/bmj/2018/05/03/eugene-milne-the-transfer-of-public-health-to-local-authorities-suggests-alternatives-are-possible/ [Accessed 1 February 2020].

ONS (Office for National Statistics) (2018) 'National life tables, UK: 2015–2017'. Available from: https://www.ons.gov.uk/people populationandcommunity/birthsdeathsandmarriages/lifeexpectancies/bulletins/nationallifetablesunitedkingdom/2015to2017 [Accessed 11 August 2019].

ONS (Office for National Statistics) (2019) 'Health state life expectancies by national deprivation deciles, England and Wales: 2015 to 2017'. Available from: https://www.ons.gov.uk/peoplepopulation andcommunity/healthandsocialcare/healthinequalities/bulletins/healthstatelifeexpectanciesbyindexofmultipledeprivationimd/2015to 2017 [Accessed 11 August 2019].

Public Health Act (1936) UK Public General Acts. Available from: http://www.legislation.gov.uk/ukpga/Geo5and1Edw8/26/49/contents [Accessed 13 August 2019].

Public Health England (2019) 'Whole systems approaches to obesity'. Available from: https://www.gov.uk/government/publications/whole-systems-approach-to-obesity [Accessed on 11 August 2019].

Raleigh, V. (2018) 'What is happening to life expectancy in the UK?' Available from: https://www.kingsfund.org.uk/publications/whats-happening-life-expectancy-uk [Accessed on 10 August 2019].

Wanless, D. (2002) 'Securing our future health: taking a long-term view'. Available from: https://www.yearofcare.co.uk/sites/default/files/images/Wanless.pdf [Accessed 13 August 2019].

Wellbeing Budget (2019) New Zealand Government. Available from: https://treasury.govt.nz/sites/default/files/2019-05/b19-wellbeing-budget.pdf [Accessed 12 August 2019].

Welsh Government (2015) 'Well-being of Future Generations (Wales) Act 2015: The Essentials'. Available from: https://futuregenerations.wales/wp-content/uploads/2017/02/150623-guide-to-the-fg-act-en.pdf.

Zenk, S.N., Schulz, A.J., Odoms-Young, A.M. (2009) 'How neighborhood environments contribute to obesity', *The American Journal of Nursing*, 109(7): 61–4. Available from: https://www.ncbi.nlm.nih.gov/pmc/articles/PMC2789291/ [Accessed 21 August 2019].

3

Health and social care systems

Anna Coleman, Jolanta Shields and Tim Gilling

Introduction

The National Health Service (NHS) has a key role in improving population health in Britain. Yet despite progress, health inequalities persist (PHE, 2018a), as noted in Chapters 1 and 2. Life expectancy has increased for some groups, including those living with complex, multiple and chronic conditions, but others have experienced a widening of the inequality gap (Raleigh, 2018); see Chapters 1 and 2 for a social determinants perspective on health inequalities. The demographic shift towards an ageing and growing population places new demands on the health care system, raising questions about its long-term sustainability (Guzman-Castillo et al, 2017). Successive governments have pursued centralisation, delegation, devolution and privatisation as means of addressing growing demands across the health and social care system (Peckham et al, 2005). Recently, in England, a clear consensus has emerged to embed (public) health in all policies (HiAP), taking into account wider determinants of health and including prevention (LGA, 2016).[1] Local Authorities (LAs) are seen to be uniquely positioned to facilitate this transformation, being close to local communities with an understanding and responsibility for issues such as environment, employment, housing and education. These socio-economic factors are seen to significantly impact on people's health and wellbeing in a way that the NHS cannot address alone. The NHS Long Term Plan (NHSE, 2019) and the earlier 'Prevention is Better than Cure' document (DHSC, 2018) set out the government's ambition to reshape the existing health care model by strengthening public health and prioritising primary medical and community health services. Central to this are Integrated Care Systems (ICSs), planned to be in place across the whole of England by April 2021, which provide a stronger basis from which the NHS, LAs and other organisations can work together on prevention, wellbeing and health. However, on average, local government spending on services has fallen by 21 per cent in real terms since 2009–10 and these cuts have not been equally distributed across the country, being greater in more deprived areas (Amin-Smith and Phillips, 2019, p 2).

Against this backdrop, this chapter offers a critical analysis of the role of LAs in relation to promoting health and wellbeing for local communities. Taking Dahlgren and Whitehead's 'rainbow model' (1991) as a starting point (see Preface to this volume), the chapter traces recent policy initiatives and illustrates the complexity involved in tackling inequalities in the newly emerging health care systems. The chapter begins by briefly outlining the relevant policy and legislative context to better understand the role of LAs in advancing the public health agenda. It then draws on the example of health and social care devolution in Greater Manchester (GM) to illustrate both the opportunities and challenges faced by local organisations in operationalising and implementing national policy in the context of austerity.

The wider policy context

The role of local government in public health functions, as detailed in Part III of this volume, can be traced to the social and economic developments in the 19th century that resulted in rapid urbanisation with poor housing and workplace provision (Gorsky et al, 2014). Since then, public health duties have expanded, conferring more responsibility for population health on local government. However, public health functions were incorporated within the NHS in 1974 and did not return until 2013 (see Chapter 16). The White Paper *Healthy Lives, Healthy People* (Department of Health, 2010), informed by the findings from the Marmot Review (Marmot et al, 2010), proposed a new approach to public health whereby 'local government and local communities […] [would be] at the heart of improving health and wellbeing for their populations' (Department of Health, 2010, p 4). This was a significant shift from prioritising clinical treatment to prevention of illness with a focus on interventions to address the wider determinants of health (identified by Dahlgren and Whitehead, 1991) seen to be closely aligned with the functions of LAs, examples of these being housing, leisure, transport and planning. The Health and Social Care Act (HSCA12, ref 195(1)) transferred responsibility for health improvement (as part of public health responsibilities) to LAs and obliged them to establish Health and Wellbeing Boards (HWBs) in their local area to work closely with Clinical Commissioning Groups (CCGs), NHS England and local communities through local

Healthwatch (the independent advocates for people who use health and social care services).

The HSCA12 also created Public Health England (PHE), an executive agency of the Department of Health and Social Care, as well as the other bodies detailed in Table 3.1. These changes echoed the wider commitment of the Coalition government, articulated under the Localism Act (2011), aimed at devolving decision-making powers from national government to the local level. The landscape is complex as, for example, responsibilities for improving the health of local populations, including a reduction in health inequalities, sit with upper tier and unitary local authorities (those with social services responsibilities), while the delivery of some public health functions, including protection and promotion of health (for example, immunisation and screening services), rests with the NHS.

The previous 20 years had seen numerous calls for health and care services and other services impacting on the wider determinants of health to become more integrated. However, in England there has long been a fundamental tension as NHS services are free at the point of use and means-tested social care is provided by local government. Policy initiatives in England have included the 2006 NHS Act Section 75 flexibilities, HWBs, the Better Care Fund (from 2013) and

Table 3.1: Selected healthcare and associated organisations introduced under HSCA12

Organisation	Description
Clinical Commissioning Groups (CCGs)	Health commissioning organisations replacing Primary Care Trusts (PCTs) in April 2013. Responsible for planning and buying of NHS healthcare. CCGs are membership organisations led by family doctors (GPs) to gain a clinical voice.
NHS England (NHSE)	Arm's-length executive body with delegated (via annual mandate) responsibility to deliver health services. It sets the priorities and direction of the NHS and encourages the national debate to improve health and care.
Public Health England (PHE)	An executive agency, sponsored by the Department of Health and Social Care, which exists to protect and improve the nation's health and wellbeing, and reduce health inequalities. It advises government and supports action by local government, the NHS and the public, and health protection.
Health and Wellbeing Boards (HWBs)	Hosted by upper-tier local authorities, bringing together the NHS, public health, adult social care and children's services, including elected representatives and others, to plan how best to meet the needs of their local population and tackle local inequalities in health. Set local strategic direction.

Integrated Care pilots (from 2013). There were also some wider public sector initiatives (including elements of health, local authorities and national government) introduced to promote place-based approaches to funding and service configuration, including Total Place Pilots in 2009, Whole Place community budgets in 2011, the 2013 troubled families initiative and latterly English devolution deals (Miller and Glasby, 2016).

The Five Year Forward View (NHSE, 2014) called for a 'radical upgrade in prevention and public health' with 'stronger public-health related powers for local government and elected mayors' giving shared responsibility for health and social care of local population (NHSE, 2014, para 4). The document consolidated earlier efforts for joint working and local health leaders were asked to come together in 44 geographically defined 'footprints' across England, to produce Sustainability and Transformation Plans (STPs) (later known as Partnerships) for transforming services using an allocated funding envelope (NHSE, 2014). It also introduced New Care Models, with 50 'Vanguards' selected to trial the development of new ways of integrated working (Checkland et al, 2019). At the same time, many initiatives focused on integrated person-centred care involving both the NHS and LAs (see Table 3.2).

The NHS Long Term Plan (NHSE, 2019) sets out the ambition for joined-up care that reduces dependency on emergency care and supports local approaches to blend health and social care budgets,

Table 3.2: Initiatives introduced to focus on integrated person-centred care

Initiative	Description
Better Care Fund	2015–16 £3.8 billion of pooled funding into a single budget for health and social care services (2015–16) to work closely together to protect adult social services while reducing demand for acute beds. Provided a context where the NHS and local authorities work together, as equal partners, with shared objectives. Plans are developed in a local area by the relevant CCG(s) and owned by the relevant HWB.
Personal Health Budgets	Part of the NHS's comprehensive model of personalised care to support healthcare and wellbeing of individuals. Planned and agreed between an individual and the CCG.
Troubled Families Programme	Administered by the Department for Communities and Local Government and funded by central government, it involves LAs identifying and working with 'troubled families' via dedicated workers, and only receiving payment on the successful completion of the case; for instance, moving a family into permanent employment.

among other initiatives (NHSE, 2019, p 4). Under ICSs, NHS organisations, in partnership with LAs and others, will take collective responsibility for managing resources and improving the health of the population they serve. The long-awaited Adult Social Care Green Paper is also expected to strengthen the approach, prioritising person-centred integrated care. Local government has a vital role to play in delivering this agenda through its public health and social care functions. Local communities are integral to the health care system and play an important part at population and individual level (often asset-based), with individuals taking greater responsibility for their health and wellbeing. However, budget pressures in adult social care present challenges across many areas.

Place based planning and integrated care systems

The strength of place-based initiatives in England is that they focus on the impact of the wider determinants of health, not just ill-health. In turn, this draws attention to the key functions of LAs, which were described by Lyons (2007, p 51) as 'place-shaping' – 'the creative use of powers and influence to promote the general well-being of a community and its citizens'. The legitimacy of LAs as 'democratically accountable stewards' is central to this approach, allowing LAs to respond and shape services in the way that these are responsive to local needs (Department of Health, 2011, p 1). As planning authorities, LAs, for instance, have an opportunity to influence the built environment so that it supports adopting healthy lifestyles (leisure, transport, housing, and so on). For example, a refreshed memorandum of understanding (PHE, 2018b) was signed by over 25 stakeholders in 2018, emphasising the importance of housing in supporting health and setting out a shared commitment to joint action across government, health, social care and housing sectors in England. Likewise, the licensing powers of LAs allow them to consider the wider impact of fast food and gambling outlets, particularly if these are to be established close to schools. For example, in Sheffield, the council adopted an innovative approach by framing tobacco and obesity as commercial determinants rather than lifestyle choices, shifting investment directly towards control and enforcement as well as interventions that sought to change public attitudes (LGA, 2019a). In 2013, Coventry City Council became a 'Marmot City', an initiative spanning seven LAs working with public and voluntary sector organisations on innovative projects that aimed to reduce inequalities by embedding six policy objectives of the Marmot Review (2010).[2] Since adopting the status, Coventry has reported a narrowing of the life expectancy gap between the most affluent and most deprived and improvements in educational, employment and health outcomes (Faherty and Gaulton, 2017). Attention has additionally been drawn to the fact that LAs are major employers as well as 'anchor intuitions' closely connected to the wellbeing of the populations they serve (LGA, 2018a). The Department for Communities and Local Government (DCLG, 2017) estimated in 2017 that the total procurement expenditure of LAs stood at over £60 billion, meaning these organisations also have the potential to indirectly impact on the lives and 'the conditions of many more workers that they do not employ' (LGA, 2018a, p 27).

The focus on 'place' as a source of problems as well as solutions is not new, and has been widely used in regeneration studies (Lawless et al, 2010). In particular, New Labour's Neighbourhood Renewal (SEU, 2001) set out to tackle inequality and social exclusion by empowering local communities and strengthening the role of LAs through Local Strategic Partnerships. These were not dissimilar to what STPs/ ICSs are trying to achieve, although the emphasis is now strongly on integration between health and social care.

For LAs, 'place' matters, although the term takes different meanings and purposes. Increasingly, though, LAs are using place-based initiatives to address complex health inequalities. Since the passing of the Social Value Act (2012) and HSCA 2012, public bodies have had to consider the wider social, environmental and health implications of their commissioning decisions, with LAs required to improve health outcomes and reduce health inequalities. HiAP, mentioned earlier, provides an important collaborative framework to achieve this 'by incorporating health considerations into decision making across sectors, policy and service areas, and addressing wider determinants of health' (PHE, 2016, p 4). In Liverpool, the council extended the approach to include Health in all Policies and Places, emphasising the role of LAs in driving this agenda forward (LGA, 2019a, p 8).

Dorling (2010), however, argues that defining inequalities in terms of LAs' boundaries is not necessarily helpful as LAs engage at different levels, including regional, national and recently system level. He also suggests that focusing on single measures such as income or population size is likely to miss important cleavages, an example being the extreme variations between areas and neighbourhoods. Purdam (2017) makes this point compellingly by using the Metrolink map in GM to illustrate, for instance, how male life expectancy at birth in Rochdale is nine years shorter than in Milnrow, areas only three tram stops apart. In this sense, the concept of place is far more nuanced and contested especially in the context of STPs/ICSs (predicted to cover populations between 1 and 3 million) with their emphasis on collaboration as a panacea for deeply entrenched structural problems. Hammond and colleagues (2017, p 225) argue that 'turning down the noise on political contestation through evoking notions of local consensus' risks obscuring the reality of austerity policies and their impact on LAs that are delivering health and social care to the local population.

According to the National Audit Office (NAO, 2018), LAs have been facing significant challenges since 2010–11 as funding has been reduced despite growing demand, particularly for social care. The fiscal stress under which LAs operate means that balancing statutory provision requirement with financial survival is likely to affect the quality of public health interventions. The NAO offers some optimism, citing cases where LAs were able to make progress by successfully commissioning for quality and best value (NAO, 2018). The Local Government Association (LGA) also reported a largely positive impact of relocating public health to LAs in England, claiming these were able to deliver 'better outcomes [in a number of areas] at less cost than the NHS did when they controlled public health' (LGA, 2019b, p 3). However, a note of caution is sounded in relation to the proper funding for LAs' public health and meaningful engagement with councils to make further progress around prevention and avoid a postcode lottery. This is particularly pertinent in the light of the recent analysis by the BBC based on the resilience index prepared by the Chartered Institute of Public Finance and Accountancy (CIPFA), which found that 11 LAs were close to fully exhausting their reserves within four years' time if no action was taken (CIPFA, 2018; BBC, 2019).

The organisational landscape around which public health functions operate is increasingly complex and changing. Commissioning in complexity is discussed in Chapter 13. The earlier development of some STPs lacked public visibility and left a legacy that has been difficult to overcome (Coleman, 2016). The absence of wider engagement of all parties (LAs, the public) in early development resulted in local priorities having to be retrofitted into the plans. Recently, Corcoran (2019) identified 11 separate governance and accountability challenges that NHS and LAs may face when seeking to work more collaboratively. For instance, the report drew attention to how LAs talk about places and residents whereas the NHS tends to talk about premises and patients. It also highlights different funding regimes, planning cycles and geographies that can be problematic for decentralisation and local integration, alongside the enduring issues of historically embedded siloed thinking and organisational focus and oversight. The NHS

Long Term Plan (NHSE, 2019), while intended to take a system-wide view, appears to be 'written by the NHS for the NHS, not for the whole health and care system, since the funding settlement excludes public health, social care, education and training' (Humphries, 2019). This resonates with the report by the Health and Social Care Select Committee, 'First 1000 days of life' (DHSC, 2019), which noted the structural problems with government financing that hinder early local interventions. Although the government claims it encourages departments 'to work across traditional boundaries to deliver improved public services', the reality can be far more complex in practice. The Centre for Public Scrutiny (CfPS), suggest that this may be because political and organisational cultures have not yet had time to adapt. Central to the process of transformation is 'good governance [...] from which councils can build and sustain the changes and respond to local needs' (CfPS, 2019, p 5). According to the CfPS, the traditional aspects of governance find themselves increasingly at odds with the emerging models, prompting calls for new forms of decision-making. This may involve, for instance, creating a 'constitution for the place' (see the Wigan and Preston model, Chapter 8) or, as the CfPS calls it, 'the community constitution', which emphasises collaboration based on transparent lines of accountability, responsibility and ownership for the agreed outcomes (CfPS, 2019).

This approach is particularly pertinent in the context of the reforms introduced by HSCA12, which resulted in territorial boundaries that do not necessarily align with developing STPs/ICSs and can cut across LAs and HWBs. The ICSs, for instance, are intended to operate at three levels simultaneously: system (working together to set priorities, plan and agree the overall level of integration, 1–3 million population), place (within the system and focused on planning localised services alongside the delivery of secondary and community care, 250,000–500,000 population) and neighbourhoods (centred around primary care networks with general practitioner (GP) networks covering populations of 30,000–50,000 and with multidisciplinary teams working together to provide primary and community care). This raises questions about levels of accountability and rights of patients, residents and communities to health and social care services. This matters if HWBs are to produce joint strategic needs assessments that look at the current and future health and care needs for their local area, allowing to better plan and commission health, wellbeing and social care services within the LA.

While the argument for developing ICSs is compelling, and Corcoran (2019) provides a series of potential enablers (e.g. joint appointments and shared objectives) that have already been used to drive the progress, this should not preclude the case for careful examination of proposals. In this context, LAs have a number of important roles through their decision-making and scrutiny arrangements. LAs with social care responsibilities have powers to review issues relating to planning and delivery of health services and in certain circumstances can refer proposals for major changes to health services to the Secretary of State (CfPS, 2017). As well as powers relating to NHS bodies, there is a key role for scrutiny committees to review the actions that LAs are taking to improve public health (Ferry and Murphy, 2018). Overview and scrutiny and other forms of local assurance have a vital role to play, providing democratic and other links between national policymakers, commissioners, providers and the communities they serve. As champions of local needs, elected representatives and others with an assurance role help to safeguard the quality and safety of health and social care as well as promoting actions on the wider determinants of health. The current challenge is for the NHS and LA scrutiny to develop agreed ways of working to facilitate effective timely scrutiny of strategic issues, outcomes expected from ICSs and people's experiences of local services.

Deloitte's (2019) report suggests nine success criteria against which to measure a more joined-up, population-oriented approach to health and care that STPs/ICSs could utilise. These include developing a common language to enable better data sharing; provision of funding, infrastructure and leadership support; agreeing appropriate performance measures (KPIs) across systems; establishing wider public engagement in prevention; and promoting patient activation and empowerment. The development of integrated ways of working is presently dependent on establishing successful local alliances rather than changes to primary legislation, meaning progress is varied and can be delayed by unresolved problems related to, for example, VAT liabilities, KPIs and exemptions that are different for NHS trusts and private providers.

The dominance of central institutional policy and regulatory frameworks plays an important role in affecting the development of STPs/ICSs. Earlier reforms introduced by the HSCA12 weakened regional structures, questioning the resilience of the health and social care system to deliver government policy (Exworthy et al, 2017).

The devolution and decentralisation agendas are problematic when LAs have no control over national funding streams, albeit increased autonomy over spending. According to the LGA (2018b), funding for adult social care faces a gap of by £3.5 billion by 2025. This is significant since much of the NHS Long Term Plan (NHSE, 2019) is centred on initiatives that aim to tackle wider determinants of health with an expectation that LAs would be able to help close the inequality gap. The increasing deficits in the acute (NHS) sector also mean that planning around long-term goals in health and social care is difficult. There is still an uncertainty about the vision for social care, and until the Green Paper is published the issue of prevention is open to debate.

Learning: health and social care devolution in Greater Manchester

An insight into devolved metropolitan authorities is presented in Chapter 5. The devolution of health and social care in GM illustrates some of the issues of establishing place-based healthcare initiatives that require the involvement of local government by referencing health and social care devolution in GM. Since 2015, local partners have taken 'devolved control' of the region's health and social care budgets (£6 billion per annum for the 2.8 million population). GM prioritised the creation of an integrated system, with distinctive local provision, and increased scope for joint commissioning, the pooling of public resources, the creation of provider alliances and promotion of new ways of working (Walshe et al, 2018).

In February 2015, plans to devolve decisions over health and social care spending in GM to a newly established strategic partnership board (GMHCP) (AGMA, 2015) were announced. This initial deal was negotiated quickly by key leaders (including the LA) across GM following wider devolution powers being granted to GM in November 2014. The new GMHCP Board brought together 10 LAs, 12 (latterly 10 owing to a merger) CCGs, 15 NHS trusts and foundation trusts, and NHS England, which set out an ambitious strategy – 'Taking Charge' (GMCA, 2015) – including reforms, governance arrangements and targets. Four high-level reform themes were proposed: upgraded population health prevention, transformed community-based care and support, standardised acute and specialist care, and standardised clinical support and back office services. Developments were facilitated by stable GM leadership and close political cooperation of the 10 LAs over 20 years, and more recently joint working by the 10 CCGs across the GM footprint.

Since the 2015 devolution agreement, much effort has gone into enhancing relationships, setting up governance arrangements and agreeing strategies and plans. The GM Partnership has embraced complexity and started tackling reconfiguration across the whole system. Walshe et al (2018) describe a 'soft' devolution due to a lack of statutory authority and formal levers for use over NHS organisations and fewer over LAs. The associated Transformation Fund (extra funding to facilitate change) has been used imaginatively to encourage change, but this is non-recurrent funding and the system still needs to operate effectively and meet national targets against which individual organisations are still measured.

The inclusion of LAs and other relevant organisations, as well as health, has encouraged change across the system. This has included delivery of integrated care via ten single commissioning functions based on the local authority footprints that work across health and social care; local single hospital services bringing together providers of hospital-based services; and a series of local care organisations to facilitate the joined up working of community health services, social care, GP services, mental health services, voluntary services and private sector providers (Walshe et al, 2018).

At the time of writing, health and social care devolution in GM remains in transition and it is too early to gauge its success (Walshe et al, 2018). In April 2019 (three years after the GMHCP went live) two interrelated initiatives have come together: the GM Model of Public Services announced in December 2018 (following on from the GM Strategy 'Our People, Our Place', GMCA, 2017), proposed that every area of public service should have health benefits as an objective: housing, education, work, digital and transport connections, environment and so on. It suggests that the complex challenge of improving the population's health is now being locally addressed in ways that national government could not accomplish. In parallel, the five-year Prospectus released by the GMHCP in April 2019 (GMHCP, 2019) sets out ambitions for a population health system, where inclusive economic growth is a main theory that focuses on upstream prevention rather than cure. Linkages to the GM industrial strategy and Northern Powerhouse initiatives will also be of great interest.

Despite progress, some historic challenges endure. The gap in health inequalities with the rest of England remains in many areas, while the health economy is struggling to meet increasing demand for services and to reach some of the national target measures, such as Accident and Emergency discharge times (Dunhill, 2019a). Recent national policy changes, integrating NHS England, NHS Improvement and PHE responsibilities, have resulted in a new regional level director for the North West being appointed, to whom the leader of GM's health and social care devolution programme will now report rather than directly to NHS England's Chief Finance Officer. While GM suggest this is no more than creating a clearer single line of reporting to facilitate ongoing change and improvement locally, others suggest a dilution of local autonomy (Dunhill, 2019b).

Discussion and conclusion

The wider determinants of population health conceptualised by Dahlgren and Whitehead (1991) as rainbow-like layers of influence illustrate the interdependence of multiple factors on the health and wellbeing of the population; see Chapter 2, Figure 2.1. The model is useful for identifying policy responses that are holistic and therefore extend beyond the narrow medical model of illness. The NHS can no longer be exclusively to treat the sick but a service that works in partnerships to address the wider determinants of health, many of which (transport, housing, worklessness, for example) are heavily influenced by LAs. In this chapter, the authors have illustrated how in the last decade the policy has shifted towards integration, where a variety of organisations are now responsible for setting strategic direction, service provision and encouraging asset-based working to reduce social inequalities together. Policymakers are looking for smarter ways of working, which focus on upstream prevention and general wellbeing as well as treating ill health, shifting the mindset from reactive to proactive developments. These initiatives bring attention to the third layer of the rainbow model, with, for example, social and community networks in association with LAs playing a greater role in facilitating conditions to ensure people stay healthy and independent for as long as possible. At the same time, to solve enduring 'wicked issues' (Rittel and Webber, 1973), organisations across all sectors (health, local government, voluntary, etc) are having to find ways of effectively working together to meet local demands within constrained budgets.

As the chapter has demonstrated, this is challenging in a system that is constantly evolving and in which organisations have unique institutional logics, governance, accountability, funding, budgets and decision-making cycles that do not align easily. Even with political will, the progress is dependent on reconciling difficult issues to do with regulation that cut across organisations and sectors and varying levels of responsibility for particular aspects of health and wellbeing. The layering of new initiatives upon old ones has also created challenges, with some programmes effectively operating in direct conflict, an example of this being integrated working and increased competition.

Changes to legislation may be required to overcome these obstacles (for example, moving funding away from being activity-based to population-based) and it had been hoped the NHS Long Term Plan (NHSE, 2019) and the long-anticipated adult social care Green Paper (still awaited at the time of writing, May 2020) would help to clarify this. The policy responses, however, need to be formulated and implemented through the meaningful engagement and intersectoral partnerships rather than driven by crisis in the acute sector. Different sectors need to be recognised as having more expertise in certain areas and, despite the cultural challenges, be included in all developments that look to integrated ways for working. Recognising where power is located in the local system and who is driving change will help to increase accountability but also inject the necessary pragmatism to ensure realistic expectations. This is important if community and social networks, in which LAs are integral, are to be fully engaged in tackling the causes of complex health inequalities.

This will be even more pertinent in the post COVID-19 pandemic landscape, with potentially different and more complex needs emerging as a result. There is already evidence that links the disease to inequality (Ahmed et al, 2020) with figures from the Office for National Statistics (Barr, 2020) suggesting that residents in areas of deprivation have experienced double the death rates of those in affluent areas. What is apparent is that the risks from COVID-19 are further exacerbated by social and economic inequalities, and issues linked to ethnicity, gender, age and underlying health conditions (Begum et al, 2020). Significantly, though, the current pandemic exposes the fragilities of the health, social care and public health systems in England that will need to be addressed to adequately respond to enduring inequalities in UK society and the increasingly global nature of health challenges.

Notes

[1] In the UK, the devolved administrations of England, Scotland, Wales and Northern Ireland have adopted different approaches to health and social care. In this chapter the authors focus on the English situation. For further information, see Part II of this book.

[2] 1) giving every child the best start in life; 2) enabling all children, young people and adults to maximize their capabilities and have control over their lives; 3) creating fair employment and good work for all; 4) ensuring a healthy standard of living for all; 5) creating and developing sustainable places and communities; 6) strengthening the role and impact of ill-health prevention.

References

AGMA (Association of Greater Manchester Authorities) (2015) 'Greater Manchester Health and Social Care Devolution: Memorandum of Understanding'. Available from: http://www.nhshistory.net/mou%20(1).pdf [Accessed 9 April 2020].

Ahmed, F., Ahmed, N.E., Pissarides, C. and Stiglitz, J. (2020) 'Why inequality could spread COVID-19' *Lancet Public Health*, 5(5): e240.

Amin-Smith, N. and Phillips, D. (2019) 'English council funding: what's happening and what's next?' Institute of Fiscal Studies. Available from: https://www.ifs.org.uk [Accessed 18 June 2019].

Barr, C. (2020) 'Deprived areas have double death rates of affluent', *The Guardian*, 1 May. Available from: https://www.theguardian.com/politics/live/2020/may/01/uk-coronavirus-live-job-cuts-end-lockdown-politics-covid-19-latest-updates?page=with:block-5eabe3278f08a459b6585968#block-5eabe3278f08a459b6585968 [Accessed 1 May 2020].

Begum, M., Verma, A. and Starling, B. (2020) 'How inequalities are affecting the response to COVID-19'. Available from: http://blog.policy.manchester.ac.uk/posts/2020/04/how-inequalities-are-affecting-the-response-to-covid-19/ [accessed 1 May 2020].

BBC (2019) 'English councils warned about "exhausting" reserve cash'. Available from: https://www.bbc.co.uk/news/uk-england-48280272 [Accessed 20 June 2019].

CfPS (Centre for Public Scrutiny) (2017) 'Accountability and scrutiny: the issues for local government in a changing political environment'. London: CfPS.

CfPS (Centre for Public Scrutiny) (2019) 'Governance, culture and collaboration'. London: CfPS.

Checkland, K., Coleman, A., Billings, J., MacInnes, J., Mikelyte, R., Laverty, L. and Allen, P. (2019) 'National evaluation of the Vanguard new care models programme: interim report: understanding the national support programme'. University of Manchester, LSHTM and University of Kent.

CIPFA (Chartered Institute of Public Finance and Accountancy) (2018) 'Measured resilience in English authorities'. London: CIPFA.

Coleman, A. (2016) 'Secrecy and service challenges in the new NHS – can STPs deliver?' Manchester Policy. Available from: http://blog.policy.manchester.ac.uk/posts/2016/12/secrecy-and-service-challenges-in-the-new-nhs-can-stps-deliver/ [Accessed 2 April 2019].

Corcoran, F. (2019) 'Delivering effective governance and accountability for integrated health and care'. London: CfPS.

Dahlgren, G. and Whitehead, M. (1991) *Policies and Strategies to Promote Social Equity in Health*, Stockholm: Institute for Futures Studies.

Deloitte (2019) *The Transition to Integrated Care Population Health Management in England*, London: Deloitte Centre for Health Solutions.

Department of Health (2010) 'Healthy lives, healthy people: our strategy for public health in England'. London: The Stationery Office.

Department of Health (2011) 'Public health in local government: commissioning responsibilities factsheet'. London: The Stationery Office.

DHSC (Department of Health and Social Care) (2018) 'Prevention is better than cure: our vision to help you live well for longer'. Crown Copyright, DHSC.

DHSC (Department of Health and Social Care) (2019) 'Policy paper: government response to the health and social care select committee report on "First 1000 days of life"'. Available from: https://www.gov.uk/government/publications/government-response-to-the-first-1000-days-of-life-report/government-response-to-the-health-and-social-care-select-committee-report-on-first-1000-days-of-life? [Accessed 27 July 2019].

DCLG (Department for Communities and Local Government) (2017) 'Local government financial statistics England No. 27 2017'. Available from: https://assets.publishing.service.gov.uk/government/uploads/system/uploads/attachment_data/file/627895/LGFS27_Web_version.pdf [Accessed 12 June 2019].

Dorling, D. (2010) 'Using the concept of "place" to understand and reduce health inequalities', in F. Campbell (ed) *The Social Determinants of Health and the Role of Local Government*, pp 16–25, London: Improvement and Development Agency.

Dunhill, L. (2019a) 'Regulators intervene in Devo Manc', *Health Services Journal* (25 February). Available from: www.hsj.co.uk/acute-care/regulators-intervene-in-devo-manc/7024502.article [Accessed 27 June 2019].

Dunhill, L. (2019b), '"Watered down" Devo Manc gets regional line manager', *Health Services Journal* (17 April). Available from: https://www.hsj.co.uk/north-west/watered-down-devo-manc-gets-regional-line-manager/7024901.article [Accessed 27 June 2019].

Exworthy, M., Powell, M. and Glasby, J. (2017) 'The governance of integrated health and social care in England since 2010: great expectations not met once again?' *Health Policy*, 121(11): 1124–30.

Faherty, G. and Gaulton, L. (2017) 'Working together to reduce health inequalities in the Marmot City of Coventry', *Primary Health Care*, 27(2): 26–9.

Ferry, L. and Murphy, P. (2018) 'What about financial sustainability of local government! – a critical review of accountability, transparency, and public assurance arrangements in England during austerity, *International Journal of Public Administration*, 41(8): 619–29.

GMCA (Greater Manchester Combined Authority) (2015) 'Taking charge of our health and social care in Greater Manchester'. Available from: http://www.gmhsc.org.uk/wpcontent/uploads/2018/05/Taking-Charge-summary.pdf [Accessed 9 April 2020].

GMCA (Greater Manchester Combined Authority) (2017) 'Our people, our place: Greater Manchester strategy'. Available from: https://www.greatermanchester-ca.gov.uk/ourpeopleourplace [Accessed 2 April 2019].

Gorsky, M., Lock, K. and Hogarth, S. (2014) 'Public health and English local government: historical perspectives on the impact of "returning home"', *Journal of Public Health*, 36(4): 546–51.

GMHCP (Greater Manchester Health and Social Care Partnership) (2019) 'Taking charge: the next 5 years. Our prospectus'. Available from: www.gmhsc.org.uk/wp-content/uploads/2019/03/GMHSC-Partnership-Prospectus-The-next-5-years-pdf.pdf [Accessed 2 April 2019].

Guzman-Castillo, M., Ahmadi-Abhari, S., Bandosz, P., Capewell, S., Steptoe, A., Singh-Manoux, A., Kivimaki, M., Shipley, M.J., Brunner, E.J. and O'Flaherty, M. (2017) 'Forecasted trends in disability and life expectancy in England and Wales up to 2025: a modelling study', *The Lancet Public Health*, 2(7): 307–13.

Hammond, J., Lorne, C., Coleman, A., Allen, P., Mays, N., Dam, R., Mason, T. and Checkland, K. (2017) 'The spatial politics of place and health policy: exploring sustainability and transformation plans in the English NHS', *Social Science and Medicine*, 190: 217–26.

HSCA12 (Health and Social Care Act) (2012) Available from: https://www.legislation.gov.uk/ukpga/2012/7/contents/enacted [Accessed 2 April 2019].

Humphries, R. (2019) 'The NHS, local authorities and the long-term plan: in it together?', London: King's Fund. Available from: www.kingsfund.org.uk/blog/2019/03/nhs-local-authorities-long-term plan [Accessed 9 April 2020].

Lawless, P., Foden, M., Wilson, I. and Beatty, C. (2010) 'Understanding area-based regeneration: the new deal for communities programme in England', *Urban Studies*, 47(2): 257–75.

LGA (Local Government Association) (2016) 'Health in all policies: a manual for local government', London: Local Government Association, Ref.1.4.

LGA (Local Government Association) (2018a) 'Nobody left behind: maximising the health benefits of an inclusive local economy', London: Local Government Association, Ref. 22.15.

LGA (Local Government Association) (2018b) 'Majority of people unprepared for adult social care costs'. Available from: https://www.local.gov.uk/about/news/majority-people-unprepared-adult-social-care-costs [Accessed 10 April 2019].

LGA (Local Government Association) (2019a) 'Public health transformation six years on: partnerships and prevention', London: Local Government Association, Ref.22.38.

LGA (Local Government Association) (2019b) 'Improving the public's health: local government delivers', London: Local Government Association, Ref.1.88.

Localism Act (2011) UK Government. Available from: http://www.legislation.gov.uk/ukpga/2011/20/contents/enacted [Accessed 27 June 2019].

Lyons, M. (2007) 'Place shaping: a shared ambition for the future of local government', London: Department of Communities and Local Government.

Marmot, M., Allen, J., Goldblatt, P., Boyce, T., McNeish, D., Grady, M. and Geddes, I. (2010) 'The Marmot review: fair society, healthy lives: the strategic review of health inequalities in England post-2010'. Available from: www.parliament.uk/documents/fair-society-healthy-lives-full-report.pdf [Accessed 9 April 2020].

Miller, R. and Glasby, J. (2016) 'Much ado about nothing? Pursuing the "holy grail" of health and social care integration under the coalition', in R. Mannion, M. Exworthy and M. Powell (eds) *Dismantling the NHS? Evaluating the Impact of Health Reforms*, pp 171–89, Bristol: Policy Press.

NAO (National Audit Office) (2018) 'Financial sustainability of local authorities 2018'. Available from: https://www.nao.org.uk/report/financial-sustainability-of-local-authorities-2018/ [Accessed 10 April 2019].

NHSE (NHS England) (2014) 'Five Year Forward View'. Available from www.england.nhs.uk/wp-content/uploads/2014/10/5yfv-web.pdf [Accessed 9 April 2020].

NHSE (NHS England) (2019) 'The NHS long term plan'. Available from: https://www.longtermplan.nhs.uk [Accessed 2 April 2019].

Peckham, S., Exworthy, M., Powell, M. and Greener, I. (2005) 'Decentralisation, centralisation and devolution in publicly funded health services: decentralisation as an organisational model for health-care in England'. Technical report. Available from: http://researchonline.lshtm.ac.uk/id/eprint/3582134 [Accessed 2 April 2019].

PHE (Public Health England) (2016) 'Local wellbeing, local growth: overview'. London: Public Health England Press Office. Available from: https://assets.publishing.service.gov.uk/government/uploads/system/uploads/attachment_data/file/560598/Health_in_All_Policies_overview_paper.pdf [Accessed 12 June 2019].

PHE (Public Health England) (2018a) 'Health profile for England report: 2018'. London: Public Health England Press Office. Available from: https://www.gov.uk/government/publications/health-profile-for-england-2018 [Accessed 2 April 2019].

PHE (Public Health England) (2018b) 'Improving health and care through the home: a national memorandum of understanding'. London: Public Health England Press Office. Available from: https://assets.publishing.service.gov.uk/government/uploads/system/uploads/attachment_data/file/691239/Health_Housing_MoU_18.pdf [Accessed 2 April 2019].

Purdam, K. (2017) 'The devolution of health funding in Greater Manchester in the UK: a travel map of life expectancy', *Environment and Planning A*, 49(7): 1453–7.

Raleigh, V. (2018), 'What is happening to life expectancy in the UK?', *The Health Foundation*. Available from: https://www.kingsfund.org.uk/publications/whats-happening-life-expectancy-uk [Accessed 20 May 2019].

Rittel, H.W. and Webber, M.M. (1973) 'Dilemmas in a general theory of planning', *Policy Sciences*, 4(2): 155–69.

SEU (Social Exclusion Unit) (2001) 'A new commitment to neighbourhood renewal—national strategy action plan', London: Cabinet Office.

Walshe, K., Lorne, C., Coleman, A., McDonald, R. and Turner, A. (2018) 'Devolving health and social care: learning from Greater Manchester', Manchester: Alliance Business School. Available from: https://www.mbs.ac.uk/media/ambs/content-assets/documents/news/devolving-health-and-social-care-learning-from-greater-manchester.pdf [Accessed 2 April 2019].

4

Strictly come partnering: are health and wellbeing boards the answer?

David J. Hunter

Introduction

Partnership working has been a long-standing objective of health and social policy, in recognition of the reality that few policy puzzles are simple and the preserve of any single agency or government department. 'Wicked issues' that display complex multiple causes in search of solutions that are intersectoral require joined up approaches at both national and local levels. Despite this awareness, in practice effective joint working remains the exception rather than the rule, and governments and their agents struggle to achieve success while remaining trapped in their silos and protecting their narrow interests (Hunter and Perkins, 2014; Perkins and Hunter, 2014).

How to do partnership working differently was behind the creation of health and wellbeing boards (HWBs) at the time of the 2012 NHS changes. At the time, there was much enthusiasm for these new entities and expectations ran high. Resources were made available to support boards and to help members consider how to create effective partnerships across local government and the National Health Service (NHS).

Sadly, some eight years later, the shine has gone off HWBs despite the fact that the issues they were set up to tackle remain as visible and deep-seated as ever. Indeed, after nearly a decade of austerity, which has contributed to a sharp rise in health inequalities and entrenched the North–South divide, and with the potential fallout from Brexit around the corner with as yet unknown but almost certainly negative consequences, the need for powerful HWBs that can bring about real change to improve the lot of ravaged communities has never been greater.

A recent study (led by the author of this chapter) of HWBs in England established in 2012, when responsibility for public health transferred to local government, found that, with few exceptions, HWBs punched below their weight and were not the powerful system leaders that had been hoped for (Hunter et al, 2017). Similar findings were reported in a series of reviews conducted by Shared Intelligence in the early years of HWBs (Shared Intelligence, 2013, 2014, 2015). With the advent of sustainability and transformation programmes (STPs) and integrated care partnerships (ICPs) following the introduction in 2014 of a major programme of reform within the NHS (NHSE, 2014), an opportunity for HWBs to become key drivers for a new integrated approach with local government at its centre has largely been missed. For the most part, they have been ignored or overlooked.

Yet, for all their failings and weaknesses, HWBs remain the only forum bringing together the main stakeholders in an area that may hold out some hope that they could still succeed. The chapter reviews recent evidence concerning the performance of HWBs and considers what fate might await them in a policy context increasingly likely to be shaped by the aftermath of the COVID-19 pandemic and its impact on public health.

The enduring appeal of partnerships

Partnerships have never been out of vogue in the United Kingdom, but arguably the need for them has never been greater. Paradoxically, despite their enduring appeal, evidence of their value and impact is negligible (Hunter and Perkins, 2014). For the most part, partnerships have proved underwhelming when it comes to their performance, and they have been unable to overcome deep-seated departmentalism and the silo mindset prevalent in government and public services.

There are a number of reasons in good currency to explain why partnerships may be undergoing something of a renaissance. In particular, the complexity of public policy given the multifaceted nature of the problems it is seeking to address is more widely acknowledged. Solutions to most contemporary public policy challenges cut across professional, service and organisational boundaries at all levels of government. Examples include confronting climate change, addressing non-communicable diseases, improving health and wellbeing (mental and physical) and tackling health inequalities. There is nothing especially new about these challenges, but they have become more acute owing to demographic and lifestyle-related changes and to the fact that they remain so persistent and seemingly impervious to efforts to tackle them.

The language has shifted to reflect and capture these changes. Whereas previously the discourse was centred on health services and health care, now it is more common to use the terms 'health system' and 'place-centred approaches' to capture and describe the complex interconnections between services affecting the health of communities. Successfully resolving pressures on the NHS in respect of acute services and bed occupancy depends increasingly on moving upstream to give higher priority to prevention and population health. At a subnational level, this can best be done through local government, which is why the return of public health to English local authorities in 2012 was widely welcomed (Hunter, 2016).

As long as public health had remained the responsibility of the NHS, from 1974 to 2012, attention was all too often focused on individual behaviour change involving clinical and other interventions. But we know that health behaviours cluster among the same social groups, which dictates that solutions are required that focus on the social determinants of health (Buck and Frosini, 2012). This requires connecting a range of different policy responses, which might include housing, education, transport, income support and employment opportunities. Therefore, so the thinking went, if public health were returned to local government it would be better placed to tackle inequalities in health and the wider social determinants of health by adopting a strong population focus in place of a narrow one confined to health service provision.

There is recognition of the need to adopt a whole systems focus in the NHS Long Term Plan (NHSE, 2019). Indeed, it is the first time in the history of the NHS and its multiple reforms since the mid-1970s that such a perspective has featured so prominently, with a whole chapter devoted to the need for a population health perspective – the NHS assuming a key advocacy role both nationally and locally. It is acknowledged that the NHS cannot lead on its own, and although the critical role of other partners, notably local government, is perhaps not as centre stage as it ought to be, there are at least the beginnings of movement on this score. Arguably, such a journey began with the introduction of HWBs, when local government regained responsibility for public health; but the story of their progress demonstrates how far there is to go.

Health and wellbeing boards: a new approach to partnerships?

With public health moving back to local government in England (see Chapter 2), there was recognition of a need to establish partnerships that connected local government with other relevant agencies notably the NHS and third sector organisations. The answer was HWBs, their title hinting at what was intended to be a broad and inclusive role in terms of connecting with all those services and professionals whose work contributed to wellbeing in the widest sense (Perkins et al, 2019).

HWBs were designed to serve as place-based hubs to ensure all the key partners in a locality were brought together in one forum and to join up what was regarded as an increasingly fragmented system as a result of changes brought about by the Health and Social Care Act 2012 (Humphries and Galea, 2013). The boards were where key leaders from the health and care system would work together to improve the health and wellbeing of their local population and reduce health inequalities. Each top tier and unitary local authority was to have its own HWB and its members would collaborate to understand their local community's needs, agree priorities and encourage commissioners to work in a more joined-up way. In addition, the boards were intended to help give communities a greater say in understanding and addressing their local health and social care needs, and to provide a forum for challenge and discussion.

HWBs were required to adopt a minimum membership of six members made up of one local elected representative, a representative of the local HealthWatch, a representative of each local Clinical Commissioning Group, and local authority directors for adult social services, children's services and public health. Boards were at liberty to expand their membership if they so wished. The accountability of HWBs to their local communities was to operate through having local councillors as board members. Implementation support for the setting up of HWBs was provided by the Department of Health (DH) together with the Local Government Association (LGA) and early implementer HWBs. An online National Learning Network brought together emerging HWBs to share their thinking and experience with peers.

How effective such implementation support was is hard to assess, since in this particular case it has not been subject to dedicated independent evaluation. In a review of the issues underlying policy design and failure, the researchers noted that within complex messy systems it is unclear how best to ensure effective implementation, although there is now greater interest by governments in demonstrating how it can be strengthened and supported (Hudson et al, 2019). While a study of implementation support of the Care Act 2014 found that it had been widely welcomed and had achieved some notable successes, a rapid review of the evidence for other policy initiatives and the implementation, including HWBs, found that the impact appeared to be negligible (Peckham et al, 2019).

With regard to the setting up of HWBs, one lesson that was learned from previous partnerships operating between the NHS and local government was avoidance of the temptation to be overly prescriptive about how the boards would operate. While there was guidance and development support on offer from the DH and LGA, as previously noted, it was not intended that this should be slavishly adhered to. The preference was for local authorities to establish HWBs that were aligned to particular contexts and with the need for central direction to be kept to a minimum. There was therefore considerable and deliberate permissiveness over how HWBs would operate and agree their governance arrangements to fit local contexts. For some, such freedom proved both liberating but also disconcerting, and it led to a desire in some places for more specific guidance – although this was resisted and kept to a minimum given the lessons from previous partnerships.

Despite their diversity, HWBs possess some common defining features that set them apart from their predecessors. To begin with, they are place-based through being located in local authorities as statutory committees of the council; see the introduction to Part III. They therefore cannot be ignored or disbanded. Moreover, within a local authority setting, HWBs are well placed to bring together a wide range of interests, including health, housing, planning, education and social care. The other statutory responsibilities bestowed upon HWBs concern the production of a Joint Strategic Needs Assessment in each locality that would form the basis of the Joint Health and Wellbeing Strategy (JHWS). Unfortunately, as we shall see, the power to produce a JHWS proved insufficient as it contained no provision to secure or track its implementation.

Another key lesson to be learned from previous, and largely ineffectual, partnership arrangements was how to ensure that HWBs actively contributed to better health outcomes for local communities. Literature reviews of the evidence on such partnerships found little cause for optimism (Hunter and Perkins, 2014). A rapid literature review conducted for the research on HWBs highlighted the main determinants of successful public health partnerships and the principal barriers to their success (Hunter et al, 2015). They are listed here.

Determinants of successful partnerships

Three factors stood out:

- clarity regarding the goals and objectives of the partnership;

- evidence of goodwill and trust between partners, especially at the frontline level;
- a clear strategic commitment to performance through robust monitoring and evaluation.

Barriers to effective partnerships

Again, three key factors were highlighted:

- conflicting agency priorities, which served to negate or limit the potential of the partnership;
- lack of vertical as well as horizontal linkages between partners; that is, absence of ownership;
- excessive bureaucracy, making participants susceptible to becoming overly focused on processes rather than outcomes.

The overall political and economic context in which HWBs were established was less than ideal if it was intended that it should help nurture them and enable them to flourish. By 2012–13, the effects of austerity had begun to be felt across the public sector in general and in local government in particular, where the squeeze on finances was felt most acutely. Despite such an inauspicious start, early studies of HWBs in their shadow and initial start-up phases showed they were displaying features that distinguished them from their predecessors. These included the engagement of general practitioners; wider relations between the NHS and local government and not just social care; ensuring local communities were able to contribute to decisions about their services, partly through the involvement of HealthWatch and the voluntary sector; and opportunities following the move of public health into local government with improved accountability and governance in place (Humphries, 2013; Coleman et al, 2016).

However, in a close-up study of the workings of HWBs in five local authorities, the findings concluded that HWBs were not after all so different from their predecessors, with many similar deficiencies on display (Hunter et al, 2017). While those working in, or with, HWBs argued that partnerships needed clear goals with ownership of these at all levels, in practice this was not generally the case. Rather than functioning as, in the jargon, 'system leaders', HWBs were more inclined to resemble a collection of leaders each accountable to their respective organisations with their own (often conflicting) priorities. As one interviewee put it, 'big people with big personalities' exerted a disproportionate influence over policies and agendas. The result was that HWBs lacked strategic direction.

Mention has been made of the limited powers at the disposal of HWBs. In regard to the JHWSs, three particular problems were evident. First, there was little ownership of these and a corresponding lack of accountability for elements of them. They were not seen as an integral part of the health and social care landscape and could end up competing with strategies produced by other agencies. Secondly, the strategies partly reflected work that was already in hand by other agencies, so risked bringing little added value to the proceedings. Thirdly, and finally, the strategies suffered from being 'motherhood and apple pie' statements, with too many priorities, no clear measures of success and few details of how implementation would occur and be tracked and monitored. So, while JHWSs were required to be produced and published, there was no stipulation that they had to be implemented nor that the HWB would be given the powers to monitor their impact. Far from being an instrument to effect change, JHWSs had no traction on the system.

When it came to developing partnerships, and despite some efforts to do things differently, the HWBs in our sample ended up largely following the practices of previous partnerships, which, as noted earlier, were regarded as defective in many respects. In particular, HWBs failed to capitalise on the experience that had been achieved of securing good attendance from board partners. Whereas a lack of commitment and poor attendance had characterised previous partnerships, it was hoped that with all the key partners present at HWB meetings this might result in a greater commitment to make the partnership work and achieve agreed goals. Instead, there was little evidence that high attendance had any positive impact. There was certainly poor progress made in tackling the wider determinants of health.

While there was encouraging evidence of trusting relationships having been developed in one of the study sites our research covered, these did not translate into much by way of achieving improvements in health and wellbeing. Elsewhere, there was a lack of engagement and trust that manifested themselves in an absence of information–sharing, personality conflicts, evidence of tensions among health sector partners, poor partnership working between the local authority and the voluntary sector, and different leadership approaches jockeying for supremacy.

With regard to involving local communities in understanding and addressing their health and social care needs, the research found that the voluntary sector and HealthWatch locally had little influence on HWBs. There was no evidence of meaningful involvement.

The problem of a lack of accountability, whereby HWBs were unable to hold partners to account for results as distinct from enjoying good relationships with them that meant little in terms of achieving change, was widely evident. This was accompanied by a lack of performance monitoring and accountability for outcomes. Tangible outcomes were notable for their absence with goals and targets set in the JHWS not followed up in terms of making progress to achieve them. Process outcomes, such as producing the JHWS and signing off on other strategies, seemed to substitute for the actual implementation of policy.

Given their lack of statutory powers, HWBs were obliged to exercise 'soft power' if they were serious about influencing and negotiating change. As was pointed out in the House of Commons Health Committee in its inquiry into public health post-2013, HWBs' 'authority does not lie in having executive powers but in their capacity to influence others through the persuasiveness of their arguments and success in building sound relationships' (House of Commons Health Committee, 2016, para 74, p 37). At best, evidence for success was limited. HWBs were yet to position themselves as the key strategic forum for driving the health and wellbeing agenda.

Systemic weaknesses of this type left HWBs vulnerable to being buffeted from all sides by competing agendas played out against a backdrop of policy tension and conflict. One such tension evident was between the meta-policy of localism and devolved authority on the one hand and the desire to ensure consistency between local authorities on the other, to avoid what might be perceived as unacceptable variation. Localism was seen as desirable by many of those who were interviewed, bringing decisions about place and personalisation to a local level. Others were less approving, believing that HWBs and the transfer of public health to local government had contributed to increasing fragmentation of the system.

The reality of institutional complexity and competing system hierarchies evident in the integration of health and social care and arrival of the Better Care Fund (BCF), which was introduced at around the same time as HWBs, resulted in the dilution of local priorities and a loss of focus for HWBs. The BCF in particular proved to be a major distraction and absorbed senior officer time that might otherwise have been available to tackle the health determinants and inequalities agendas that were ostensibly the main business of HWBs. Indeed, the problem of integrating health and social care was regarded as being of such high and urgent priority politically at national level that HWBs felt under considerable pressure to respond. In such a context, HWBs tended to be regarded as bodies to ratify decisions in the absence of any challenge from partners.

The conflicting pressures to which HWBs were subjected were confirmed in the evidence submitted to the Health Committee's inquiry mentioned above. This showed clearly that the performance of HWBs was mixed, with boards addressing the challenges they faced with 'variable success. Progress is slow and subject to constant changes in, and demands from, national policy' (House of Commons Health Committee, 2016, para 76, p 37). A review of the state of HWBs by Shared Intelligence commissioned by the LGA at around the same time found that in such a context boards could all too easily lose focus, 'with 'mission creep' a real and present danger' (Shared Intelligence, 2016).

Despite these difficulties and weaknesses, the committee concluded that there is 'cautious optimism' over the future of HWBs and their 'ability to bring and hold the health system together thereby reducing the fragmentation that threatens it in many places' (House of Commons Health Committee, 2016, para 76, pp 37–8). In its response to the committee's report, the government made no reference to HWBs, which may suggest that they are no longer, if they ever were, seen as pivotal bodies with regard to system leadership (Department of Health, 2016).

It is not only in respect of HWBs where partnership working among health system agencies remains problematic. The evidence from other areas on its overall failure, and the reasons for this, reflects the findings from studies of HWBs referred to earlier: the complex configuration of partnerships, their focus on process over outcomes and the difficulty of measuring the impact of collaboration. In any complex system, attributing causation to a single factor will always be fraught with difficulty. It is also the case that partnerships, regardless of their purpose and location, have been subject to frequent disruption as successive waves of reform have swept over the system. A fixation on structural upheaval has resulted in trust being weakly developed, constant churn as staff movements take place and an absence of long-term thinking. Such factors have been at work, for example, in respect of delivering the national immunisation programme in England (Chantler et al, 2019). The researchers found that partnership working facilitated information-sharing (in contrast to what the study of HWBs revealed) but was less effective at promoting shared action (in keeping with the finding from the HWB study). The study found a key barrier to partnerships working was a lack of an allocated budget, leading the researchers to conclude that 'partnership working has been mandated without any recognition that it is not a cost neutral activity' (Chantler et al, 2019, p 9).

Where next for partnerships?

All the findings reported here make for rather depressing reading, and it is difficult to remain optimistic that things are going to improve significantly (Buck, 2020). Of course there will be exceptions, and these should not be overlooked or ignored. Indeed, we need to capture these success stories and build on them in order to replicate the lessons where possible. But if past practice is any guide, they are likely to remain exceptions, and transforming the way partnerships operate across a whole system will remain an aspiration without major investment (human and financial) in their future.

Those interviewed for our study of HWBs were asked for their views on what the future might hold in the wake of the appearance of STPs during the final stages of the research. They were not optimistic about the future of HWBs, fearing that they would become irrelevant and be subsumed or, worse, bypassed by STP boards or their emerging successors in the shape of ICPs. One interviewee suggested that either HWBs should be made more powerful or they should be abandoned. The alternative was a 'lingering death' that was in no one's interest.

So, while HWBs still exist, their role and place in the architecture being put in place in the NHS are unclear. At the same time, there are encouraging signs that many local authorities, including a number in the north-east of England where there is a history of effective collaboration owing to the size of the region and its general stability in terms of public sector employees, are refreshing their boards and looking in particular at how to give them more traction in the system. The findings from the research reported earlier and related studies are being heeded in some quarters. While encouraging, there remains the issue of where HWBs fit into the new system, and how they can add value when up until now they are rather been sidelined.

This is a matter of unfinished business, and is an important conclusion to draw at a time when the NHS is undergoing major renewal from within by adopting a place-based approach to health and wellbeing that is centred upon ICPs. These are in the process of replacing STPs, which began to emerge in around 2016 as the *NHS Five Year Forward View* was implemented. But the governance of ICPs remains weak and lacking in legislative clarity, although there is no stomach for rectifying these deficiencies at the present time – a view endorsed by the House of Commons Health Committee in its inquiry into the NHS Long Term Plan (House of Commons Health and Social Care Committee, 2019). The committee concluded that they are a pragmatic set of reforms, which remove barriers to integrated care. This evolutionary and consultative approach to health reform was welcome, particularly given the challenge of legislating in a hung parliament and the fact that there remains little appetite for another large-scale top-down reorganisation of the NHS.

But the committee was critical of the NHS Long Term Plan as being too NHS-centric, with too little consideration for the wider system with which the NHS seeks to integrate. It sought more clarity about the role of HWBs in ICSs. The LGA argued that HWBs could be used in place of joint committees, rather than as separate entities alongside them which on the face of it would appear to make a lot of sense.

These conclusions and recommendations from the Health Committee echo the reflections from the study of HWBs featured in this chapter. Indeed, the committee could and perhaps should have gone further by critiquing the surprising absence of HWBs from the discourse about ICPs and how they should be implemented. While the NHS Plan has much to say about ICPs, it has virtually nothing to say about HWBs and, as the committee notes, not much more about the centrality of local government to a place-based and whole-systems approach to improving health. Indeed, instead of HWBs being at the centre of such moves and serving as the forum to drive a systems approach, they have for the most part been overshadowed by efforts to establish new partnerships, which appear to make no sense and run the risk of creating partnership overload and the confusion that might ensue.

Key lessons for successful partnership working remain as valid today as they have always done and are applicable to HWBs as they consider their future (Hunter and Perkins, 2014; Edmonstone, 2019):

- Policies and procedures need to be more streamlined – focus on outcomes, not process and structure.
- Those at higher strategic levels could learn from frontline practices that operate in a more organic and integrated way.
- Partnerships in practice can be rather messy constructs.
- There is a tendency to over-engineer partnerships, often to the exclusion of being clear about purpose and achievement, should be resisted.
- Structures are less important than relational factors such as trust and goodwill.
- Leadership styles are important – they should be collaborative, integrative and adaptive.

As the literature on partnership working demonstrates, partnerships are hard to make work at the best of times. In the current landscape of organisational and policy fragmentation, austerity-driven cuts in staffing and services, together with uncertainty over the impact of Brexit, it is hard to see how any partnership arrangement could be made to work successfully. Blaming HWBs for their failure may be misplaced when wider contextual forces and constraints are at work. Looking back at the origins of HWBs and the good intentions surrounding their creation, it may prove to be a case of the right solution but the wrong time. To that extent, HWBs became something of a poisoned chalice, and while they are clinging on, their fate remains uncertain and insecure. At the same time, and acting in their favour, they remain currently the one forum with legislative force where all the key agencies impacting on health and wellbeing in a community come together. That surely makes them worth defending, as well as offering hope that they could occupy a pivotal role as system leaders pursuing a mission to tackle health inequalities and improve health and wellbeing. But for that to happen, the boards themselves will need to show they are capable of rising to the challenge. It may not be too late for that, although time is running out.

Whether the impact of COVID-19 will be a factor in the fate of HWBs remains unknown at the time of writing. However, if we are to put the crisis arising from the pandemic to good use then ensuring HWBs are empowered to become effective place-based change agents in their local communities must be a priority. We know the virus has hit deprived communities, such as those located in the North-East of England, hardest. Their health status is already poor, made worse by a decade of austerity that has stalled life expectancy and increased the amount of time people spend in poor health (Marmot et al, 2020). If the UK's response to COVID-19 was severely hampered by successive governments since 2010 seeking to shrink the state and hollow out the public realm, the failure of HWBs to make much of an impact on health outcomes is part of the toxic mix of social policies and programmes to which the country has been subjected. Only when we learn 'to think the state again' will intersectoral collaborative mechanisms like HWBs stand a chance of success (Judt, 2011). In particular HWBs can serve as a bulwark against a return to an NHS that is dominated by buildings, beds and hospitals. Ensuring that public health in the widest sense, with a focus on the social determinants of health, is at the forefront of policy is essential. HWBs ought to be the driving force to make that happen.

Conclusion

If there were a strictly come partnering contest, how would one judge the performance of HWBs? On the basis of the evidence reviewed in this chapter it would not be a high-scoring or memorable one. HWBs would not score highly on the leadership board. But is a comeback possible? Perhaps, although for that to happen HWBs would need to learn the lessons that explain what has gone wrong and why.

It seems that HWBs are at a crossroads with two possible future scenarios lying ahead of them. The first envisages boards continuing to be talking shops and being regarded as increasingly irrelevant as a consequence, with other types of partnership eclipsing or even replacing them altogether. Most likely, HWBs will simply wither on the vine with few noticing their fate. The alternative scenario sees a bright future for boards as 'the anchors of place in a sea of new initiatives', to quote the former Chair of the LGA Community and Wellbeing Board, Councillor Izzi Seccombe, speaking at a conference in Durham in September 2017.

For this second scenario to have any chance of being realised in a context where the fallout from COVID-19 will impact on all aspects of health and wellbeing, a window of opportunity beckons as the NHS Long Term Plan is implemented, but it will be a brief one and there is no time to lose on the part of those who believe that HWBs could yet become the system leaders envisaged by their architects back in 2012.

References

Buck, D. (2020) *The English Local Government Public Health Reforms: An Independent Assessment*, London: The King's Fund.

Buck, D. and Frosini, G. (2012) *Clustering of Unhealthy Behaviours Over Time*, London: The King's Fund.

Chantler, T., Bell, S., Saliba, V., Heffernan, C., Raj, T., Ramsay, M. and Mounier-Jack, S. (2019) 'Is partnership the answer? Delivering the national immunisation programme in the new English health system: a mixed methods study', *BMC Public Health*, 19(1): 83. Available from: https://doi.org/10.1186/s12889-019-6400-6 [Accessed 9 April 2020].

Coleman, A., Dhesi, S. and Peckham, S. (2016) 'Health and Wellbeing Boards: the new system stewards?', in M. Exworthy, R. Mannion and M. Powell (eds) *Dismantling the NHS? Evaluating the Impact of Health Reforms*, Bristol: Policy Press, pp 279–99.

Department of Health (2016) *Government Response to the House of Commons Health Committee Report on Public Health Post-2013*, London: Department of Health.

Edmonstone, J. (2019) *Systems Leadership in Health and Social Care*, London: Routledge.

House of Commons Health Committee (2016) *Public Health Post-2013*. Second Report of Session 2016–17. HC140, London: House of Commons.

House of Commons Health and Social Care Committee (2019) *NHS Long-Term Plan: Legislative Proposals*. Fifteenth Report of Session 2017–19. HC2000, London: House of Commons.

Hudson, B., Hunter, D. and Peckham, S. (2019) 'Policy failure and the policy-implementation gap: can policy support programs help?', *Policy Design and Practice*, 2(1):1–14. Available from: https://doi.org /10.1080/25741292.2018.1540378 [Accessed 9 April 2020].

Humphries, R. (2013) 'Health and wellbeing boards: policy and prospects', *Journal of Integrated Care*, 21(1): 6–12.

Humphries, R. and Galea, A. (2013) *Health and Wellbeing Boards: One Year On*, London: The King's Fund.

Hunter, D.J. (2016) 'Public health: unchained or shackled?', in M. Exworthy, R. Mannion and M. Powell (eds) *Dismantling the NHS? Evaluating the Impact of Health Reforms*, Bristol: Policy Press, pp 191–210.

Hunter, D.J. and Perkins, N. (2014) *Partnership Working in Public Health*, Bristol: Policy Press.

Hunter, D.J., Visram, S., Brown, S., Finn, R., Gosling, J., Adams, L. and Forrest, A. (2015) 'Interim report no 1: scoping the evidence base on health and wellbeing boards and similar partnership arrangements', Durham: Durham University.

Hunter, D.J., Perkins, N., Visram, S., Adams, L., Finn, R., Forrest, A. and Gosling, J. (2017) 'Evaluating the leadership role of health and wellbeing boards as drivers of health improvement and integrated care across England'. NIHR Policy Research Programme Project PR-XO-1113-11007.

Judt, T. (2011) *Ill Fares the Land*, London: Penguin Books.

Marmot, M., Allen, J., Boyce, T., Goldblatt, P. and Morrison, J. (2020) *Health Equity in England: The Marmot Review 10 years on*. London: Institute of Heath Equity and The Health Foundation.

NHSE (NHS England) (2014) *NHS Five Year Forward View*, London: NHS England.

NHSE (NHS England) (2019) *The NHS Long Term Plan*, London: NHS England.

Peckham, S., Hudson, B., Hunter, D., Redgate, S. and White, G. (2019) Improving Choices for Care: a strategic research initiative on the implementation of the Care Act 2014. Draft final report. NIHR Policy Research Programme Project PR-R14-1215-21006.

Perkins, N. and Hunter, D.J. (2014) 'Health and wellbeing boards: a new dawn for public health partnerships?', *Journal of Integrated Care*, 22(5/6): 220–9.

Perkins, N., Hunter, D.J., Visram, S., Finn, R., Gosling, J., Adams, L. and Forrest, A. (2019) 'Partnership or insanity: why do health partnerships do the same thing over and over again and expect a different result?', *Journal of Health Services Research & Policy*, 25(1): 41–8.

Shared Intelligence (2013) *Change Gear! Learning from the pilot health and wellbeing peer challenges*, London: Shared Intelligence.

Shared Intelligence (2014) *Great Expectations. A Review of the Health and Wellbeing System Improvement Programme*, London: Shared Intelligence.

Shared Intelligence (2015) *Stick with It! A Review of the Second Year of the Health and Wellbeing Improvement Programme*, London: Shared Intelligence.

Shared Intelligence (2016) *The Force Begins to Awaken: A Third Review of the State of Health and Wellbeing Boards*, London: Shared Intelligence.

PART II

The role of local authorities in promoting health and wellbeing in the community

Introduction

Lord Graham Tope

Local authorities have a key role in shaping public services, and to a large extent this is influenced by the approaches to commissioning and infrastructural arrangements within the local authority. The establishment and effectiveness of health and wellbeing boards (HWBs), working with Clinical Commissioning Groups, should provide leadership in culture change leading to effective integration health and social care. However, there was a mixed performance of HWBs across England, as reported in Chapter 4.

The role of local authority commissioning is the focus of Part III of this book. Bridging these two parts of the book is Part II, which provides insights into local authority responses from a 'place-based' perspective.

The Localism Act and the Care Act, conceived by the Coalition government in 2010, were well intentioned legislative changes which have brought a major cultural shift in thinking, and planning. However, their implementation has been undermined by austerity budgeting by Central government which has resulted in a continued reduction of funds available for local authorities. An example of this is the Revenue Support Grant [for local authorities] which has been reduced to 50% of the 2010 value in 2019, and will be abolished by 2020. Local authorities now find themselves in a bind of having greater responsibilities for their communities but with decreasing funding to support their responsibilities. The Chartered Institute of Public Finance and Accountancy (CIPFA) has indicated, in May 2019, that 11 of the 152 English councils are at risk of running out of cash reserves. The Local Government Association, reporting on the 'systematic underfunding' of councils, pointed to 'children's services at breaking point' (see Chapter 11). A 'resilience' index of councils, published by CIPFA, highlighted those councils that had the fastest depletion rates of their reserves. 'Reducing reserve levels means that local authorities have less scope to support "invest to save" programmes [such as health prevention; see Chapter 4] and any delays in delivering savings or unexpected cost pressures have a greater impact on their financial position' (NAO, 2018); see Figures 18.1 and 18.2 in Chapter 18.

A council that was highlighted in the media in May 2019 was Nottingham County Council, which was considering merging with smaller district councils owing to overspending by millions of pounds (BBC News, 2017). The London Borough of Sutton reported that 'with reserves of £33m in 2018, reserves were actively managed according to our consideration of risk and programme of work' (see Chapter 6).[1]

With councils working under increasing financial stresses and increasing needs emerging in their local communities, concerns are being raised nationally with regard to crises in housing, children, mental health particularly of young people (Chapter 15), and the rise in preventable deaths (Chapter 1). So what are the legal responsibilities of local councils?

Councils undertake a wide range of services, some of which they are legally obliged to undertake. These include:

- **Adult social care.** The population over the age of 85 is expected to rise by 1.3 million people, many of whom will require care and support in their daily lives. Councils have a legal duty to ensure care is available for people who are unable to get out of bed, dress, cook and take medication (see Chapter 12).
- **Children's services.** These are in addition to duties to assess and provide services for children with special educational needs and disabilities, and young people previously in care. There are approximately 200 legal obligations relating to the support of children. These include safeguarding and, in extreme cases, intervention to remove a child from its parents (see Chapter 11).
- **Collection of household waste.** Although there are no rules on frequency of collection, councils are responsible for the removal of household waste. Targets for recycling rates, to at least 50 per cent, are required.
- **Roads.** The maintenance of local streets, including surfacing, lighting and traffic signals, are the responsibility of local councils, which must ensure that they have taken 'all reasonable care' to

prevent people being injured. This includes action to reduce harm caused by snow, ice and potholes.

- **Housing.** Free advice for people at risk of becoming homeless, accommodation for homeless people in priority groups, facilities for disabled people in their homes and work with the fire service, to ensure that buildings comply with general health and safety regulations, are all requirements to be undertaken by local authorities (see Bonner, 2018, pp 211–24).
- **Libraries.** Unlike the provision of parks and leisure activities, councils must provide and maintain a 'comprehensive and effective' library service 'within available resources'. The running of the service may be passed to volunteers, which would bring about savings (LGA, 2017).
- **Public health**. New responsibilities to improve the public health of their local communities were passed to local authorities in 2013 (Chapter 2). Sexual health, alcohol and other drug misuse and smoking cessation services must be provided. The wider dimensions of health and wellbeing, including lifestyle choices, healthy eating, exercise and reducing environmental risks, including poor housing, all fall within the responsibility of local councils. These responsibilities are in addition to health protection, including strategies for addressing infectious diseases, environmental hazards and extreme weather.

In addition to the above responsibilities, local councils have many other obligations, including the registration of births and deaths, managing planning applications and the issuing of licences for the sale of alcohol and street trading. However, the core requirements, listed above, have direct bearing on the social determinants of health.

The Improvement and Development Agency, part of the Local Government Association group, has reviewed the Social Determinants of Health and the Role of Local Government (I&DeA, 2010; LGA, 2017). This review addresses health inequalities from the perspective of the World Health Organization Global Commission on Social Determinants of Health, subsequently commissioned by the Secretary of State for Health to provide guidance for the UK. The I&DeA review contained various insights including the role of local government (Hunter), the concept of place (Dorling), evidence for developing strategies by local authorities (Kelly and Moore) and the roles of the directors of public health (Maryon-Davis). The conclusion of this review was that local government has the potential to have a direct impact on its citizens as a major employer and through its role in providing the psychosocial and physical environments that are key factors in morbidity and quality of life.

The Localism and Care Acts, together with reviews of the health service published in the Wanless report (Hunter, 2003) and the review of the NHS by Lord Darzi (DHSC, 2008) all laid the foundation for the current approaches to the integration of health and social care. Health inequalities are significantly influenced by austerity and geopolitical factors, as presented in Bambra et al (2018).

Austerity policies have resulted in family budgets being significantly squeezed and social mobility has decreased, with the potential for distrust in the political system and alienation of people at the lower end of the social gradient. Many local councils have cut and reduced services, impacting on health and wellbeing, the unintended consequence of which is the paradoxical effect of increasing acute health costs in the long term.

The control of financial resources is fundamental to past and current support for people and their communities. There have been major changes in the control of financial capital from the 19th to the 21st century.

There are distinct geosocial responses to these challenges faced by local authorities. Regional responses in Wales and Scotland are reviewed in Chapters 20 and 21. In England, local responses by a London borough (Chapter 6), the North-East (Chapter 7) and the North-West (Chapters 5 and 8) demonstrate some common themes and region-specific responses to these challenges. Geosocial and culture change, for instance in Wigan (Chapter 8), an area historically dependent on the coal-mining industry, and also Sunderland and Middlesbrough (Chapter 7), appears to be benefiting from a concerted community involvement in council planning via the 'Wigan Deal', and also from its geographic location within the devolved Manchester Metropolitan Authority (Chapter 5).

Note
[1]   In July 2020, local councils were in a precarious financial state due to expenditure incurred in addressing COVID-19 and significant loss of income (from car parking income, business rates, etc) due to the lockdown (LGA, 2020).

References
Bambra, C., Garthwaite, K. and Greer Murphy, A. (2018) 'Geopolitical aspects of health and wellbeing', in A. Bonner (ed) *Social determinants of health: an interdisciplinary approach to social inequality and wellbeing*, Bristol: Policy Press, pp 281–98.

BBC News (2017) 'Nottingham City Council plans to axe 200 jobs by April 2019', 19 December. Available from: https://www.bbc.co.uk/news/uk-england-nottinghamshire-42412504 [Accessed 28 July 2020].

Bonner, A. (ed) (2018) *Social Determinants of Health: An Interdisciplinary Approach to Social Inequality and Wellbeing*, Bristol: Policy Press.

DHSC (Department of Health and Social Care) (2008) 'High quality care for all: NHS next stage review final report', Norwich: TSO. Available at: https://assets.publishing.service.gov.uk/government/uploads/system/uploads/attachment_data/file/228836/7432.pdf [Accessed 13 May 2020].

Hunter, D. (2003) 'The Wanless report and public health', *The BMJ*, 327 (7415): 573–4. Available at: https://www.ncbi.nlm.nih.gov/pmc/articles/PMC194071/ [Accessed 13 May 2020].

I&DeA (Improvement and Development Agency) (2010) 'The social determinants of health and the role of local government', London: I&DeA. Available at https://www.local.gov.uk/sites/default/files/documents/social-determinants-healt-c8f.pdf [Accessed 13 May 2020].

LGA (Local Government Association) (2017) 'Delivering local solutions for public library services: a guide for local councillors', London: LGA. Available at: https://www.local.gov.uk/sites/default/files/documents/12.6_LGA%20Cllr%20handbook_Delivering%20local%20solutions%20for%20public%20library%20services.pdf [Accessed 13 May 2020].

LGA (Local Government Association) (2020) 'LGA responds to Covid-19 council funding package', 2 July. Available at: https://www.local.gov.uk/lga-responds-covid-19-council-funding-package [Accessed 28 July 2020].

NAO (National Audit Office) (2018) 'Financial sustainability of local authorities 2018 visualisation', available at: https://www.nao.org.uk/other/financial-sustainability-of-local-authorities-2018-visualisation/ [Accessed 13 May 2020].

5

Devolution and localism: metropolitan authorities

Paul Dennett and Jacquie Russell

Introduction

Public services, nationally and locally, face an unprecedented set of financial pressures, as well as challenges to quality, performance and persistently poor population health outcomes. In April 2016, Greater Manchester (GM) signed an historic devolution deal with central government. Through this deal, GM became the first, and still only, city region with health and care devolution. Decisions about how to deliver greater, faster improvements to the health and wellbeing of the residents are now made locally.

Devolution has led to the development of detailed plans focused on people and local communities; new infrastructure to build on local strengths and assets; stronger relationships across sectors and across the city-region, in turn breaking down some of the traditional silos and structural barriers that have got in the way of policymakers and financial decisions in the past. Devolution, and the way it has been implemented in GM, has provided the foundations for reforming public services. Devolution has also been accompanied by budgetary reforms. A £6 billion devolution deal brought together health and social care, and a £450 million Health and Social Care Transformation Fund was agreed to support the development of this new integrated system. The GM strategic health and social care plan sets out how these challenges will be met. A £30 million Transformation Fund has also been secured to support delivery of the first GM Population Health Plan, setting out how the opportunities of devolution will be used to help ensure that all residents will have the best start in life, to live well and to age well.

Good health is vital for confident, prosperous and ambitious places – these ambitions are inseparable. At the heart of devolution in GM is a long-held belief that decisions are best made locally, by local leaders (democratic and professional) who know their communities and are able to bridge the organisational, professional, and sector boundaries that can often drive public decision-making. Localism is at the very heart of the devolution journey.

In this chapter, the context for devolution in GM, and why it matters in terms of residents' health and wellbeing, is briefly explored. The authors set out some of the changes they have seen – the integration of health and social care, and the creation of local care systems; the bringing together of health and care commissioning; and the crucial role of partnerships across health, care, the voluntary and community sector, housing, police, fire and others.

Of course one of the arguments for local authority leadership on devolution is that good health is about more than the National Health Service (NHS) – it is about good food, warm homes, decent jobs, good education, close friends and open green and safe public spaces (to name just a few). Devolution is about connecting all these agendas, through local leadership and local action. Devolution is complex, as are the relationships between Greater Manchester and local democratic leadership in each of the ten boroughs. Throughout this chapter, the authors set out how that works in their own city of Salford. Finally, there are some observations about the future challenges for local leadership if sustained good health for residents is to be sustained.

The health context and devolution

First, for those unfamiliar with Salford and possibly even Greater Manchester (GM), health issues should be set in context. Salford is based within the GM conurbation and wider labour market of around 2.7 million people. Salford is one of two cities that, alongside the neighbouring borough of Trafford, are the central drivers of the wider GM economy.

GM as a city-region and the City of Salford itself – have changed dramatically over the past 30–40 years. Decades of population decline have been reversed. High levels of public and private investment have delivered high levels of growth, new housing and new jobs, and are driving the city-region's economy. From 2010–20, Salford's economy grew by almost £1 billion, almost 3,000 more businesses were added to the city's business base and almost 2,000 extra jobs were created. At the same time, Salford's population increased by almost 12 per cent, and by 2018 it was approaching 250,000. The city is now seeing the return on a 30-year regeneration programme, kick-started by the regeneration of Salford Quays led by Salford City Council (SCC). The city's urban transformation is expected to continue over the next 20 years, 2020–40. In 2011 a review of the city's own development pipeline suggested that the city would grow substantially in the decade up to 2020, by almost 20,000 people, over 15,000 jobs and £1.64 billion in the value of its economy (Alexander, 2011); however, in view of the current COVID-19 pandemic, employment and economic growth forecasts for Salford and the UK are uncertain.

There remains much to do, though. Notwithstanding the economic success, there continue to be long-standing and deep-rooted challenges. The data for 2016 shows that inequalities in health and wellbeing persist – across GM, over 1 million residents live in areas that are among the 20 per cent most deprived in England. To put this in context – that is 36.3 per cent of GM's population, compared with an England average of 20.2 per cent. Men in GM die almost two years earlier compared with the England average (77.8 years against an England average of 79.5). Both men and women tend to get sick sooner than elsewhere, at 60 years for men and 60.4 years for women (compared with an England average of 63.4 years and 63.8 years respectively); in some areas of GM, the people get sick as young as 50 years. Each year 12,000 children (around 1 in 3) start school not ready to learn; while 236,000 residents are out of work. These inequalities create a significant additional demand for public services – with a £7 billion gap between annual income and expenditure on the services that are required to support the people (GMHSCP, 2017b, p 10).

The City of Salford's crest reads 'the welfare of the people is the highest mission'. Since their very creation, local authorities have been tackling the determinants of health, championing better sanitation, jobs for all and decent homes.

Locally, public leaders have long held that collaboration, partnerships and local leadership lie at the heart of the solution to these public policy challenges. If 'the welfare of the people' is truly 'the highest mission', then local leaders, vested in the communities they serve, are best placed to make those complex policy and investment decisions. The Association of Greater Manchester Authorities (AGMA) has its roots in this belief, and has built a 40-year track record of collaborative working between local government, the private and business sectors, the voluntary, community and social enterprise sector, and partners across the wider public sector. Strong democratic leadership through the elected membership of the ten GM districts was and still is the cornerstone of this voluntary partnership. AGMA laid the foundations for the Greater Manchester Combined Authority (GMCA) – the first nationally when it was formally created in 2011.

The GMCA created a formal legal framework for collaboration among the ten districts, and its establishment was quickly followed by the first set of City Deals. The first Devolution Agreement with central government was agreed in 2014 – underpinning the principal of local leadership on transport, business support, employment and skills, housing and investment. The appointment of an interim GM mayor in 2015, and the election of the first directly elected GM mayor in 2016, continued this journey towards enhanced local leadership of critical areas of public services and public investment.

The foundations for the formal devolution agreement with central government in February 2016 on health and care was the next stage in the journey to take control locally of the crucial services that residents need. This agreement formally brought the NHS – in all its constituent parts – and the services it delivers, into the GM partnerships.

What has been done with devolution of health and care? Are there clear improvements in health and wellbeing outcomes as a result? We will now turn to these questions.

Starting well, living well, ageing well

Prevention – together with system-wide action on wider determinants – is a long-established principle in health and in promoting wellbeing. Dahlgren and Whitehead (1991) argue that socio-economic, cultural, and environmental forces provide a framework through which health outcomes develop for individuals, alongside social and community networks, individual lifestyle factors and genetic predisposition. The NHS Long Term Plan for England published in January 2019 is clear that 'wider action on prevention will help people to stay healthy and also moderate demand on the NHS. Action by the NHS is a complement to – not a substitute for – the important role of individuals, communities, government and businesses in shaping the health of the nation' (NHS, 2019, p 33). A system-wide commitment to prevention sits at the heart of GM's Health and Social Care Prospectus (GMHSC, 2019).

Prevention is increasingly being accompanied by a focus on wellbeing, as an alternate or complementary measure of health and service impact. The Care Act 2014 cites wellbeing as the preservation of areas such as personal dignity; physical, mental and emotional health; protection from abuse and neglect; control by the individual over day-to-day life, participation in work, education, training or recreation; social and economic wellbeing; domestic, family and personal wellbeing; suitability of living accommodation; and an individual's contribution towards society (HMSO, 2014). Similarly, the All Party Parliamentary Group on wellbeing noted that wellbeing impacts heavily on priority areas related to health, employment and educational outcome. Positive levels of wellbeing were related to positive impacts on productivity, reduction in benefit dependence, reduced absenteeism, reduction in physical illness and higher rates of educational attainment (APPG, 2019).

It is self-evident that the NHS alone cannot bear the full responsibility, nor does it have the skills, expertise or powers, for outcomes in employment, education, domestic and family life, housing, transport or other areas of public life.

In GM, devolution, underpinned by a system-wide approach to prevention, the promotion of wellbeing and the integration of health and care, is driven by the Health and Social Care Partnership and the GMCA. This partnership brings the NHS together with local authorities, schools, public sector anchor institutions, businesses, and the voluntary and community sector so as to wrap around all stages of an individual's life – from birth until death. The specific commitments and actions are set out in *Taking Charge*, the GM Strategic Health and Social Care Plan (GMHSC, 2019), the GM Population Health Plan (GMHSCP, 2017a) and the parallel GM White Paper for Public Service Delivery (GMCA, 2019b).

Locally this is translated through the Locality Plan 'Start well, live well, age well: our Salford' (SCC, 2017), which sets out the vision and strategy for the health and social care system in Salford. The Locality Plan is shared by the local authority, health and wider partners, and by both commissioners and providers. The vision laid out in it is that 'people across Salford will experience health on a parallel with the current "best" in Greater Manchester (GM), and the gaps between communities will be narrower than they have ever been before'. The Locality Plan also sets out a series of service transformations that will change the way in which care is delivered and the relationship between statutory organisations, and between statutory organisations and the public. It sets out how the SCC, commissioners and providers in the NHS, the wider public sector and the voluntary, community and social enterprise sector will build on what is already in place so that services work better and cost less.

This chapter sets out some of the structural, organisational and practical developments that have taken place in GM and in Salford to deliver on these commitments.

Integrated care – needs some examples of success

Integration of health and care was one of the primary drivers for devolution. Each of the ten localities in GM has created its own local care system – working to a framework of organisational, quality and safety standards set and agreed in GM.

Salford's own journey towards integrated delivery of health and care has been underway for some time, tracking back to 2002, and the first of our pooled budgets for services for adults with learning disabilities. In 2011, the council and the primary care trust (the clinical commissioning group, CCG, from 2013) created a joint integrated commissioning team, overseeing the integrated commissioning of services for adult mental health, learning disabilities, older people, carers and physical and sensory disability. 2012 saw the formation of Salford Together – a formal partnership between SCC, Salford Clinical Commissioning Group (SCCG), Salford Royal NHS Foundation Trust (SRFT) and Greater Manchester Mental Health NHS Foundation Trust – and the Integrated Care Programme for Older People. In 2014, the Older People's pooled budget was established, with a value of £112 million. This was followed in 2016 by a significantly increased Adults Pooled budget to the value of £240 million, and covering a range of services and service providers. In July 2016, the Integrated Care Organisation (ICO) was formally created – bringing together staff from both the NHS and council, and with SRFT the lead provider for social care in the city. An Integrated Adult Health and Social Care Commissioning Committee was formed to govern this pooled budget, ensuring decisions were taken jointly by the council and the CCG, and ensuring both democratic and clinical leadership. Salford's ICO was among the first in England to formally integrate health and adult social care in this way.

The second element of the integrated care system is commissioning. The framework for the approach was set out in the GM Commissioning Review – a single commissioning function between local authorities and CCGs; integrated neighbourhood leadership systems, which includes political, clinical leadership, asset- and strength-based community development, and resident and community engagement; a single pooled budget across health, social care and wider public services; and an investment-based approach focused on prevention and early intervention (GMHSCP, 2017b). The exact arrangement in each locality reflected local variation in relationships, institutions, communities and needs.

In April 2019, SCC and SCCG agreed to establish a single Integrated Health and Care Fund, bringing together funding for services supported by budgets for children, adults, primary care and public health – thereby creating an Integrated Health and Care Fund of almost £600 million per year for the delivery of health, wellbeing and care.

In Salford, the funding and commissioning arrangements have not been integrated lightly. Rather, the process reflects a genuine commitment to deliver better outcomes and experience for residents. Integrating commissioning and funding will mean bringing planning, decision-making and budget decisions closer together to directly affect residents' experience – ensuring they are able to see the right people, in the right place, with the right skills and experience. Of greatest importance, integrated decision-making will ensure that people receive the coordinated and proactive care essential to achieve improved population health outcomes, and meet the health and care needs of the city's growing and ageing population. It will also protect front-line services – the joint approach to adult social care, through a pooled budget and integrated commissioning team, has already protected at least £20 million of social care services in the city every year. These are services that otherwise would have been lost to residents.

The city's joint approach also ensures that Salford is able to have a clear strategic role and act with a single voice in shaping the health and care services available to people in the city in the future. This enables influence to be exerted at a GM level and nationally. For example, Salford has led the commissioning of a substance misuse service that operates across Salford, Bolton and Trafford – taking the best elements of Salford's lead provider model and applying common standards across a number of areas. Salford is consistently the best performer across GM for both opiates and non-opiates treatment, and the successful completion rate is double the national level.

The quality, safety and outcomes of the patient experience has never been more dependent on systems working well together. This includes enhanced democratic and clinical leadership in a wider range of decisions. Elected members and general practitioners have strong local insight and understanding, alongside professional and clinical expertise. The integration will ensure all resource and service decisions benefit from this combined perspective.

While devolution and integration have led to organisational and system changes, the real test is in the outcomes these changes deliver for people living in Salford and other areas of GM. We will now turn to some of the more practical changes that local leadership has helped to achieve.

Why localism matters

In a number of policy areas, the strengthened partnership between health and local government is beginning to pay dividends.

Devolution, together with local leadership and action, has helped to overcome some of the policy silos that exist in national government and Whitehall – none more so than in the area of health and housing.

Health and housing

Shelter is fundamental to a person's health and wellbeing. The importance of a decent home cannot be underestimated and has been widely understood since the Victorian social reformers of the 1880s. At the foundation of the NHS in 1948, Nye Bevan was initially made Health and Housing Minister. Unfortunately, this connection was broken in 1951. Devolution, local leadership and integrated partnership models are enabling new innovative models to be developed in GM and Salford, bringing these critical public policy areas back together.

Structurally, Salford's elected mayor is the GM portfolio lead for Housing, Planning and Homelessness. A Housing and Health Programme Board has recently been established. This brings together 15 different local organisations, representing local authorities, CCGs, housing associations, citizen's advice, hospital trusts, and voluntary, community and social enterprise organisations. It will form part of the oversight and governance arrangements for delivery of the GM Housing Strategy, which clearly includes a commitment to further integrated working between health and housing partners.

The results from bringing these agendas closer together can already be seen. The GM Joint Commissioning Board has recently agreed to allocate £1.5 million for the flagship 'A Bed Every Night programme'. Introduced by Andy Burnham, the GM mayor, this guarantees a bed every night for anyone sleeping rough on the streets of GM. It is the largest ever NHS investment in homelessness prevention, and is a clear indication of the gains in wider system functionality of new devolved and locally led decision-making models that operate across GM. This additional funding will help people using the scheme to better access health care services. It is hoped that the Ministry of Justice and Probation Services may also consider making contributions.

The GM Housing Strategy calls for 'greater integration between social housing providers and the health and social care system', stating the need for 'a more strategic approach to the commissioning of new social housing, particularly an appropriate mix of supported housing' (GMCA, 2019a). Specifically it calls for collaborative action between local government and the NHS to meet demand for an extra 15,000 units of much needed supported accommodation for older people by 2035 (GMCA, 2019a). One of the guiding principles of the Housing and Health Programme Board will be to 'health check' all housing policies as they are developed and implemented.

In Salford, there are some very practical examples of joint responses to health and housing issues. The council's public health and regulatory services teams are currently working together to reduce fuel poverty through affordable warmth schemes. The council's Helping Hands service provides support and adaptations to homes for older people and families. Salford's forthcoming local housing strategy will have a renewed focus on affordability, improved connectivity, design quality, space standards and access.

Mental health

Britain is facing a wider mental health crisis, and when so many wider determinants of health are heavily influenced by mental health issues, it is something to be taken seriously. Mental health is a second area where there has been real progress through local leadership, and specially the approach to both integrated care and integrated commissioning, planning and decision-making. The commitment and actions are set out in Salford's Mental Health Strategy (SCC, 2019).

An estimated 36,357 people in Salford are likely to have mild to moderate mental health problems; 22 people died from suicide in Salford in 2018; 213 children and young people accessed Child and Adolescent Mental Health Services in 2017/18; and only 9.3 per cent of people with a secondary mental health problem in Salford are also in employment (SCC, 2019, p 4). The city also has a crisis of loneliness and isolation, with an estimated 32–40,000 Salford residents aged between 35 and 64 affected. Working age unmarried adults between the ages of 35–64 with long-term health conditions are amongst the hardest hit, alongside those living alone (26,500 residents), those who have recently experienced divorce (6,000 Salford residents in the past 12 months), those living in poverty or financial insecurity with a mental health issue, or carers for those with mental health problems (SCC, 2019, p 17).

As a city, Salford spends around £48.4 million on mental health services each year, and this number is expected to increase by £1.5 million over the next three years. Outside Manchester, Salford invests more in mental health services per head of population than any other area in the North West – and is the only non-Manchester area in GM to invest more than the national average.

In Salford, integrated planning and decision-making by the council, CCG and the mental health trust, has driven a single approach to the design and delivery of improved mental health provision across the city. Community psychiatric nursing, in-patient provision, supported accommodation, intermediate support and 24/7 home-based treatment is more effective as a result. This means more people are being supported at home, and carers are now contacted within 72 hours of in-patient or home-based treatment.

Similarly, until recently there were five different commissions and contracts for five different types of advocacy across health and social care – Independent Mental Capacity Advocacy, Independent Mental Health Advocacy, Care Act Advocacy, NHS Complaints Advocacy and non-statutory advocacy. These have been brought together into one, delivered through a single joint budget, meaning patients now keep the same advocate as they progress through treatment, meaning consistency of relationships and better experience and outcomes for patients.

Social prescribing and public spaces

Social prescribing is an important part of the reforms that are being introduced, supporting a focus on holistic wellbeing, rather than just treating ill health. Through the Wellbeing Matters programme, people and patients in primary care services are being connected with community organisations, linking them to local assets where they can be assisted and signposted to local activities. Wellbeing Matters is an ambitious programme rooted heavily in the principles of cross-sector working, building on people's own assets and strengths to make best use of the assets within a community. The council and its partners across the city are actively investing in and supporting a range of local assets and activities to ensure a rich range of local assets is available to support this social prescribing model.

There are very good health reasons for supporting this approach. We know that green space has a huge impact on personal and community wellbeing, as it is associated with lower levels of general distress and reduced levels of anxiety. Evidence points to 'green exercise' – exercise out and about in nature – being more effective than other forms. Communities within walking distance of green space have higher life expectancy (even when studies are controlled for age, sex, marital status and socio-economic status). Green space promotes physical activity and the participation of children in physical activity, and it is particularly effective when combined with access to recreational facilities. People who live close to green space feel healthier, and positively associate their proximity to the space as good for their health. These positive associations could well be linked to the enhanced weight management associated with green space (high levels of which correlate with roughly a 40 per cent reduction in overweight and obesity-related ill health). Cardiovascular health is improved in proximity to green space, and general health inequalities are lowest in the areas with greatest access.

Public Health England has claimed that the NHS spent around £6.1 billion on overweight and obesity-related ill health in 2014/15. The social costs of obesity are estimated at £27 billion a year, and green space is vital to combating it (PHE, 2017). And, of course, preserving green space is the best mechanism we have to fight climate change.

Through neighbourhood teams, early interventions models are being pioneered to support children, young people and their families. This means assisting them in developing and tapping into networks in their local community, developing a sense of self-worth through community participation and engagement, while strengthening their existing skills and promoting self-reliance.

The Sport England local pilot provides investment to tackle the causes of children and young people's inactivity. The scheme currently sits between five connected work programmes that are building additional capacity in the system – and is run in partnership with schools, Salford Council for Voluntary Services, sports clubs, Salford Community Leisure, SCC youth services and the Health Improvement Service. By working with existing community organisations such as Little Hulton Big Local, this partnership allows a whole system approach to collaborative working, co-producing physical activity initiatives.

The Local Spatial Plan elaborates specific policies to improve the environment, create healthier places and check all new developments against a Health Impact Assessment.

Substantial funds have been invested into green space in Salford over the past decade, bringing disused space to life as well as reclaiming wasteland and restoring parks. The most high-profile investment has been made by the Royal Horticultural Society (RHS), with the RHS Garden Bridgewater, the society's fifth national garden. This will cover a vast 154 acres of land and will potentially attract an estimated 700,000 visitors per year, thereby becoming the largest RHS garden both in size and in use.

As part of this development, a new Horticultural College and Learning Centre is to be opened, forging links with regional educational bodies running higher-level RHS courses. This will mean training and apprenticeship opportunities for Salford residents and a wide range of activities for the general public. Ideas currently include the provision of a therapeutic garden and the opportunity to develop personal green space for individuals and groups.

Between 2010 and 2019, over £7 million will have been invested in improvements to the Bridgewater Canal, providing one of the largest single investments in Salford's green infrastructure over the past few years. The 4.9 miles of towpath are to be upgraded to create a pedestrian- and cycle-friendly route for residents, providing access to a variety of employment sites, recreational sites and other green spaces.

Significant investment has also gone into the local parks along the canal, managing the woodland, upgrading the paths, installing seating and more. A five-year programme of activities and events is currently in place to encourage learning about the canal and involvement from local residents.

In Cutacre Country Park, comprising 40 hectares of land extending into neighbouring Bolton, former surface-mining areas are currently being restored to provide new and improved wildlife habitats and recreation facilities (including lagoons, ponds, footpaths and more). In Castle Irwell, our second largest flood basin is nearing completion increasing our levels of protection from the River Irwell. New Community Sports pitches will be made available within the basin, and a new wetland and recreation area has been created towards the north. This work began in 2016, but the completion date will depend on the council's financial status after the COVID-19 crisis.

Historic Peel Park – one of the oldest in the country – underwent a complete renewal in February 2015, funded by Parks for People and the Heritage Lottery Fund. Improvements included heritage interpretation, rediscovered paths and walks, new play areas, a new ranger's office and formal gardens. The park also began to host and promote events and activities in connection with Salford Museum and Art Gallery. Currently, in May 2020, all public buildings have been closed and public events cancelled due to the COVID-19 lockdown.

The West Salford Cycle Network has also been created to link the Bridgewater Way, Port Salford Greenway and the former loop lines together.

All these investments have been carefully considered in collaboration with health teams and are fully integrated into the SCC agenda for social prescribing and the promotion of wellbeing. The Salford Population Health Plan outlines these ambitions, recognising the explicit links between the environment we live in and the health of the local population. In particular, it is recognised that green space is a community asset with potential roles for social prescribing and the prevention of long-term disease. The Greenspace Strategy

Supplementary Planning Document also brings forward policies and guidance from the council's plan that are related to recreation standards, public health, design and development, with the aim of protecting and improving open spaces.

Conclusion

This chapter outlines the devolution journey in GM, how it has been implemented and illustrates some of the work done locally to deliver on the system changes that were part of the devolution vision. Devolution has led to investment as well as substantial organisational and system changes. These have only been possible because of the local relationships that existed before devolution, and because of the ongoing investment in the development and maintenance of those relationships – at GM and locally, and across sectors and organisations; relationships that are based on trust and a mutual respect for each other's professional, clinical and democratic expertise. There is also a mutual commitment to provide the best possible public services and experiences for the people who live in local communities and rely on those services.

Despite the achievements – only some of which have been discussed here – there remains much to do. There is still a £7 billion funding gap in GM between public spend and tax income. Notwithstanding the growth that has been created, there are 65,700 unemployed people in the city-region, including a quarter of all 16- to 19-year-olds. In addition, 12,000 children each year are not ready for school, life expectancy is nearly two years below the national average for both men and women, and 18,000 of all residents are in the homelessness risk category.

The ongoing government commitment to a policy of austerity continues to deplete our public services. Due to uncertainty of the UK allocation of funds to local councils, anticipated reductions in council income from business rates and other income such as car parking, a revision of council budgets will be undertaken at a later stage of the COVID-19 pandemic. Reductions in the administrative budgets of health clinical commissioning groups will not be reinvested in local front-line services, but will be returned to government nationally. It is one thing to understand the crisis facing our populations and city-regions, quite another to make the long-term investment decisions needed when faced with choices between early intervention and prevention that we know are crucial for sustainable good health in the future and services for ill-health treatment today.

The whole system approach enabled by devolution, including a whole system focus on wider determinants, has allowed many services to avoid total collapse – and there have been huge and positive steps in an overwhelmingly challenging situation. Despite devolution, policy and funding for health and local government remains highly centralised. In this policy and funding context, hard decisions will continue to be necessary. But in GM, we will continue to lobby for even greater local control and leadership of the critical public services that our residents need. Devolution and local leadership remain the only viable solution.

References

Alexander, R. (2011) 'Manchester Local Economic Assessment; Summary and Conclusions', a report for AGMA. Available from: https://www.trafford.gov.uk/planning/strategic-planning/docs/greater-manchester-local-economic-assessment-summary.pdf [Accessed 9 April 2020].

APPG (All-Party Parliamentary Group) (2019) 'A spending review to increase wellbeing', APPG on Wellbeing Economics. Available from: https://wellbeingeconomics.co.uk/wp-content/uploads/2019/05/Spending-review-to-ncrease-wellbeing-APPG-2019.pdf [Accessed 14 May 2020].

Dahlgren, G. and Whitehead, M. (1991). *Policies and Strategies to Promote Social Equity in Health*, Stockholm: Stockholm: Institute for Futures Studies.

GMCA (Greater Manchester Combined Authority) (2019a) 'Greater Manchester Housing Strategy'. Available from: https://www.greatermanchester-ca.gov.uk/media/2257/gm-housing-strategy-2019-2024.pdf [Accessed 9 April 2020].

GMCA (Greater Manchester Combined Authority) (2019b) 'The Greater Manchester model'. Available from: https://www.greatermanchester-ca.gov.uk/media/2302/gtr_mcr_model1_web.pdf [Accessed 9 April 2020].

GMHSC (Greater Manchester Health and Social Care) (2019). Taking Charge: The Next 5 Years: Our Prospectus (http://www.gmhsc.org.uk/wp-content/uploads/2019/03/GMHSC-Partnership-Prospectus-The-next-5-years-pdf.pdf [Accessed 9 April 2020].

GMHSCP (Greater Manchester Health and Social Care Plan) (2017a) 'Greater Manchester population health plan'. Available from: https://www.gmhsc.org.uk/wp-content/uploads/2018/05/Population-Health-Plan-2017-2021.pdf [Accessed 9 April 2020].

GMHSCP (Greater Manchester Health and Social Care Plan) (2017b) 'Greater Manchester health and social care plan – commissioning review', July. Available from: https://www.gmhsc.org.uk/wp-content/uploads/2018/05/Population-Health-Plan-2017-2021.pdf [Accessed 24 June 2020].

HMSO (2014) Care Act, 2014 (London), Chapter 1.

NHS (National Health Service) (2019) 'The NHS long term plan'. Available from: https://www.longtermplan.nhs.uk [Accessed 2 April 2019].

PHE (Public Health England) (2017) 'Health Matters: Obesity and the Food Industry'. Available from: https://www.gov.uk/government/publications/health-matters-obesity-and-the-food-environment/health-matters-obesity-and-the-food-environment--2 [Accessed 9 April 2020].

SCC (Salford City Council) (2017) 'Start well, live well, age well: our Salford'. Available from: https://www.salfordcvs.co.uk/sites/salfordcvs.co.uk/files/u26/Salford-Locality-Plan-A4-trifold-leaflet_0.pdf [Accessed 9 April 2020].

SCC (Salford City Council) (2019) 'Salford Mental Health All Age Commissioning Strategy 2019–2024'. Available from: https://extranet.salfordccg.nhs.uk/application/files/2615/5412/4803/Salford_Mental_health_All_Age_Integrated_Commissioning_Strategy.pdf [Accessed 9 April 2020].

6

A place-based approach to healthy, happy lives

Ruth Dombey and Adrian Bonner

Introduction

The London Borough of Sutton, in south-west London, has had stable political leadership for the last 34 years. During this time, the population has become increasingly diverse and continues to grow. The last ten years of reduced central government funding have resulted in budgetary planning that has presented many challenges. In this chapter, Ruth Dombey, leader of the council, outlines innovative approaches to maintain a healthy, happy and safe community. Place-based approaches, involving integrated health and social care integration and outcome commissioning, have been developed with a view to a consideration of 'health' in all council planning.

> I was standing in a queue at my local pharmacy, listening to the pharmacist chatting to the elderly man in front of me while she made up his prescription. She clearly knew him well and he felt at ease with her. I noticed much of the conversation revolved around his wife and her health – and understood why when it transpired that he was the carer for his wife and was getting up several times during the night to see to her needs. His physical and mental exhaustion was due to his caring responsibilities and the wider context of his life. The pharmacist understood that and was able to give him useful advice. (Ruth Dombey)

So often, people are categorised by their specific needs and problems. What is your housing need, your medical need, your financial need? What can I do to help you with that one aspect of your life? What services can I offer to help you address that particular need? But life is not linear – it is messy and complicated and interconnected. What if we were to ask what you would like in order to lead an active, healthy and happy life?

People are not just patients, service users, passive recipients of public services. People have a right to a say in their own lives, a right to be involved in decisions that affect everyone and a right to decide their own priorities. We have a responsibility to be active citizens of the world we live in and help to shape that world for the better. We are bound by one common factor – the place where we live. It may not be the place where we work or study or even where we spend most of our time. But 'place' plays a huge role in determining our health outcomes – the air we breathe, the way we travel, how safe we are, how we spend our leisure time, the education we give our children.

The wider determinants of health – housing, environment, leisure, income and education – are well recognised and are just as important as access to good health care. If we want to develop long-term strategies to enable social and cultural change with new models of care, more community-based responsibility for our neighbours and more freedoms and flexibilities to help us make better choices, then the role of place is key. This reflects the place-based approach that is being promoted by the London Borough of Sutton as it delegates its statutory duties across the range of services it manages, collaborating with other statutory and third sector organisations within and beyond the two parliamentary constituencies of Sutton and Cheam, and Carshalton and Wallington.

A place-based approach to health and wellbeing – in its widest sense – can bring together all parts of the public sector to focus on positive outcomes. In 2016, one of the authors of this chapter, Ruth Dombey, was pleased to be part of a National Commission set up by National Local Government Network (NLGN) and Collaborate and chaired by Lord Victor Adebowale to address some of these challenges. In our Final Report – Get Well Soon, Reimaging Place-Based Health (NLGN, 2016) – the need for increased funding for health and social care and the need to shift from treatment towards prevention was highlighted. Instead of asking people 'what health services do you want?', a very different response would be elicited if the question was 'what would help you to enjoy life more?'. To address this question, partnerships based around the skills and expertise of local government, the third sector, community and enterprise sector, housing providers, health services and community pharmacies should be promoted. This is described as 'place-based health'. The approach is based around internationally recognised high-quality evidence on integrated personal commissioning from health systems. Support for the view that early intervention and prevention (in health and social care) is vital has been generated from studies in Greater Manchester (see Chapter 5). These indicate that early intervention and prevention not only improves outcomes but it also potentially saves money in the longer term (Nesta, 2015). Active partnerships involving local government and the National Health Service (NHS) have been developed through Vanguard sites and devolved budgets in Greater Manchester and Cornwall, but a systematic shift in culture is needed. To explore the wider determinants of health and 'place-based health', the NLGN commission reviewed four geographical areas, the London Borough of Sutton, Sunderland (see Chapter 7), Birmingham and Suffolk, as the process of change had already begun, and these were places appropriate to be selected for this review. A recognition from these socio-geographic insights suggested that a new vision for place-based health would realise a reversal of the current balance of funding and energy in the system away from crisis management and towards prevention. This will require three fundamental shifts in thinking and working:

- **From institutions to people and places.** To move towards prevention and embedded health as a social movement, power and control should be transferred from health and care institutions to the capacity (positive assets) of people and local resources integrated to support place-based health.
- **From service silos to outcomes for people.** The development of horizontal place-based systems from the vertical silos of health and social care involves cultural and behavioural change. The recognition of enablers of this change is important in order that these can be developed and supported at every level, leading to the creation of a new system from the inside out.
- **Enabling change from national to local.** While national bodies should focus on creating a long-term environment for prevention, they must recognise place-based approaches rather than reinforcing silos and remove blockages for local practitioners.

The commissioners, including the author of this chapter, Ruth Dombey, concluded that:

> Our vision for place-based health, centres on three core principles:
> - People must be empowered to take greater control over their own lives, to influence personalised services and to take greater responsibility for their wider health outcomes;

- All resources and assets in places must be used to support wider determinants of health and wellbeing outcomes;
- A system shift towards preventative and early intervention will require services to organise and professionals to behave in very different ways.

At a national level, there is growing recognition that the role of place is key. The King's Fund has recently published a report, introducing the work of NHS England's Healthy New Towns (Naylor and Buck, 2018), a three-year programme:

> to look at how health and wellbeing can be planned and designed into new places. It brings together partners in housebuilding, local government, health care and local communities to demonstrate how to create places that offer people improved choices and chances for a healthier life.
> The programme's three priorities are:
> - planning and designing a healthy built environment;
> - creating innovative models of health care;
> - encouraging strong and connected communities.

The final report from NHS England, entitled 'Putting Health into Place' (NHS England, 2018), sets out national recommendations for change and provides practical tools for everyone involved in creating new places. Based on ten principles as a route to creating healthier places, it talks about the importance of partnerships across the whole spectrum and how local communities need to be involved in early engagement to help develop the places in which they live.

In local authority management of local resources, there are often constraints owing to the drivers of funding and targets of separate organisations; decisions are based on what is best for the particular organisation and not the people who are being served. Working within service silos leads to a failure in understanding the complexities of people's lives. A traditional approach is to find ready-made, one size fits all solutions, and attempt to adapt them to the local context, rather than understanding the local context and working with local people to find solutions. A more effective strategy is to listen to what people are saying and what will make a difference to them.

The London Borough of Sutton regularly consults its constituents in the development of policies and strategies. An example of this is in the development of the Sutton Health and Care Plan. This has been developed from an evidence base, an extensive consultation over a two-year period involving residents, voluntary and community groups, businesses, health and social care services, housing associations, schools and colleges, police and fire services and many other representatives of the public and private sector. The pivotal question in this work was 'What sort of place do we want Sutton to be, and how can we work differently to build it together?'.

In developing new ways of working between Sutton Council and the Sutton Clinical Commissioning Group (CCG), the Sutton Health and Care Plan aims to support 'better health and wellbeing outcomes for local residents by working closely with a range of stake holders, local people and carers who use services in Sutton'. Within the borough and with other boroughs in South London there is a good history of partnership working. These active partnerships are with the community and voluntary sector and HealthWatch Sutton. The South West London Alliance provides a communication channel across Sutton, Merton, Croydon and Kingston (NHS, 2019).

The joint approach being developed in the Sutton Health and Care Plan not only provides a framework for NHS long-term planning through integrated care plans, working with the community and voluntary sector, but addresses health inequalities from a social determinants of health perspective. The main priorities of the plan are:

- a better quality of life and opportunity for all residents;
- places underpinned by inclusive and sustainable growth;
- a coherent system of health and care that is shaped around the needs of Sutton's residents.

To achieve good outcomes from these aims, transformational change will be brought about by the following partnership principles:

1. Think Sutton.
2. Work across sectors.
3. Get involved early.
4. Build stronger, self-sufficient communities.
5. Provide coordinated, seamless services.

In supporting Sutton residents across the lifespan, there are a number of challenges and opportunities that are being addressed in implementing the Sutton Health and Care Plan, to enable people to start well, live well and age well.

Start well

One of the key recommendations of the Marmot Review (Marmot, 2010) is to 'Give every child the best start in life'. Although Sutton is a safe, supportive community, not every family and child is thriving. School readiness, mental health and supporting children with special educational needs and disability are priority planning issues being considered by Sutton Council. Supporting parents of children and young people with special educational needs is part of the council's statutory responsibility.

In line with national data published in a recent *Lancet Psychiatry* study in which 6 per cent of young people aged 16–24 years had self-harmed (Borschmann and Kinner, 2019), a report from HealthWatch Sutton (HealthWatch, 2019), surveying 5,000 young people aged 11–18, indicated that 6 per cent of the interviewees had experienced self-harm and 25 per cent had felt lonely in the last month prior to the interview. There was a decline in wellbeing between 12 and 18 years. This decline in wellbeing was linked to time spent using a phone/computer screen. This issue has been reviewed by Critchlow (Critchlow, 2018). The HealthWatch report noted that 40 per cent of the students had sleep problems, with a direct correlation between sleep hours and improved wellbeing. Furthermore, lesbian, gay, bisexual and transgender young people were four times more likely to have suicidal thoughts compared with those who identified themselves as heterosexual.

Within the work of the Sutton Health and Care Plan, a Suicide Prevention Strategy has been developed (LBS, 2019). Collaborative working between the council and Child and Mental Health Services is being supported by funding from NHS England so a Trailblazer programme can be run; this involves the training of mental health support workers at the Institute of Psychiatry, King's College, in order to provide low-level interventions in a number of local schools (South West London Health and Care Partnership, 2019).

Live well

Eating well, taking exercise and generally making 'healthy' life choices are not new concepts in the area of public health. However, in addition to popular interest in healthy living choices, as reflected in the number of broadcast and digital media outputs, personal responsibility for our wellbeing is at the centre of the social determinants of health (rainbow) model, the subject of this book. In Sutton, 65,000 people have developed long-term conditions such as diabetes and/or high blood pressure.

The traditional view that these 'medicalised' conditions can be solely addressed through general practitioner (GP) prescribing is being challenged in the implementation of the Sutton Health and Care Plan. 'A system shift towards preventative and early intervention will require services to organise, and professionals to behave in very different ways.'

Nearly 13 per cent (12.8 per cent) of adults smoke in Sutton, in line with the national average. A lower proportion (1.7 per cent) of adults in Sutton, compared with the national average, cycle for travel at least three days a week. This might be related to heavy 'London' traffic and the hilly terrain in some parts of the borough. These challenges are being addressed through council-led cycle routes and rental schemes, including folding bicycles and electric bikes available for use in the community. Currently, Go Sutton, a local minibus scheme aimed at reduced short car journeys that can be reserved via an app is on trial. This place-based health and wellbeing strategy is not only good for residents and their families, but it also has significant economic benefits when the council adapts its spending priorities at a time of decreased funding from central government.

For those people with learning disabilities, Sutton Council is committed to addressing inequalities by acknowledging the need for meaningful employment, accessibility and a diverse range of support. Overall, 64.1 per cent of adults with a learning disability have an annual health check with a GP, a higher take-up than the national average (PHE, 2018).

Age well

Employing a team of Admiral Nurses who are trained to give support to people living with dementia and their families, the council is able to offer support, increase coping techniques and improve understanding of the condition – which allows people to stay longer in their own homes and be more independent (Dementia UK, 2019). This is one of a number of initiatives to address the issues of older people. Older people, with multiple health problems including diabetes, hypertension and depression, receive support from GPs. However, frequently the primary factor mitigating against health and wellbeing is loneliness. Nationally, 59 per cent of people who use social care do not get as much social contact as they would like (PHE, 2019). The lack of social contact is reported in 71.8 per cent of carers. Combating loneliness and social isolation among older people is an important component of managing the challenges faced by elderly people as their care needs become more complex with age. Age well is a key component in the Sutton Health and Care Plan, which aims to reduce social isolation, increase physical and mental health outcomes, promote intergenerational relationships, improve non-medical support (including extending the provision of social prescribing), integrate Sutton Health and Care At Home Service, redesign the 'falls model' and expand delivery of the End of Life Care model.

Local government has a key role to play in health and wellbeing across all activities in the borough. By exercising its role of leadership of place, we can work with the NHS and all the other community and voluntary sector partners to develop a more sustainable and joined-up health and care system that puts wellbeing and personal choice at its heart. This needs dedicated and committed leaders who understand the different systems and can influence outcomes. It means breaking down organisational silos and putting the person at the centre. It means shifting resources and funding towards prevention and early intervention. Entrenched ways of thinking and ways of working need to be challenged. Courage to take risks and trust the intuition and experience of the people we are working with and working for is needed.

Council responses to austerity budgeting by central government

In response to the unprecedented financial pressures and increased needs being experienced by Sutton Council, a number of statutory obligations are under threat. These include support for the homeless, special educational needs provision, homecare and looked after children services. A rethink of the way in which council financial structures are organised, and starting to judge success by joint outcomes rather than organisational outputs, was needed to deliver the £70 million of savings to date, with another £17 million saving planned over the next three years (2019–2021).

The efficiency plans show a movement from service by service commissioning to an outcome commissioning approach. Based on historical data, consultation and a major review of the council's budgeting structure, five outcome areas have been identified for cross-service commissioning and monitoring. These are used by the council to commission and monitor effectiveness of the use of public money (see Figure 6.1).

Political leadership is vitally important. Elected members can lead and challenge because they have democratic accountability and answer

Figure 6.1: Five outcome areas used for outcome commissioning by the London Borough of Sutton

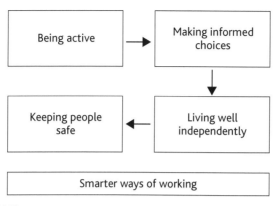

Source: LBS, 2018

to their residents. Local government has the necessary expertise to enable this to happen, the council owns large tracts of housing and is building more, development and regeneration is taking place, and work to improve air quality and encourage active, healthy lives continues. Town planning, licensing, environmental health, building control and education services are all provided. Help is being given to generate jobs and income, the council is working with the private sector to encourage vibrant town and district centres, as well as supporting local communities and voluntary groups. The council also tends its parks, playgrounds and open spaces.

Despite diminishing funds from central government restricting the activities of local councils, they are in a powerful position to manage locally owned land and control its use for the public good. This is exemplified by the significant socio-economic collaborative work between Sutton Council, the Institute of Cancer Research (ICR), the Royal Marsden Foundation Trust and the Greater London Authority (ICR, 2019).

The masterplan, the London Cancer Hub, is based around an innovation district. It is attracting talented researchers and experts from different fields of science, with a 'Knowledge Centre combining laboratories, business space, an auditorium and leisure facilities'. The Hub is planned to become a leading edge centre for cancer detection, monitoring, treatment and research, as well as promoting medical education. Through the investment of more than £1 billion and the creation of more than 13,000 new jobs, local, national and international health needs are being addressed.

Additionally, in response to increased needs for school places in the borough, a new academy school has been being built in the grounds of a now disused hospital adjacent to the Cancer Hub. This innovative project will proactively link the Cancer Hub with the academy school, which will specialise in medical and health sciences (see Figures 6.2 and 6.3).

Figure 6.2: The government awarded Sutton Council £300,000 to support the development of the London Cancer Hub. The photo shows Cllr Ruth Dombey OBE, Mayor of London Sadiq Khan and the Chief Executive of ICR, Professor Paul Workman, discussing plans.

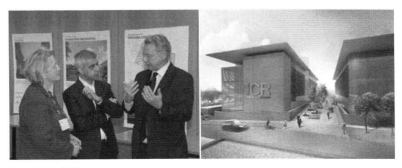

Source: ICR, 2016

Figure 6.3: Architect's impressions of the planned London Cancer Hub, planned to become one of the world's top life-science campuses, and an example of an 'innovation district'

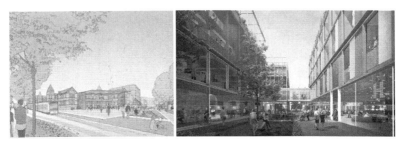

Source: ICR, 2016

Local business enterprises are being linked to these research and health technologies. Related activities on Sutton High Street will be encouraged and linked to other high street developments.

Partnership working

The strategic planning of borough-wide management of public assets and the addressing of statutory obligations is being integrated with the Sutton Health and Care Plan. Local community leaders are needed to provide an insight into local needs and work with local people. This place-based approach to healthy communities is driven by the huge amount of time that is spent listening to local people, engaging with local groups, understanding how the different services impact on their lives and encouraging them to get more involved with the decisions that affect them and the place where they live. Good leaders don't deliver change on their own; they have the ability to make real connections and take people on a journey with them. They develop the relationships and trust that underpin success and allow the building of strong partnerships that bring about lasting change.

The council's intention is that a shared vision for the borough will embrace collective ideas on how to tackle some of the big issues facing people (see the discussion on 'wicked issues', in the Conclusion of this book). Decisions, planning and delivery of services will be shaped, governed and delivered through a partnership that links public, private, voluntary and community sectors and allows them to work together. Improving the lives of people who experience inequality will form the bedrock of the partnership's work. The role of the partnership will be to provide leadership and oversight, commit organisational time and resource to the initiatives, unblock barriers and consider the lessons learnt and their relevance to future change.

The council recognises that asking all partners to radically change their way of working is a lot to ask. During discussions with the partners, there was an agreement that initially three priorities would be identified, with a view as to how working together in partnership would make a difference to those people most affected. It has been important to ensure that this is real trusted partnership working and not driven by local government, with everyone else following on behind. The agreed common issues to be jointly tackled are:

- tackling domestic abuse and its causes;
- providing early help to young families at risk of disadvantage;
- supporting older people.

While the domestic abuse work is being coordinated by the council, the local NHS is leading on the work with early help to young parents and perinatal mental health, and Age UK Sutton is leading on the third strand, supporting older people to lead more independent and fulfilling lives and developing an age-friendly borough. This partnership between the statutory sector and third sector is supported by more than 300 voluntary groups that are working with Community Action, previously called Sutton Council for Voluntary Services (CAS, 2019).

Social prescribing is a non-medical approach to dealing with health issues. It enables primary care services to refer people with social, emotional or practical needs to a range of local, non-clinical services, such as financial, pastoral and community support. Sutton CCG and the council are exploring how social prescribing might be provided locally as part of a partnership between GPs and a range of public, voluntary and community organisations.

Better Contacts is a partnership between Sutton Council and the local fire brigade, aimed at providing preventative support to vulnerable residents across the borough. To begin with, the project is concentrating on reporting potential issues regarding fire prevention, safeguarding, alcohol and drug misuse, housing and employment needs. Fire officers are visiting people at risk and helping them to identify the support they need.

An example of the work being done to tackle domestic abuse is the setting up of a domestic abuse housing operational group, to share knowledge across all housing professionals in the borough and cascade best practice. With support from the nationally recognised Domestic Abuse Housing Alliance (DAHA, 2019), a consistent and effective housing response to domestic abuse in Sutton – with Sutton Housing Partnership (which manages the council's housing stock) and other housing providers working towards DAHA accreditation – is ensured.

According to the report, loneliness increases the likelihood of death by 26 per cent, and people with strong relationships are 50 per cent more likely to survive life-threatening illness. The creation of strong and cohesive communities, based on place, can make a huge difference to people's health and wellbeing.

It is still early days in implementing this new place-based approach to the local authority's management of local assets for the benefit of a healthy community. However, differences are becoming apparent as the various agencies work together. A better understanding of the different organisations and the worlds in which they operate is developing. By putting the person at the heart of what is being done, and understanding the wider context of their lives within their families and their communities, greater knowledge is being gained of how to work together and come up with solutions that reflect the needs and aspirations of Sutton's inhabitants. It is being learnt that strong, reliant and interconnected communities – the social assets of those living around us – can provide the social networks and support mechanisms that individuals need in order to thrive.

Every place is different. We can all learn from each other – what works and what doesn't and why. But local diversity is crucial and to be welcomed because it is a direct response to the diversity of place and the people living there. Relationships are key, as is strong leadership and a shared vision of our place.

The first female GP, Dr Elizabeth Blackwell, said: 'We are not tinkers who merely patch and mend what is broken […] we must be watchmen, guardians of the life and the health of our generation, so that stronger and more able generations may come after.'

> Local government needs to step up to this challenge, recognise the vital role we have to play in the social determinants of health and use our enabling and persuading powers to bring everyone to the table. Now, as never before, we owe it to our residents and our neighbours, the people we share this place with, to break down organisational barriers, pool our resources, listen to and learn from each other and strive together to create places where people can live happy, healthy lives and thrive. (Cllr Ruth Dombey, Leader of Sutton Council)

References

Borschmann, R. and Kinner, S.A. (2019) 'Responding to the rising prevalence of self-harm', *Lancet Psychiatry*, 6(7): 548–9. Available from: https://www.thelancet.com/journals/lanpsy/article/PIIS2215-0366(19)30210-X/fulltext [Accessed 9 April 2020].

CAS (Community Action Sutton) (2019) Available from: https://www.suttoncvs.org.uk/ [Accessed 9 April 2020].

Critchlow, N. (2018) 'Health and wellbeing in the digital society', in A. Bonner (ed) *Social Determinants of Health: An Interdisciplinary Approach to Social Inequality and Wellbeing*, Bristol: Policy Press, pp 103–17.

DAHA (Domestic Abuse Housing Alliance) (2019) Available from: https://www.dahalliance.org.uk/ [Accessed 9 April 2020].

Dementia UK (2019) 'Admiral nurses: the specialist dementia support that families need'. Leaflet. Available from: https://www.dementiauk.org/wp-content/uploads/2019/06/Admiral-Nurse-leaflet-new-style-web.pdf [Accessed 14 May 2020].

HealthWatch (2019) 'Young people's mental health survey report'. Health Watch Sutton (January). Available from: http://www.healthwatchsutton.org.uk/children-and-young-peoples-mental-health [Accessed 9 April 2020].

ICR (Institute of Cancer Research) (2016) 'London cancer hub cited in report on innovative districts in capital'. Available from: https://www.icr.ac.uk/news-archive/london-cancer-hub-cited-in-report-on-innovation-districts-in-capital [Accessed 9 April 2020].

ICR (Institute of Cancer Research) (2019) 'The London cancer hub'. Available from: https://www.icr.ac.uk/our-research/centres-and-collaborations/strategic-collaborations/london-cancer-hub [Accessed 9 April 2020].

LBS (London Borough of Sutton) (2018) 'Outcomes-based commissioning plan'. Available from: https://moderngov.sutton.gov.uk/documents/s57009/6%20Appendix%20A%20-%20Outcomes%20Based%20Commissioning%20Plan%202018-19.pdf [Accessed 9 April 2020].

LBS (London Borough of Sutton) (2019) 'Suicide Prevention'. Available from: https://www.sutton.gov.uk/info/200152/children_and_young_people/1759/suicide_prevention [Accessed 9 April 2020].

Marmot, M. (2010) 'Fair society, healthy lives', The Marmot Review, Institute of Health Equity. Available from: http://www.instituteofhealthequity.org/resources-reports/fair-society-healthy-lives-the-marmot-review [Accessed 8 April 2020].

Naylor, C. and Buck, D. (2018) 'Supporting the healthy new towns programme'. Available from: https://www.kingsfund.org.uk/projects/supporting-healthy-new-towns-programme [Accessed 9 April 2020].

Nesta (National Endowment for Science, Technology and the Arts) (2015) 'At the heart of health: realising the value of people and communities'. Available from: https://www.nesta.org.uk/report/at-the-heart-of-health-realising-the-value-of-people-and-communities/ [Accessed 9 April 2020].

NHS England (2018) 'Putting health into place', NHS England Publications, Ref 08473. Available from: https://www.england.nhs.uk/wp-content/uploads/2018/09/putting-health-into-place-v4.pdf [Accessed 9 April 2020].

NHS (2019) 'South West London Health Care Partnership', NHS South West London. Available from: https://www.swlondon.nhs.uk/ [Accessed 9 April 2020].

NLGN (New Local Government Network) (2016) 'Place-based health', The Place-Based Health Commission. Available from: http://www.nlgn.org.uk/public/2016/get-well-soon-reimagining-place-based-health [Accessed 9 April 2020].

PHE (Public Health England) (2018) 'Learning disabilities profile'. Available from: https://fingertips.phe.org.uk/profile/learning-disabilities [Accessed 9 April 2020].

PHE (Public Health England) (2019) 'Productive healthy ageing'. Available from: https://fingertips.phe.org.uk/profile/healthy-ageing [Accessed 9 April 2020].

South West London Health and Care Partnership (2019) 'CYP emotional wellbeing programme: whole schools approach and trailblazer – programme update February 2019'. Available from: https://moderngov.sutton.gov.uk/documents/s64822/9a%20 Presentation%20on%20Wave%20One%20Trailblazer%20 arrangements.pdf [Accessed 14 May 2020].

7

Inequalities in health and wellbeing across the UK: a local North-East perspective

Edward Kunonga, Gillian Gibson and Catherine Parker

A City by the Sea
Yes I come from a city by the Sea
And its shores and its water have become a part of me
And when I die it's where I want to be
In a grave in that city by the Sea

I was born, I was raised upon the tide
And the salt, and the sea, yeah, it warms me up inside
Upon the sand, there is no place to hide
From the view where the ocean meets the sky

Yes it's cold and it's hard where I come from
And you do what your dad did or you don't quite belong
Forget all that 'cause we'll do as we please
There is life in my city by the Sea

Martin Longstaff, 2012

Introduction

Chapter 2 of this book, by the Association of Directors of Public Health, provides a review of the system changes of public health, moving from the National Health Service (NHS) back to management by local authorities. The authors of that chapter also point to the major concerns about the limited potential for delivery upstream of health prevention and promotion that was due to reductions in funding from central government to local authorities. The Association of Directors of Public Health has long championed taking a whole-system and long-term view about how we create, enable and sustain the health and wellbeing of everyone in society.

This chapter will identify the challenges facing the North-East from a population health perspective, and the implications for the area of the contemporary context of the reductions in funding that widen health inequalities and create challenges in the labour market. It will consider the potential benefits of building new approaches that address these challenges using community assets, place-based, targeted, collaborative approaches and are based heavily on community ownership, participation and voice.

The chapter will review the responses of local authorities (LAs) in the North-East to reduced central government funding, examine key issues such as supporting vulnerable groups (children/young people, older people, homeless, unemployed and so on), then highlight LA and community responses and innovation approaches to supporting people via health and wellbeing strategies.

As with other chapters in the book, this review will take account of the critical socio-economic issues arising from the Brexit process and during the 'end of austerity', particularly with respect to the North-East region of the United Kingdom (UK).

It has been acknowledged for a long time that there are inequalities in health outcomes across the UK (Department of Health and Social Services, 1980; Black et al, 1999; Whitehead and Dahlgren, 2006; Marmot et al, 2020). The widely recognised north–south divide described a massive difference in life expectancy, healthy life expectancy and a number of health indicators between the north and the south of England. Previous policies and national initiatives have sought to address these inequalities with limited success. The latest data highlights that these inequalities are widening, with the northern areas witnessing a reversal of year-on-year improvements in life expectancy at birth, a decline in the rate of progress in reducing premature deaths from cardiovascular diseases, cancer and respiratory conditions, and a significant increase in drug-related deaths and suicides.

It is not a coincidence that these patterns of poor outcomes and slow progress in improving population health mirror the patterns of deprivation. Health inequalities are a result of complex interactions between a wide range of factors, with the conditions in which one is born, live, work and age having a significant impact on health and wellbeing. The 2018 King's Fund Report summarises the impact of various factors on health and wellbeing outcomes (Buck et al, 2018). They conclude that socio-economic factors contribute up to 50 per cent of health and wellbeing, lifestyle-related risk factors about 30 per cent and health care at best 20 per cent of population health outcomes.

Health inequalities have been defined as unfair, unjust, socially produced (and therefore modifiable) and avoidable variations in outcomes between population groups (Whitehead and Dahlgren, 2006). These population groups can be defined by geography or by common interest or circumstance, such as protected characteristics (ethnicity, sexuality and disability), vulnerability (mental health status, homelessness, substance misuse) and socio-economic deprivation. National research and reports have highlighted the poor life expectancy compared with the general population for certain vulnerable groups, such as:

a. *People with serious mental illness* die 15 to 25 years earlier than the general population. The majority of these deaths are linked to poor physical health and preventable causes (Saxena, 2018).
b. *People with learning disabilities* die, on average, 14 years younger than the general population (Lodge, 2019). The causes of death for this population group are preventable long-term conditions such as diabetes, obesity, heart failure, chronic kidney disease or stroke and cancers.
c. *Minority ethnic groups* generally have poorer health and greater premature deaths than the White British ethnic group (Evandrou et al, 2016). The social determinants of health are unequally distributed across ethnic groups, leading to health inequalities.

The scale of the challenge in Middlesbrough

The north–south divide in health and wellbeing outcomes in the UK can mask the variations that exist within local areas. After decades of progress, since 2011 the improvement in age-standardised mortality rates and life expectancy has slowed down considerably for both males and females in Middlesbrough. The gap in life expectancy between the most and least deprived areas within Middlesbrough is 9.4 years for males and 7.4 years for females. This gap is widening as a result of slower and in some cases static progress in more deprived areas than in less deprived areas (PHE, 2019).

In Middlesbrough, a relatively small unitary local authority in the North-East of England with a population of approximately 140,000, there are inequalities in length and quality of life. Life expectancy at birth in Middlesbrough is 76.2 years for males and 79.8 for females, and this is lower than the England average (79.5 for males and 83.2 for females). The year-on-year improvements in life expectancy have halted and are showing a concerning downward trend.

Healthy life expectancy for both males and females in Middlesbrough is significantly lower than the average for England. There is a difference in healthy life expectancy within Middlesbrough of over 20 years between the most deprived and the most affluent neighbourhoods. The most deprived areas of the town have significant gaps between healthy life expectancy and overall life expectancy. There is a challenge of premature deaths, while a greater proportion of the population spends most of their adult life living with poor health – an issue the Office for National Statistics termed a 'double jeopardy' (ONS, 2017). A large proportion of residents in Middlesbrough begin to have poor health before retirement age.

The major causes of premature deaths and preventable illnesses in Middlesbrough are cancer, heart and respiratory diseases, which account for a large number of premature deaths. Deaths from suicides, drug-related deaths and accidents are the second largest cause of the gap in life expectancy for males between Middlesbrough and the rest of England. This is because most of the suicide, drug-related and accident deaths occur among younger men (Middlesbrough Director of Public Health, 2017).

Sunderland: a city by the sea

Like Middlesbrough, Sunderland has many challenges that impact on the health of its residents. As shown in Figure 7.1, people live for fewer years than the average for England and more years of their lives are spent dealing with poor health and disability (PHE, 2019). The reasons for such poor health outcomes are complex. The loss of the industries that were the prime source of employment in the city in the second half of the 20th century was significant, and certainly played its part. Since then, however, the jobs lost have been replaced, and yet still poor health outcomes remain.

Again, like Middlesbrough, more people die prematurely from chronic diseases such as cancer, heart disease and respiratory conditions (IHME, 2018). These diseases are also, along with issues in relation to mental health and musculoskeletal conditions, major causes of poorer *healthy* life expectancy (IHME, 2018). When we start to consider why this might be the case, the answer can take us straight to some of the modifiable risk factors – many of which are largely linked to behaviours, in particular high levels of smoking, poor diets and harmful consumption of alcohol and inactivity (IHME, 2018). Drug misuse also has an impact on both ill-health and early death. For most of these risk factors, there are stark inequalities in behaviours,

Figure 7.1: Sunderland life expectancy and healthy life expectancy

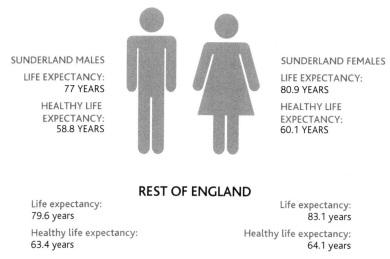

SUNDERLAND MALES

LIFE EXPECTANCY:
77 YEARS

HEALTHY LIFE
EXPECTANCY:
58.8 YEARS

SUNDERLAND FEMALES

LIFE EXPECTANCY:
80.9 YEARS

HEALTHY LIFE
EXPECTANCY:
60.1 YEARS

REST OF ENGLAND

Life expectancy:
79.6 years

Healthy life expectancy:
63.4 years

Life expectancy:
83.1 years

Healthy life expectancy:
64.1 years

Source: PHE, 2020a

with those that are less healthy more often found among the most disadvantaged populations. Even where there are fewer inequalities in behaviours, such as consumption of alcohol, the harm resulting from the behaviour tends to have less impact on the most affluent.

Research has shown that mental wellbeing has been associated with a range of behaviours that are known to improve health, such as exercise (Chanfreau et al, 2018) and diet (Pressman and Cohen, 2005), as well as not smoking (Steptoe and LaMarca, 2012). The association between poor mental wellbeing and behaviours that damage health has led some to suggest that they may be 'survival strategies' in the face of multiple problems (Friedli, 2009).

There is now compelling evidence that the social determinants of health have a greater impact on health outcomes than either individual behaviours or the services we have in place to address poor health. We also know that there are stark inequalities of outcomes in relation to many of those social determinants of health – be they access to employment, income, education, housing or even living in a neighbourhood you can be proud of among people who will support you when you are in need. Unfortunately, the impact of austerity on local services and national changes to welfare means that support is often unavailable at a time when people need it most (ILG, 2013; Cheetham et al, 2017).

Although jobs previously lost within the city have been replaced, these have not always benefited those living in Sunderland and are not always well paid. This means that income remains relatively low (ONS, 2018), leading to high levels of child poverty (PHE, 2019). Work is not always 'good work', and there are still lower levels of employment and young people not in education, employment and training than in many other parts of England (PHE, 2019). One of the key determinants of health is having a good job, yet, anecdotally, there are parts of Sunderland where there are families who have not been in work for generations. There are certainly high levels of workless households when compared with England as a whole, 19.4 per cent compared with 13.9 per cent (ONS, 2019). Before austerity, jobs in public sector organisations were often a bridge to a better life. These so-called 'anchor institutions' are often invested in local communities and unlikely to move to another area. While this is still the case, taking this route has become more difficult as many organisations, such as local government, police forces, fire and rescue services and schools, have been required to shed jobs to operate within reducing budgets that take little account of need and demand. Such institutions can not only provide direct employment, but they can also procure and commission for social value, use their buildings and estates in a way that will support local communities, consider environmental sustainability when making key decisions and work as a partner in developments that go beyond their core business (Reed et al, 2019).

Since the Equality Act 2010 came into force, these anchor institutions have also had a significant duty in relation to inequalities. The public sector 'equality duty' ensures that 'public bodies play their part in making society fairer by tackling discrimination and providing equality of opportunity for all' (Government Equalities Office, 2011). However, despite a socio-economic duty being included in the Act, this element has never been enacted, although arguably this does not mean that organisations cannot consider the needs of people who are impacted by such inequalities when they are taking decisions and developing policies.

In Sunderland, there is clear evidence that people impacted by socio-economic disadvantage and those who share one of the protected characteristics continue to suffer health inequalities. This includes poorer life expectancy in more disadvantaged areas, poorer mental wellbeing and more unhealthy behaviours for people with a physical or learning disability (PHE, 2020a), higher levels of smoking among those who are unemployed or in routine and manual occupations (PHE, 2019) and gaps in employment rates for those with a long-term health condition, a learning disability or in contact with secondary mental health services when compared with the overall employment rate (PHE, 2019).

The growing health and care gap in the North-East

The growing gap between years spent in good health and those spent with long-term conditions, ill health or disability is a major concern, particularly in the North-East. This is exacerbated by low property prices, which encourage the movement of older people to live in lower priced areas, such as Sunderland (by the sea); however, they bring with them health costs associated with an ageing population. This has been referred to as the window of need or the health and care gap, as it represents the time between the onset of ill health and the resolution of that ill health, which for most long-term conditions is present throughout the rest of the individual's life. It is estimated that despite the shorter life expectancy in women and men living in deprived areas, their higher burden of disease results in 22 per cent and 16 per cent more costs for the NHS per person respectively compared with women and men in affluent areas. This results in an additional spend of £4.8 billion per year, almost 20 per cent of the total hospital budget, without taking into account additional costs, including social care provision.

Addressing the health and care gap requires joined-up action to achieve healthier lives for longer, as well as supporting individuals with long-term conditions and co-morbidities to achieve independent living as long as possible. Achieving these improvements requires a balance in approaches that has prevention at the forefront of strategy, policy and resource allocation, and values and builds community assets as well as strengthening approaches to health care, care and support. The next section describes the action that is required at national and local level to address these challenges.

National level action

The impact of national level action on health and wellbeing and health inequalities is significant in terms of policy development, implementation and review as well as resource allocations.

Policy development and implementation

There are a number of national policies that have an impact on health and wellbeing, ranging from education, housing, industrial and economic regeneration policies to welfare reforms and changes to the benefit system that disproportionately affect vulnerable people, families and communities. The welfare reforms have impacted negatively on the poorest and most vulnerable, with reports that the process of reviewing benefits has been linked to suicides, drug-related deaths and self-harm. The impact on emotional wellbeing and mental health is very significant. It is important that government policy decisions and reforms are subjected to robust health impact assessment to ensure that intended and unintended consequences do not lead to a widening of health inequalities. The impact of government policies and other levers has been reported and celebrated as among the key achievements of the last century, examples being the impact of legislation on reductions in smoking prevalence and the impact of seatbelt legislation on the number of people killed or seriously injured in road traffic accidents.

It is important for the government to utilise national policies as key levers for achieving improvements in public health outcomes. The evidence base for the impact of minimum unit pricing on reducing alcohol-related harm and alcohol control is very compelling, and so is the impact of legislative control on the food industry in tackling obesity. However, these have not been reflected in government policy and legislation to date, which has slowed down the scale and pace of improvements in tackling alcohol-related harm and obesity – leading to questions about how seriously these issues are being taken by national government.

Another significant challenge is the development and reforms of national policy in government departmental silos. A number of public sector reforms are taking place at a national level, and these are creating different pressures for local implementation as they generate new pressures or conflict. These range from welfare reforms, housing reforms, education reforms and NHS reforms to policing reforms and immigration reforms. In many cases, at the local implementation phase of these reforms there is often a complex interaction of factors that leads to poor outcomes for individuals, families and communities at the receiving end. There are often unintended consequences as some of the policies lead local organisations to work against each other or create perverse incentives and unnecessary competition. It is important that policy development at a national level occurs across government departments and across sectors to ensure alignment and coordination of recommendations and reforms. There is a key role for Public Health England as the national public health organisation to engage across government departments and sectors, thereby ensuring that the protection and improvement of the public's health is an important consideration in policy reviews, developments, monitoring and evaluations.

Central government cuts and the impact of austerity

Since the beginning of austerity, local government and a number of other government departments have witnessed a significant reduction in resources. This has an impact on resources available at a local level as departments respond to these funding reductions by making cuts to services.

The Institute of Fiscal Studies (IFS) estimates that between 2002 and 2015 local government spending on services fell by over a quarter, with a greater percentage of cuts being borne by local authorities in the more deprived areas compared with affluent areas. Almost similar to the inverse care law described by Tudor Hart, the cuts have been greatest in the areas where the need is greatest. This has resulted in a significant reduction in spend on the non-statutory services that have a greater preventative and wider wellbeing focus as councils prioritise the spend on statutory provision of public health, health care, children's and adult social care.

This phenomenon was first described by Barnet Council in 2012, through the Barnet 'Graph of Doom' (see Chapter 10, Figure 10.1). It was a presentation of the future if there was no mitigation and if demands from children's social care and adults social care increased, a situation that would result in the council struggling to protect vulnerable people and not having the ability to deliver other non-statutory services, especially non-statutory services. Barnet Council's 'Graph of Doom' was dismissed by the Department for Communities and Local Government (DCLG) at the time as not being a true depiction of the future funding arrangements, At the time, the DCLG's response was, 'We don't suggest this is not a challenge, which it is, we're quite up front with that, but we don't believe it is as apocalyptic as the "Barnet graph of doom" indicates.' (See also Chapter 10, Figure 10.2.)

However, this scenario is now being played out in a number of local authorities across the country. The IFS reports that cuts to local government spending have not been uniformly applied, with an average reduction of 5 per cent for social care spend and a growth of 10 per cent for children's social care. In contrast, there have been massive reductions in council spend on children and youth centres of up to 60 per cent, reductions in cultural and leisure services of up to 40 per cent and reductions in planning and development and housing of up to 50 per cent.

By 2019, Middlesbrough Council's spending power had been reduced by around 35 per cent. This is higher than the 29 per cent average reduction for local authorities across England. Meanwhile, there continues to be a rise in demand for children's social care and adult social care cases. In an update to the health and wellbeing board for Middlesbrough in 2019, it was reported that the local clinical commissioning group was in special measures for its financial position in 2018, the local tertiary hospital, South Tees Acute NHS Foundation Trust, was carrying a significant financial deficit and Cleveland Police had witnessed a 36 per cent reduction in funding since 2010 – despite having the fifth highest crime rates nationally.

Reforms and reductions in the NHS, police, education, social care and other sectors have a direct impact on service delivery and indirect impact, given that the public sector is the biggest employer in our region. These reforms and reductions limit the local area's ability to tackle the root causes of ill health and reducing health inequalities. This is against the backdrop of the wider poverty and deprivation that continues to be faced by the borough. Middlesbrough is the sixth most deprived local authority in the country. Ten wards in the town are in the top 1 per cent most deprived areas in the country and half of neighbourhoods in the town are in the top 10 per cent most deprived areas in the country. Child poverty rates continue to increase and stand at 31.3 per cent, an increase of 3.3 per cent since 2013.

Sunderland has seen similar reductions in public funding. Northumbria Police has seen reductions in its budget of £142 million since 2010, Sunderland City Council has dealt with reductions of more than 30 per cent, and the Fire and Rescue Service has similarly had significant budget reductions. While the NHS has fared slightly better, Sunderland Clinical Commissioning Group has, in recent years, had one of the lowest percentage growths in budget in the country.

Community centred approaches

Community-centred approaches are key for sustainable improvement in public health outcomes, as discussed in Chapter 8 (PHE, 2020b). The asset-based approaches recognise that communities have assets and resources, and if mobilised these can go a long way towards supporting health and wellbeing. These assets range from tangible resources to informal networks and social capital. However, it is important to ensure these assets are not seen as replacements for services and functions that should be delivered by statutory and other agencies.

In order to deliver community-centred approaches, the following paradigm shift is required:

1. Shifting from a focus on deficits and what's wrong in communities to what asset can we build upon, *from what's wrong* to *what's strong*.
2. A change in dialogue with communities, individuals and families, from a *what's the matter* to a *what matters* approach.
3. A shift from focusing on the things we can measure to what matters to communities, *from what we can count* to *what really counts* for individuals and communities.
4. A shift in services being configured for the convenience of service providers to models that are based on a meaningful understanding of the communities served.
5. Active participation by citizens through co-production and giving communities and local people power to make decisions about plans for their area and services.
6. Building on the recent developments in social prescribing to ensure communities are provided with the support that will meet their needs without over-medicalising social issues.

In achieving this shift, it must be acknowledged that the historically assessed indicators and the successful markers of service delivery (numbers through the service, waiting times and so on) tell us little about the impact of the services on the health and wellbeing of the community and even less about their impact on health inequalities. Two notable studies conclude that connectivity and positive relationships are at the heart of human wellbeing (Waldinger, 2016; Stocks-Rankin et al, 2018). The question of how this can be built in (and not bolted on) through planning processes and delivery of services and interventions must be answered by the creation of partnership with communities and across organisational boundaries. This is the only way in which health and wellbeing systems can be accountable for focusing on what matters to our communities (see Chapter 13).

Integrated approaches to improving health and wellbeing

Since the publication of the NHS Long Term Plan in May 2020, there has been an increasing interest in population health and population health management with the expectation that each integrated care system will have a clear population health plan. Failure to invest in prevention and wellbeing approaches has long been recognised as a threat to the sustainability of the NHS (Hunter, 2019). While this focus is very welcome and desperately required, there is a risk that these approaches will be seen as new rather than building on the work of directors of public health and health and wellbeing strategies and systems that are already in place.

Supporting people with complex needs and multiple vulnerabilities

In many local authority areas, individuals with complex and multiple vulnerabilities receive care and support from a wide range of services that are often not joined up, meaning that care is not effectively coordinated. For example, an individual might misuse substances, have a family and dependants who are at risk or classed as vulnerable, have no stable accommodation, be a victim or perpetrator of domestic violence and have mental health issues. Current arrangements for individuals with such complex lives often involve support and care that is delivered through a wide range of disjointed services. Traditionally, provision of support services has been based on the issue rather than on specific support for individuals and their families.

There is a need to move from an approach that provides disparate support for individuals with complex needs or multiple vulnerabilities to a more joined up and coordinated offer. These 'wicked issues' are discussed in Chapters 4, 10 and 13.

In Middlesbrough, work is under way, informed by the Plymouth model, to develop a vertically integrated model for substance misuse, homelessness prevention and domestic violence prevention and support services that will ensure coordinated care and support. The integrated model will, if successful, ensure that individuals and their families have the following:

1. Easy access to comprehensive, effective and efficient services that can support them from crisis through to recovery, at the right time and in the right place regardless of entry point, using the no wrong door approach.
2. A more efficient system through a collaborative model of support that reduces duplication and delivers an improved client experience with positive outcomes;
3. The making every contact count approach will be achieved by integrating those key, common components of services for vulnerable people with shared processes, pathways and outcome targets within the specialist services as well as delivering wider prevention and early help support.

4. Cross-agency support and multidisciplinary working will include statutory services such as early help, mental health, primary care, criminal justice partners, and adult and children's social care.

Integrated approaches to wellness

When public health transferred from the NHS into local government in April 2013, the majority of public health teams novated contracts to councils for delivery of a wide range of public health programmes, some of which were issue specific. The evidence suggests that most people have more than one risk factor, and in most cases these risk factors cluster. In their report, the King's Fund made recommendations for a shift from traditional silo-based interventions to integrated approaches for improving wellness. Local research in the North-East of England has also concluded that such 'Single-issue lifestyle services have made little impact on health inequalities' (Cheetham et al, 2017).

Further to the consideration of integration of services, there is also the need for a shift in public health approaches from the traditional focus on commissioned lifestyle-based services to approaches that address the underlying causes of poor health and wellbeing. The lifestyle and behaviour change services, while having their place in addressing lifestyle risk factors, are not sufficient on their own. This is because of the level of reach they have into communities, the inherent inequalities in access and the prevention paradox (the people with the greatest need and ability to benefit from preventative services are the least likely to access them).

Addressing public health challenges requires a different approach when services are more integrated and targeted, and supplemented by wider interventions at civic and community levels as well as through direct service provision (PHE, 2019). There needs to be a recognition that the commissioning of public health services has not delivered the public health outcomes commensurate with the level of resources that draw from public health teams. They have disproportionately drawn resources (financial, human and technical expertise) away from these civic and community level approaches, which have greater benefit at a population level, to time-limited and labour-intensive commissioning and procurement processes for lifestyle interventions. These services are often commissioned in isolation and achieve minimum levels of population coverage, often with higher uptake from the populations with the least needs. It is important for public health teams and professionals to recognise the following:

1. Public health improvements will not be driven through commissioned services alone (see Chapter 10). Public Heath England's Population Intervention Triangle (see Figure 7.2) provides a useful framework through which to assess the balance of interventions at civic, community and service levels in addressing health inequalities (PHE, 2019).

There is a need to apply the public health core skills and approaches (such as health impact assessment, health needs assessment, health equity audit, partnership working, application of evidence and being intelligence driven) and learn from public health successes that have not been based on commissioned service delivery.

2. Public health is not restricted to people within the specialist public health team – there is need for the development of a wider public health network that acknowledges the role of other professional groups, organisations and communities in addressing inequalities.

Figure 7.2: Population Intervention Triangle

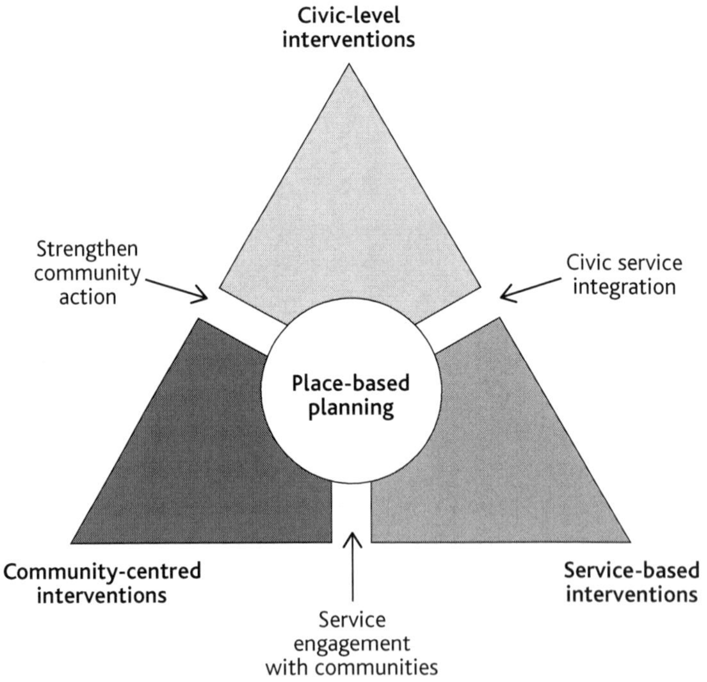

Source: PHE, 2019

Implications for the public health workforce

According to the Public Health England Fit for Future report, in order to drive improvements in population health, the public health workforce needs to be fit for the future, *an increasingly agile, flexible, multidisciplinary workforce that retains many current public health skills and develops new ones.* The NHS Interim people plan also makes similar observations with regard to the need for greater system leadership, with more people working across organisational, professional and sector boundaries with the ability to influence outside positional authority. Through the Health and Social Care Act 2012, directors of public health must be system leaders and the advisors to politicians and senior leadership teams on all health matters. This can include working through health and wellbeing boards and other similar partnership structures.

Health and wellbeing boards have not always delivered on the expectations held when they were first implemented in shadow form in 2012 (see Chapter 4). They were meant to be a strategic forum where local agencies worked together to have a joint understanding of local population need and to ensure that the planning, delivery and improvement of local health and wellbeing services was informed by that understanding. The review of health and wellbeing boards carried out by the Local Government Association (LGA) has identified a number of issues with a number of health and wellbeing boards, ranging from 'being talking shops' to being stifled by requirements to complete mandatory returns, sign off local plans and carry out performance management for local health and wellbeing systems. The LGA recommended that for health and wellbeing boards to achieve their full potential, a senior leader needs to take a strong interest in shaping and driving the agenda. .Directors of public health are very well positioned to drive this forward. It is important that the public health profession continues to take stock of the changes in the local government arrangements, NHS, Public Health England and other sectors to ensure the public health workforce remains relevant and fit for the future.

Other workforce opportunities that the public health team needs to embrace and further develop include:

1. Development of career paths in public health from apprenticeships all the way to senior public health leadership roles.
2. Workforce planning needs to be carried out in collaboration with other parts of the system to enable sharing of expertise and

development of joint appointments and posts that work across the system and across organisations.
3. Public health capacity-building across organisations and sectors. An example of how this can be achieved is the use of the making every contact count approach.
4. Public health leaders to take opportunities for system leadership roles outside traditional public health careers. The Public Health England Fit for Future report recommended the need for public health leaders to consider career progression outside traditional career pathways.

An asset-based response

Sunderland has many assets. As a 'city by the sea', it has a beautiful coastline that often astounds visitors as well as many green spaces. Often, however, it is the people and the relationships between them that are its greatest strengths. This includes the relationships between people who lead organisations, particularly in those anchor institutions.

Organisations in Sunderland have traditionally worked well together to improve outcomes for residents of the city. The impact of austerity has stretched some of these partnerships, and on occasion this has led to the stalling of health improvements. One such area has been outcomes in relation to teenage pregnancy. This is an important public health issue as it can impact on the life chances of both young parents and their babies. Babies born to teenage mothers have a 60 per cent higher rate of infant mortality than average and a 63 per cent higher risk of living in poverty. Mothers have a 30 per cent higher risk of poor mental health two years after giving birth and are more likely not to be in education, employment or training by the age of 20. Young fathers are twice as likely to be unemployed aged 30, even after taking account of deprivation. Teenage pregnancy also has an impact on the public purse at a time when budgets are shrinking: every £1 spent addressing it is estimated to save £4 (PHE/LGA, 2018).

What works to reduce teenage pregnancy is now well documented (detailed in Figure 7.3), and in Sunderland these factors were largely addressed, resulting in annual decreases in teenage conceptions. As the impact of austerity began to take effect, however, many of the interventions that had proved to be successful in the past were either stopped or cut back. The impact this had can be seen in Figure 7.4. What can also be seen, however, is the impact of a new partnership that was established in 2015. This worked to re-establish interventions that were known to work and to improve and integrate others. After

Figure 7.3: What works to reduce teenage pregnancies

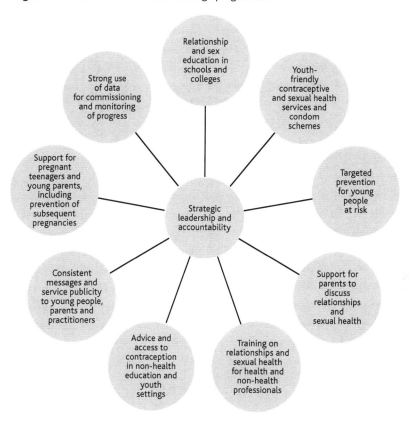

Source: PHE/LGA, 2018

the stalling in outcomes when evidence-based interventions were stopped or reduced, teenage conceptions began to fall again, reducing the gap between Sunderland and both the North-East and the rest of England.

The approach taken did not, however, only rely on partnership working and evidence-based practice. Young people were actively engaged in and influenced much of the work, including developing a new brand for the c-card, the scheme that provides young people with free condoms, and developing a radio campaign with the local radio station SunFM.

There is clearly still some way to go before the Sunderland rate of under 18 conceptions reaches the national average. However, the impact of this approach does give some cause for optimism. The experience suggests that, even at a time of substantial challenge, if partners work together to implement what is known to work for

Figure 7.4: Under 18 conceptions in Sunderland (rate per 1,000 population)

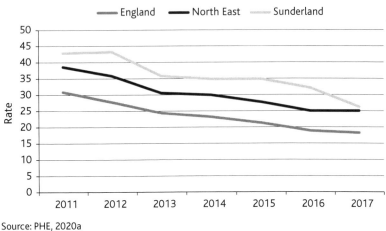

Source: PHE, 2020a

the benefit of their residents, taking account of the context they are working in and involving local communities, they can have a significant impact on inequalities in health outcomes.

What next – a whole-city approach?

Figure 7.5, an approach to prevention and addressing health inequalities adapted from a framework for addressing health inequities developed by the Bay Area Regional Health Board (Bay Area Regional Health Inequities Initiative, 2015), demonstrates the multiple domains a city such as Sunderland needs to operate in if it is to make a step change in its efforts to improve health and reduce inequalities.

It is clear from the framework that sustained improvement will only be achieved if organisations, communities and individuals take every opportunity to improve people's life chances. This cannot be just the responsibility of the local NHS or the council, with its responsibilities for social care and, more latterly, improving health. It needs to be a whole city approach that takes every opportunity to prevent people from becoming ill or, should they already have a health condition, ensure that they are supported in staying as healthy as possible and keeping their independence.

This has been recognised in a new City Plan that has been developed. This is not for the council but for the whole city, and addresses the challenges Sunderland has – such as migration out of the city, lack of home-grown businesses, qualifications and skills of residents not meeting the needs of city industry and poor health behaviours and outcomes.

Figure 7.5: Prevention and inequalities framework

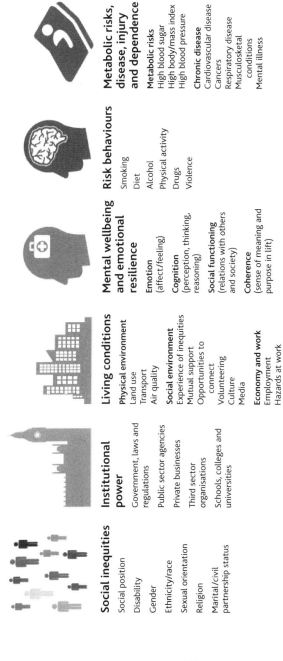

Social inequities

Social position

Disability

Gender

Ethnicity/race

Sexual orientation

Religion

Marital/civil
partnership status

**Institutional
power**

Government, laws and
regulations

Public sector agencies

Private businesses

Third sector
organisations

Schools, colleges and
universities

Living conditions

Physical environment

Land use

Transport

Air quality

Social environment

Experience of inequities

Mutual support

Opportunities to
connect

Volunteering

Culture

Media

Economy and work

Employment

Hazards at work

Income

Access to healthy food

Opportunities for
physical activity

Services

Health care

Social care

Welfare support

Leisure services

**Mental wellbeing
and emotional
resilience**

Emotion
(affect/feeling)

Cognition
(perception, thinking,
reasoning)

Social functioning
(relations with others
and society)

Coherence
(sense of meaning and
purpose in lift)

Risk behaviours

Smoking

Diet

Alcohol

Physical activity

Drugs

Violence

**Metabolic risks,
disease, injury
and dependence**

Metabolic risks

High blood sugar

High body/mass index

High blood pressure

Chronic disease

Cardiovascular disease

Cancers

Respiratory disease

Musculoskeletal
conditions

Mental illness

Death

Life expectancy

Healthy life
expectancy

Infant mortality

Source: PHE, 2020a

The plan has three key themes: a dynamic city, a healthy city and a vibrant city. A 'dynamic city' will have more and better jobs and housing, improved qualifications and skills, and a lower carbon environment with digital connectivity. These all chime with the framework in Figure 7.5. A 'healthy city' will give people access to the same opportunities and life chances; they will lead longer and healthier lives and remain independent for longer. Neighbourhoods will be more attractive and there will be improved transport links, supporting active travel. A 'vibrant city' will see more residents participating in their communities, this including cultural events and activities, more people feeling safe, and more resilient individuals and communities.

If these ambitions are met, there is every likelihood that there will start to be improvements in people's health in Sunderland. However, key to this is a shift in the relationship with local residents and communities. This is best expressed through the values described in the City Plan, in which the commitment is made that 'We innovate, we enable and we are respectful.'

Treating people with respect is fundamental if we want to improve residents' health. They need to be taken seriously, with their knowledge and skills appreciated, as well as their expertise in relation to what works in the context of their lives. This ensures that those who suffer from systematic inequalities are not further disadvantaged by new services, policies or other interventions. Finally, treating people with respect is also good for their mental wellbeing; it has been said that 'the public mental health equivalent of sewers and clean water are respect and justice' (Friedli, 2009).

Organisations that are respectful will almost certainly enable people rather than 'doing for' or 'doing to' them. This helps to build not only individual resilience but also, through building on community assets, community resilience.

Finally, if organisations connect with people and better understand their lives and their needs, innovations are more likely to be successful, and when they are not there is a better understanding of why they have failed. While community asset-based approaches are crucial and can build community resilience, considerations of 'New Power', which can allow people to connect and participate with institutions, thereby gaining an enabling function, is another way in which local people can take ownership of a problem and help to find ways to resolve it.

While it would be disingenuous to suggest that increased public resources are not needed to improve a range of outcomes for people in Sunderland, working in new ways across partner organisations and with local residents for those things that really matter has the potential to achieve much more than working in isolation and ignoring the knowledge that local people have. It is difficult to think of something that matters more in Sunderland than improving health – this could be the issue that allows people to connect with each other and many of the organisations in the city. Although creating new and better jobs and improving skills will undoubtedly improve people's lives and ultimately their health, by connecting organisational partners and the wider community of our residents so that they are able to work together, it might just be possible to achieve even more – a shared sense of purpose and control.

Uncertainty over future funding arrangements

There are uncertainties over future funding arrangements for local government, public health and wider public sector arrangements. The recent announcement of a funding settlement for the NHS, while aimed at providing stability for the NHS, presents a significant risk if there is not a similar settlement for public health and social care. There is a need to ensure planning, and resource allocation is based on an understanding of the complex interplay between public health preventative programmes and social care's early intervention, while approaches to support independent living and the developing place-based approaches should have public health at their heart.

Public health and prevention budgets are often the first victims of any budget reductions, efficiency programmes and cuts. The funding levels for public health remain sub-optimum and recently the Health Foundation called for the government to reinvest at least £1 billion to reverse the cuts made to the public health grant to local government (see Chapter 2).

In 2013, public health transferred into local government with a ring-fenced allocation. In 2014, in-year cuts to the public health grant of 6.2 per cent were implemented, and the subsequent comprehensive spending review recommended an additional 16.2 per cent over the four-year cycle of the review. At the time of transfer, concerns were raised regarding the level of funding for public health, as this varied across the country. An attempt was made to develop an allocation formula for public health through the Advisory Committee on Resource Allocation, and the recommendations from the committee received mixed reactions. According to the formula, deprivation and premature mortality were taken as indicators of public health need. This did not consider the burden of ill-health in deprived communities and the related costs of looking after an unhealthy population. In addition, the formula did not seek to address the issues around the level of resources available for prevention.

Currently, in May 2020, with less than a year left for confirmed public health allocations, there still remains no certainty on the future funding arrangements for public health or the levels of funding available to local authorities. Findings from a proposal that was consulted on, that public health would be funded from business rate retention, have yet to be reported. This lack of certainty makes long-term planning for preventative public health programmes very challenging. The next spending review will need to ensure there is a sustainable funding package for local public health if the ambitions in the Prevention green paper and the NHS Long Term Plan are to be realised.

Local-level action

The transfer of public health from the NHS to local government that occurred in April 2013 provided an opportunity for a significant shift in approaches to public health improvements. Hailed as public health coming home, this transition allowed directors of public health and their teams to be embedded within local authorities – which are key organisations responsible for places and local people. Despite the ongoing reductions in funding, local government has at its disposal a number of levers and instruments that can be utilised in order to improve health gains.

Population level interventions

Public health is defined as the art and science of improving health and wellbeing, reducing health inequalities through the organised efforts of society. For a long time, the focus has been on commissioning of lifestyle-related interventions, whereby public health acknowledged the role of social determinants of health and their importance, and yet the interventions, strategies and action plans are more focused on addressing lifestyle risk factors and challenges (Carey et al, 2017; Powell et al, 2017).

The recently launched resources from Public Health England and the Department of Health provide very good frameworks and approaches into the development of robust local public health systems and place-based approaches (PHE, 2019). There has been a wider recognition of the role of social determinants of health on health and wellbeing outcomes and reducing health inequalities. The Marmot Review, through its six policy recommendations, identified the key areas for achieving a fairer society and provided a framework for coordinating local work to achieve improvements in health and wellbeing outcomes. In a number of areas, including Middlesbrough, these recommendations formed the basis of the health and wellbeing strategies. Examples from work in Middlesbrough include the consideration of alcohol-related harm in the Statement of Licensing Policy, consideration of problem gambling in the Gambling Policy, health objectives in the Local Plan, involvement in the development of a housing plan and a transport plan, and the inclusion of health considerations in hot food outlet applications as well as broader economic growth considerations. However, a number of local authorities have established themselves as Marmot Cities, to embed the recommendations into their local approaches. These cities include Stoke, Newcastle, Gateshead, Bristol and Coventry, and evaluations are currently under way to review the progress this approach has facilitated.

Anchor organisations in local areas include NHS organisations, councils, colleges, universities, police, registered social landlords, big private sector organisations and in some cases voluntary and community sector organisations. There is a great opportunity for these organisations to play a greater role and contribute to the health and wellbeing of the local population through employment opportunities, purchasing power, social value, spending some of their resources locally, sustainability and reducing carbon footprint, and wider corporate social responsibility (Health Foundation, 2019). The collective power of these organisations needs to be harnessed in each local area, and partnerships such as the health and wellbeing boards will provide a forum for discussions and coordination.

Conclusion

While it is widely acknowledged that health inequalities are stubborn and persistent, we also know that they are not inevitable. Local government has a lead role to play, and throughout the country there are numerous examples of how local authorities have embraced these responsibilities and used the levers at their disposal to improve the health and wellbeing of their populations. However, local government requires support from national government in terms of national policy and creating the right levers for local action – secure and long-term settlements to provide much-needed resources so leadership and coordination can be provided at a local level. There are four key reflections with which to end this chapter, informed by local knowledge and emerging evidence:

1. **The power of place in addressing health inequalities**. In order to address stubborn and pervasive inequalities, seen in particular in the North-East of England, we need to build on the increasing evidence of the importance of system leadership and coordinated societal efforts working across civic, community and service level interventions. This aligns with the definition of public health that emphasises the role of organising and harnessing societal efforts in order to improve population health.

2. **The important and undeniable role of national policy in supporting local action**. Without national policies prioritising health and health inequalities, local areas are very limited in what they can achieve. There are numerous examples of this, such as the overwhelming evidence about minimum pricing for alcohol units, and the effect this can have on tackling alcohol-related harm and availability for the most vulnerable in society, the absence of health as an objective in planning, licensing and gambling policy, the lack of consideration of health impact in recent welfare reforms – to name but a few. These examples demonstrate how, without national policy, local areas are often powerless in addressing some of the root causes of the poor public health outcomes they are trying to address.

3. There is an **urgent need to secure long-term settlements for public health**, and more importantly local government and other key anchor institutions such as policing, education, and housing. This will enable local areas to work as a system to develop sustainable investment in preventative approaches that address inequality. Financial certainty and sustained investment are crucial both for public health directly and for the wider infrastructure of which it is part. While the rhetoric for prevention has never been stronger across many national policy documents, this is yet to be matched by investment and resource allocation decisions.

4. There is need for a different paradigm that shifts the focus from deficit approaches that count illness, develop quantitative data dashboards and inform biomedical models to **approaches that value connections as a key determinant of a good life** and a fundamental characteristic of longer lives. Though it is often described as being more difficult for systems to hold themselves to account for subjective and fluid issues, there is an urgent need to find meaningful ways to focus on what matters to people and communities, and not what is the matter with them.

144

References

Bay Area Regional Health Inequalities Initiative (2015) 'Framework'. Available from: http://barhii.org/framework/ [Accessed 28 July 2020].

Black, D., Morris, J.N., Smith, C. and Townsend, P. (1999) 'Better benefits for health: plan to implement the central recommendation of the Acheson report', *British Medical Journal*, 318(7185): 724–7.

Buck, D., Baylis, A., Dougall, D. and Roberston, R. (2018) 'A vision for population health: towards a healthier future', The King's Fund, London.

Carey, G., Malbon, E., Crammond, B., Pescud, M. and Baker, P. (2017) 'Can the sociology of social problems help us to understand and manage "lifestyle drift"?', *Health Promotion International*, 32(4): 755–61.

Chanfreau, J., Lloyd, C., Byron, C., Roberts, C., Craig, R., De Feo, D. and McManus, A. (2018) 'Predicting wellbeing', prepared for the Department of Health. Available from: https://www.natcen.ac.uk/media/205352/predictors-of-wellbeing.pdf [Accessed 24 June 2020].

Cheetham, M., Visram, S., Rushmer, R., Greig, G., Gibson, E., Khazaeli, B. and Wiseman, A. (2017) '"It is not a quick fix": structural and contextual issues that affect implementation of integrated health and well-being services: a qualitative study from North-East England', *Public Health*, 152(November): 99–107.

Department of Health and Social Services (1980) 'Inequalities in Health: Report of a Research Working Group'. London: DHSS. Available from: http://www.sochealth.co.uk/history/black.htm [Accessed 10 April 2020].

Evandrou, M., Falkingham, J., Feng, Z. and Vlachantoni, A. (2016) 'Ethnic inequalities in limiting health and self-reported healthy in later life', *Epidemiology and Community Health*, 70(7): pp 653–63.

Friedli, L. (2009) 'Mental health, resilience and inequalities', WHO/Europe Regional Office. Available from: http://www.euro.who.int/__data/assets/pdf_file/0012/100821/E92227.pdf [Accessed 10 April 2020].

Government Equalities Office (2011) 'Equality Act 2010: Specific duties to support the equality duty. What do I need to know? A quick start guide for public sector organisations'. Available from: http://www.pfc.org.uk/pdf/specific-duties%20Nov%202011%20(2).pdf [Accessed 24 June 2020].

Health Foundation (2019) 'Building healthier communities: the role of the NHS as an anchor institution'. Available from: https://www.health.org.uk/sites/default/files/upload/publications/2019/I02_Building%20healthier%20communities_WEB.pdf [Accessed 29 April 2020].

Hunter, D. (2019) 'Looking forward to the next 70 years: from a national ill-health service to a national health system', *Health Economics, Policy and Law*, 14(1): 11–14.

IHME (Institute for Health Metrics and Evaluation) (2018) 'Global burden of disease 2017'. Population Health, November. Available from: https://www.washington.edu/populationhealth/2018/11/26/ihme-releases-the-global-burden-of-disease-2017-study/ [Accessed 10 April 2020].

ILG (Institute for Local Governance) (2013) 'The Impact of Welfare Reform in the North-East'. A research report for the Association of North-East Councils by the Universities of Durham, Northumbria and Teesside and the North-East region of Citizens' Advice. Available from: http://nrl.northumbria.ac.uk/14925/1/ILG_WR_report.pdf [Accessed 10 April 2020].

Lodge, K.-M. (2019) 'Premature deaths among people with a learning disability – what will it take for things to change?', *BMJ Opinion* (16 July). Available from: https://blogs.bmj.com/bmj/2019/07/16/premature-deaths-among-people-with-a-learning-disability-what-will-it-take-for-things-to-change/ [Accessed 10 April 2020].

Marmot, M., Allen, J., Boyce, T., Goldblatt, P. and Morrison, J. (2020) 'Health equity in England: the Marmot review 10 years on'. London: Institute of Health Equity. Available from: http://www.instituteofhealthequity.org/resources-reports/marmot-review-10-years-on/marmot-review-10-years-on-full-report.pdf [Accessed 10 April 2020].

Middlesbrough Director of Public Health (2017) 'Dying before our time?', annual report. Available from: https://www.middlesbrough.gov.uk/sites/default/files/DPH%20Annual%20Report%202016-17.pdf [Accessed 10 April 2020].

ONS (Office for National Statistics) (2017) 'Health state life expectancies by national deprivation deciles, England and Wales: 2015 to 2017'. Available from: https://www.ons.gov.uk/peoplepopulationandcommunity/healthandsocialcare/healthinequalities/bulletins/healthstatelifeexpectanciesbyindexofmultipledeprivationimd/2015to2017 [Accessed 10 April 2020].

ONS (Office for National Statistics) (2018) 'Overview of the UK population, November 2018'. Available from: https://www.ons.gov.uk/releases/overviewoftheukpopulationnovember2018 [Accessed 10 April 2020].

ONS (Office for National Statistics) (2019) 'Working and workless households in the UK statistical bulletins'. Available from: https://www.ons.gov.uk/employmentandlabourmarket/peopleinwork/employmentandemployeetypes/bulletins/workingandworklesshouseholds/previousReleases [Accessed 28 July 2020].

PHE (Public Health England) (2019) 'Place-based approaches for reducing health inequalities: main report'. Available from: https://www.gov.uk/government/publications/health-inequalities-place-based-approaches-to-reduce-inequalities/place-based-approaches-for-reducing-health-inequalities-main-report [Accessed 10 April 2020].

PHE (Public Health England) (2020a) 'Public Health Outcomes Framework/North East England'. Available from: https://fingertips.phe.org.uk/profile/public-health-outcomes-framework/data#page/3/gid/1000042/pat/6/par/E12000001/ati/102/are/E08000024/iid/20401/age/173/sex/2/cid/4/page-options/car-do-0 [Accessed 28 July 2020].

PHE (Public Health England) (2020b) 'Community-centred public health: taking a whole system approach: Report'. Available from: https://www.gov.uk/government/publications/community-centred-public-health-taking-a-whole-system-approach [Accessed 10 April 2020].

PHE/LGA (2018) 'Good progress but more to do. Teenage pregnancy and young people'. Available from: https://www.local.gov.uk/sites/default/files/documents/15.7%20Teenage%20pregnancy_09.pdf [Accessed 24 June 2020].

Powell, K., Thurston, M. and Bloyce, D. (2017) 'Theorising lifestyle drift in health promotion: explaining community and voluntary sector engagement practices in disadvantaged areas', *Critical Public Health*, 27(5): 554–65

Pressman, S.D. and Cohen, S. (2005) 'Does positive affect influence health?', *Psychological Bulletin*, 131: 925–71.

Reed, J.E., Howe, C. and Doyle, C. (2019) 'Successful health improvements from translating evidence in complex systems (SHIFT-evidence): simple rules to guide practice and research', *International Journal for Quality in Health Care*, 31: 238–44.

Saxena, S. (2018) 'Excess mortality among people with a mental disorder: a public health priority', *Lancet Public Health*, 3(6): 264–5.

Steptoe, A.P.A. and LaMarca, R. (2012) 'The biopsychological perspective on cardiovascular disease', in S. Waldstein, W. Kop and L. Katzel (eds) *Handbook of Cardiovascular Behavioural Medicine*, New York: Springer.

Stocks-Rankin, C.-R., Seale, B. and Mead, N. (2018) 'Healthy communities research: the Bromley by Bow model'. Available from: https://www.bbbc.org.uk/wp-content/uploads/2018/06/Unleashing-Healthy-Communities_Summary-Report_Researching-the-Bromley-by-Bow-model.pdf [Accessed 24 June 2020].

Waldinger, R. (2016) 'What makes a good life? Lessons from the longest study on happiness'. TED talk (January). Available from: https://www.ted.com/talks/robert_waldinger_what_makes_a_good_life_lessons_from_the_longest_study_on_happiness/discussion [Accessed 10 April 2020].

Whitehead, M. and Dahlgren, G. (2006) 'Concepts and principles for tackling social inequities in health' *Levelling up Part 1*. WHO Collaborating Centre for Policy Research on Social Determinants of Health. University of Liverpool Studies on Social and Economic Determinants of Population Health, No. 2. Available from: http://www.euro.who.int/__data/assets/pdf_file/0010/74737/E89383.pdf [Accessed 10 April 2020].

8

Cultural change and the evolution of community governance: a North-West England perspective

Kate Arden, Keith Cunliffe and Penny A. Cook

Background

In 2010, the United Kingdom Coalition government gave increased decision-making power to local authorities, in a move towards 'localism'. Local authorities were then able to determine their consultation processes with communities and citizens on the governance, service delivery and funding of local public services (Ferry et al, 2019). However, at the same time, the government imposed a policy of austerity, which meant that the decisions local authorities could make were restricted by substantial cuts in funding.

Under austerity, local authorities in England had to make unprecedented financial savings in response to dramatic cuts in funding from national government. The impact of these cuts has not been felt equally, with the areas of greatest need having suffered the greatest cuts. This was because central government allocation had previously been the biggest instrument of redistribution; without it, local authorities were forced to rely to a greater extent on local sources of income (for example, local tax revenue, sale of assets), which, for the most economically deprived areas, was less lucrative. Analysis by Gray and Barford (2018, p 550) shows that 'across-the-board austerity cuts in local government spending have fallen most heavily on those local areas with greatest need'. It is likely that this period of austerity has been responsible for England's health getting worse for people living in more deprived areas; health inequalities increasing; and, for the population as a whole, a decline in health, as revealed in the 'Marmot Review 10 years on' report (Marmot et al, 2020). Here it is considered how utilising the newly allowed methods of democratic deliberation and the localism agenda can mitigate some of the negative effects of austerity, in a case study area where there appears to have been a genuine redistribution of power.

Assets-based approaches at a community level

In order to develop a process of communities sharing in decision-making power, communities need to be mobilised. This involves recognising a community's assets, known as an 'assets based' or strength-based (rather than deficit-based) process. A community's assets are individual (for example, the gifts and skills of community members) or delivered through citizens' associations (for example, religious, cultural, athletic organisations) and physical/formal institutions and facilities (for example, libraries, parks) (Kretzmann and McKnight, 1996; Russell, 2011; McKnight and Russell, 2018). 'The central thrust is that communities should drive the development process themselves though identifying and mobilising existing – often unrecognised – assets and, in the process, respond to and create local economic opportunities' (Roy, 2017, p 456). A classic example often given of dramatic change from the bottom up is the creation and development of the Bromley by Bow Centre in the mid-1980s (Davis-Hall, 2018), when a local community formed a charity to meet the health needs of a population living in stark inequality. The assets-based approach is therefore not new; many social enterprises have been doing this work for a long time, and adopted the 'assets based' terminology to fall in line with the current policy discourse (Roy, 2017). The criticisms of the asset-based approach have been discussed by Roy (2017) and include that the focus on strengths can be an excuse for withdrawing public sector support and making communities responsible for their own health. However, as noted by Taylor and Baker (2018, p 55), 'Poor communities know how to be "resilient". But they cannot be expected to go it alone, especially if they are expected to take on more responsibilities'.

Four overarching themes give insight into the principles and practices of asset-based community development: 1) relationships and trust are mechanisms for change, 2) that it is based on reciprocity and connectivity: 'people not services', 3) that there is accountability and reducing dependency, and 4) having a socially sustainable model (Harrison et al, 2019).

The realisation of assets and power

In an analysis of how communities can have more power, it is noted that poverty prevents individuals from having any power at all when the struggles of daily life and survival are all-consuming and sap resilience (Taylor and Baker, 2018). In fact, in this analysis by Taylor and Baker, it is very difficult to move beyond the need for employment and income. It is observed that local enterprises can play a part in building a local area's economic resource, but without stability from public sector services the results can be limited. Moreover, the current lack of social housing leads to housing instability and transient communities. Austerity leads to a decline in social infrastructure, such as loss of parks, libraries and community centres. While 'many communities in the past have benefited from access to support, resources and infrastructure – spaces to meet, community development and other support workers, and funds' (p 55), Taylor and Baker conclude that 'resources for community engagement and development have fallen victim to these cuts in many authorities and the expertise to engage with the community has gone' (p 48). Box 8.1 gives the conditions required for communities to develop real power.

Box 8.1: Essential prerequisites for communities to become more powerful

The Local Trust report 'The Future for Communities: Perspectives on Power' (based on research funded by the Joseph Rowntree Foundation) investigated factors that prevent communities reaching their potential, and what support is needed from the rest of society to release their potential. Four essentials were identified. Communities need:

- Spaces to come together: to meet, learn, debate, plan, and act – this is called the 'social infrastructure'. These may be face-to-face or digital, ideally both.
- Financial support: from seedcorn funding that will cover basic costs to larger-scale investment.
- Access to support from community development workers or others who can link communities with developments elsewhere, share information, learning and skills, alert them to new possibilities and challenge them where necessary.
- Skills and the will on the part of decision-makers to recognise the assets and knowledge within communities and work alongside them to create change.

Source: Taylor and Baker (2018)

The assets-based approach and individual health

When considering health interventions at the level of the individual, the asset-based approach resonates with a salutogenic paradigm. Salutogenesis focuses on factors that support human health and wellbeing, rather than on those that cause disease (that is, pathogenesis) (Antonovsky, 1979; Lindström and Eriksson, 2005). The asset-based approach focuses on the strengths rather than the health needs of the individual (or patient). Therefore, an assets-based approach, embedded in the salutogenic paradigm, recognises and nurtures the skills, attributes and resources (assets) of individuals and communities to develop resilience and a sense of purpose, ultimately leading to improved health outcomes. If there is a structured attempt to link a person with a health need to an intervention that is salutogenic, assets-based and non-medical, this can be known as a 'social prescription' (Husk et al, 2020).

Aim of this chapter

The aim of this chapter is to use the example of the response of a local authority in Greater Manchester, Wigan Metropolitan Borough Council, to the opportunities afforded by localism, implemented in the face of austerity. The impact of austerity measures imposed by central government amounted to an effective reduction in Wigan Council's budget of 40 per cent phased in over 10 years, and a loss of around a fifth of its workforce. Wigan experienced the fifth highest cut in spending out of all local authorities (Gray and Barford, 2018). Despite these huge challenges, 'Wigan appears on some measures to have achieved a minor miracle ... several key metrics tell a story of improvement over the same period' (Naylor and Wellings, 2019). The response, the creation of the 'Wigan Deal' is a major transformation programme, still ongoing at the time of writing. The transformation started in 2012 and is both an approach to manage demand for services as well as a positive change in the understanding and relationship between citizens and public servants. In this chapter, Wigan's journey to date is described.

Wigan and Greater Manchester context

Wigan is a metropolitan borough in the north-west of England, it is the second largest borough in the Greater Manchester conurbation and is therefore one of the ten Greater Manchester boroughs involved in

Greater Manchester devolution. As part of the devolution settlement, Greater Manchester – comprising 12 National Health Service (NHS) Clinical Commissioning Groups, 15 NHS providers and ten local authorities – and NHS England agreed a historic Memorandum of Understanding to develop a framework for joint decision-making on integrated care that brought together health and social care budgets of £6 billion. This represented a significant shift back to local determination of how resources, previously commissioned nationally or regionally, are most effectively deployed to work with local citizens to improve health and reduce long-standing health inequalities. This was set out in the Greater Manchester Health and Social Care Partnership 'Taking Charge' Plan, within which there was a focus on wellbeing and prevention at the heart of the agreement. The Memorandum of Understanding with Public Health England made it possible to realise both Wanless's (2002) vision of the 'fully engaged scenario' and Marmot's 'Fairer Society, Healthy Lives' recommendations (Marmot et al, 2020). The agreement with NHS England afforded the ability to pursue a whole system approach through local government's wider remit for civic leadership, and greater freedom to pursue local objectives with a predominantly local, rather than national, performance regime. It also harnessed the potential of the wider Greater Manchester devolution framework and Greater Manchester's well-established political and strategic governance to implement a place-based approach to public health leadership. Marmot et al's (2010) vision of addressing interlinked health determinants, employment, planning, housing, transport, skills, education and leisure as well as integration of health, social care and wellbeing services, became a reality. Health could be firmly embedded in every policy and health outcomes could be improved at pace and scale, through evidence-based transformation of core business rather than small stand-alone projects.

Wigan has a population of 320,000. It is the ninth largest metropolitan authority in England, the second largest council in Greater Manchester – and has significant health challenges (Box 8.2). The council is responsible for an annual revenue budget of £231 million. Adult Social Care accounts for around a third of the council's net resource and over 7,000 people are supported within Adult Social Care each year. The total annual Health and Social Care spend across the borough is £669 million. Wigan has been at the heart of the devolution programme, but its Wigan Deal journey started well before Greater Manchester devolution was on the agenda; it goes back to 2010, when the council had to face some difficult decisions in relation to the introduction of austerity and year-on-year significant reduction to its revenue grants.

Box 8.2: Wigan in facts and figures

- Nearly 98 per cent of Wigan's population is White British.
- 65 per cent of the borough population is of working age.
- 23 per cent of residents have long-term illness.
- There are nearly 34,000 carers, of whom 3,000 are likely to be children.
- Nearly 100,000 people in the borough are living in the most deprived quintile.
- Rates of homelessness are high: 3.63 per 1,000 households compared with 2.48 per 1,000 for England.
- There are higher than average rates of obesity.
- There are 16 excess cancer deaths each for women and men under 75 years against the England rates 2012–14 (the majority are lung cancer deaths).
- Wigan's population aged 65+ will increase by 30,000 between 2018 and 2040 (ONS, 2020).

Transformative change

Transformational change involves widespread change at all levels of an organisation, impacting processes, culture, organisational perception and power relations (Doebbeling and Flanagan, 2011). It has also been defined as leading to an entirely new state (Dougall et al, 2018). In Dougall et al's analysis, transformative change in health and care systems is highly context dependent and is 'multi-layered, messy, fluid and emergent' and involves 'shifting mindset, changing relationships and re-distributing power' (p 84).

Since 2010, Wigan Council has achieved £134 million in savings, which is, according to the Institute for Fiscal Studies, the third largest proportionate reduction in funding across the country through government austerity (Naylor and Wellings, 2019). Wigan Council still has further savings to make (see Figure 8.1). An independent analysis by the King's Fund set out to discover how Wigan had achieved transformational change and brought about positive changes to the health of the residents of Wigan while simultaneously making very substantial savings (Naylor and Wellings, 2019). The report reveals how local political and executive leaders recognised that it was going to require upfront investment in prevention and early intervention.

Figure 8.1: Wigan Council financial savings, 2011–21

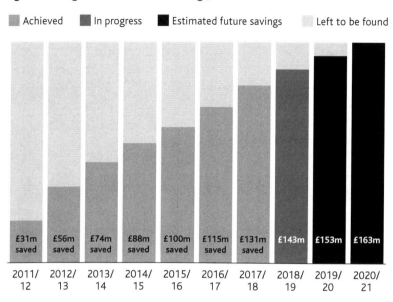

Source: Wigan Metropolitan Borough Council

At the beginning: the creation of the Wigan Deal

Wigan Council acted quickly and decisively, taking the opportunity to do things differently and initiate a programme of transformative change. This built on the borough's involvement as one of six local authorities to be awarded Creative Councils funding supported by Nesta (an innovation foundation) and the Local Government Association to test new ideas about how public services are delivered. Politicians and senior management took the opportunity to fundamentally think about a new relationship with residents and communities. This process took on the lessons from the Creative Councils' work in the urban area of Scholes (east Wigan), which had a powerful impact and challenged the way the council works with service users and the wider community. This was, crucially, coupled with a commitment to invest in local people and civic society at scale. Even more crucially, it took an invest-to-save approach, prioritising community, prevention and early intervention, while it also 'frontloaded' and 'over programmed the internal savings plan' with the focus on cash flow not just savings. This meant that more cost reductions were put in place than were needed, so there was a contingency if planned savings took longer to achieve.

The development of the Wigan Deal (see Figure 8.2) was therefore based on a different approach to financial planning and management.

Figure 8.2: The original Wigan Deal

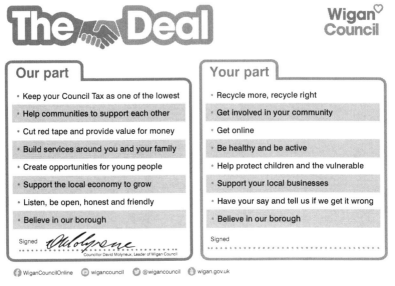

Source: Wigan Metropolitan Borough Council

It built upon the principles of community wealth-building (Centre for Local Economic Strategies [CLES], 2019). The central tenets of this approach are: plural ownership of the economy (for example, by small enterprises, cooperatives and municipal ownership); fair employment (for example, the living wage); socially just use of land (so that citizens benefit from financial and social gain); increasing flows of investment in local economies (recirculating wealth that exists); and progressive procurement (for example, local supply chains, social enterprises). Box 8.3 shows the essential components of the Wigan Deal. It was based on a key set of public service reform principles:

- A new relationship between public services and citizens, communities and businesses; in other words 'Do with, not to'.
- An asset-based approach that recognises and builds on the strengths of individuals, families and our communities rather than focusing on the deficits. Having a 'blank mind' during conversations and treating citizens as full of strengths to be revealed.
- Behaviour change in communities that builds independence and supports residents' control.
- A place-based approach that redefines services and places individuals, families and communities at the heart. Stay close to neighbourhoods and mobilise people around them.

- A stronger prioritisation of wellbeing, prevention and early intervention.
- An evidence-led understanding of risk and impact to ensure the right intervention at the right time.

Box 8.3: The essential components of the Wigan Deal

- **Strong narrative** – a simple concept that everyone can understand but is profound in its implications.
- **A belief that this is a movement not a project** – rooting the approach in public service values: 'sense of vocation'.
- **Leadership at every level** – commitment and senior sponsorship.
- **Workforce culture change** – training and core behaviours that define how we work, whatever the role.
- **A different relationship with residents and communities** – building self-reliance and independence.
- **Permissions to work differently** – leadership backing: 'we will support you'.
- **Redesigning the system** – testing our systems, processes and ways of working against our principles: 'do they make the culture and behaviours we want more or less likely?'
- **Enabling staff with the right tools and knowledge** – using new technology to support new ways of working and new roles.
- **A new model of commissioning and community investment** – market development and new arrangements for commissioning.
- **Supportive enabling functions** – breaking down barriers to progress and facilitate the change.

Early implementation

In Adult Social Care, where the Deal transformation began, the case for change was irrefutable. In 2011/12, there was a projected overspend of £6.9 million, with rising demand for services. At the time, Adult Social Care was a traditional service model with a care management focus. There was a lack of leadership and direction, accountability issues throughout the service, disengaged and risk-averse staff and bureaucratic processes with multiple assessments. The newly appointed Director of Adult Social Care and Health had, in his previous role, been instrumental in developing the People at the Heart of Scholes work that underpinned the development of the 'different conversation' approach of the Deal. The King's Fund analysis reveals that the council had agreed to draw on its financial reserves only for short-term enabling of transformation (and not for day-to-day costs), in order to invest to save. This was used to fund extra social workers temporarily while care packages were assessed and targeted effectively to individual needs (Naylor and Wellings, 2019).

Essentially, the service aimed to connect people to individually tailored, meaningful activities, allowing them to grow in skills, relationships and ambitions, and reducing their dependence on the service. This connected the assets of the individual (their existing skills and interests) with the assets present in the community (existing opportunities and facilities). It also helped to foster and build community wealth, health and civic pride. The successful elements of the redesigned adult social care offer were:

- know your community (community map and resources);
- Community Book (a website with meaningful activities in the neighbourhood www.communitybook.org);
- market shaping (understanding the market and ensuring that the needs of the local population are met, Institute of Public Care, 2015; CLES, 2019);
- new commissioning models;
- new roles:
  - community knowledge workers – knowing their patch;
  - volunteer community connectors;
  - community link workers within primary care.

The Deal for Health and Wellness

In 2013, two years after the original Wigan Deal was developed and with the impending transfer of public health back to its original home in local government from the NHS, the Deal for Health and Wellness (Figure 8.3) was developed. This built on the overall principles of the Wigan Deal and applied them within the context of transforming the health and wellbeing of the population and the health, care and wellness system across the borough. It is an asset-based, application of 'different conversations' between citizens and health and social care staff, and targeted investment in building community resilience for health and wellness. The approach has been integral to the development of the integrated care organisation.

One element of the Transforming Population Health programme is Heart of Wigan, which promotes physical activity, through the

Figure 8.3: The Deal for Health and Wellness

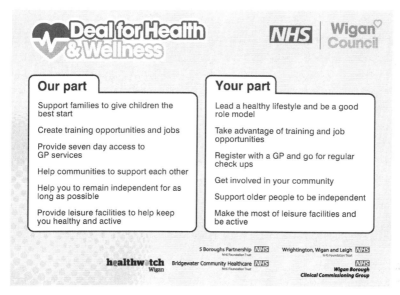

Source: Wigan Metropolitan Borough Council

utilisation of green spaces and active travel, to improve the health of Wigan residents. As described in Figure 8.4, it was built on learning from the North Karelia project in Finland, which was the first well-documented community intervention programme (starting

Figure 8.4: Development of the Heart of Wigan, Royal Society for Public Health

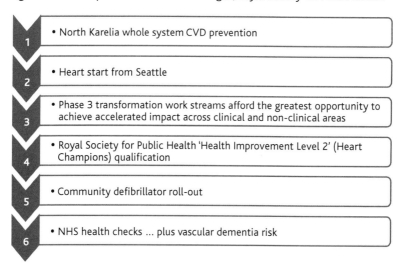

Source: Wigan Metropolitan Borough Council

in the 1970s) that aimed to influence health behaviour changes on several levels in the community (Vartiainen, 2018). This successful programme demonstrated that population risk factor changes as well as improvements and new treatments caused a substantial decline in mortality. This was supplemented by learning from Heart Start Seattle, another programme from the early 1970s, where out-of-hospital defibrillation was demonstrated to greatly improve outcomes in those with cardiac failure (Cobb et al, 1975). Using this learning, several elements were put in place: transformations in services; training of Heart Champions; and rollout of defibrillators in the community and NHS. The success of Heart of Wigan has been built on strategic leadership and collaboration from across all partners. The programme encompasses the commissioning of all health improvement services.

The formation of the Healthier Wigan Partnership

In 2018, under the programme of transformation, services that had never previously been integrated, such as community nursing and adult social care, were brought together under robust governance structures. The Healthier Wigan Partnership, which is a partnership of health and care providers and commissioners bound together by an Alliance Agreement, was formed to have the responsibility for service redesign and to bring together groups. The key aim was to organise health services in a way that allowed individuals to look after their own wellbeing, to receive early interventions and be looked after locally where possible. This partnership enabled the council, NHS and its partners to deliver their part of the Deal for Health and Wellness, while empowering and enabling individuals to look after their own wellbeing, and thus deliver the citizens' part of the deal.

The 'service delivery footprint' (SDF) is the geographical unit for the organisation of public services in the borough. There are seven SDFs and they are coterminous with the 14 townships. This recognises the natural geography (two townships per SDF) and also aligns with the seven primary care networks. There is therefore a single, coherent, sub-borough geography. SDFs are also the geography of integration for wider public services, including Greater Manchester Police and schools.

The key service components are:

- reformed primary care in clusters focusing on local populations of 30,000–50,000 persons;
- integrated community services;

- implementation of the Start Well offer;
- public health interventions wrapped around general practitioner (GP) surgeries;
- community-based mental health alignment to SDFs;
- shift of hospital activity (diagnostic and treatment) to community;
- place-based working across health and care and a full range of public and voluntary sector services.

Philosophy and behaviours throughout the integrated services and organisations are reflective of Wigan Deal principles – for example, all staff from all organisations attend a common and immersive Be Healthier Wigan experience. The King's Fund's analysis found that 'the most remarkable features of this process have been a striking consistency of approach, highly effective leadership and a sense of self-belief and pride among people working in a wide range of services' (Naylor and Wellings, 2019, p 8). This effective leadership allowed all levels of staff in the council to be confident in taking risks, gave them support and encouraged innovation. The culture become one of support for this new way of working and there was a 'no blame' culture if things did not work out; instead, staff were encouraged to learn from their mistakes and move on. The partnership's work fits into the wider notion of place, working locally with other sectors such as education and wider public services.

Impacts in Wigan

The King's Fund report (Naylor and Wellings, 2019) documents some of the impacts in Wigan, and describes the achievement of a 'minor miracle' (p 5). It describes how Wigan Council saved more than £140 million (including losing a fifth of its workforce) while key outcome measures improved over the same period.

One of the impacts in Wigan is the increase in community engagement as a result of the transformation. Box 8.4 gives examples of citizens who are getting involved through health champion activities in a 'movement for change'. Another illustration of citizen engagement and co-development with citizens was the work that went into developing the New Deal 2030. A strong commitment was made to speak to as many people as possible about what their ambitions were for the place they live. A Big Listening Project was launched (September to December 2018), in which the team used a bright green sofa to 'pop up' across the borough, visiting 83 locations and speaking to more than 6,000 people in high streets and GP surgeries, and outside the

Box 8.4: Wigan's 'Health Movement for Change'

There are now **23,000 citizens engaged**, including:

- **1,350** Health Champions
- **495** Heart Champions
- **856** Cancer Champions
- **10,000+** Dementia Friends
- **200+** Young Health Champions

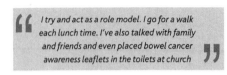

> I try and act as a role model. I go for a walk each lunch time. I've also talked with family and friends and even placed bowel cancer awareness leaflets in the toilets at church

> Most of the group of young Mums had disengaged from school. They had poor literacy, no qualifications and an absence of praise.
>
> The qualification is the first one she has got. That's a real achievement. She left the course much more confident and with a qualification she can put on her CV

The Community Health champions are

- Embedded within existing programmes,
- Made up of members of the community, front line staff and volunteers from across the public voluntary and private sectors.

Developments at the time of writing include the roll-out of Autism Friends, In Mind Champions and the recently-launched Communities in Charge of Alcohol programme led by the residents of Hag Fold

Wigan was the Alzheimer Society Dementia Friendly Town of the Year 2016 and aims to be the first Autism Friendly Borough

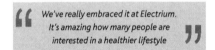

> We've really embraced it at Electrium. It's amazing how many people are interested in a healthier lifestyle

hospital and supermarkets. There was no set list of questions; the aim was an informal conversation about what was important to individuals for the future, during which ideas were captured on paper. Other activities included an online survey and use of a video booth. Findings were organised into key themes and incorporated directly into the new Deal 2030 strategy, which included the best start in life for children and young people; happy healthy people; communities that care; vibrant town centres; an environment to be proud of; embracing culture, heritage and sport; economic growth that benefits everyone; a well-connected place; to be confidently digital; and a home for all. From this, an Our Town campaign was launched, to give people more say on what goes on in their local area.

Positive outcomes have also been seen across a range of health indicators. For example, routinely collected data on cancer mortality (Figure 8.5) show that Wigan's rates of cancer mortality are dropping faster in Wigan compared with the England average (Figure 8.5a) and that the drop has been more rapid and greater than in areas that are

Figure 8.5: Indexed under-75 mortality from cancer: (a) compared with England and (b) compared with Wigan's statistical neighbours

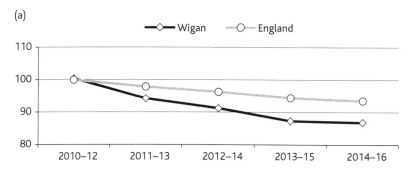

(a)

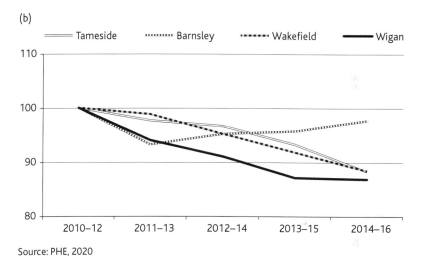

(b)

Source: PHE, 2020

otherwise similar (and would be expected to perform similarly; that is, Wigan's 'statistical neighbours', Figure 8.5b). In the past six years, early deaths attributed to cancer have reduced by 16 per cent for males and 9 per cent for females. Wigan's rates are now similar to the national rate (previously Wigan had a significantly higher rate).

Similarly, 2016–18 figures show that healthy life expectancy among males and females has increased since 2009, by 26 months for males (to 61.1 years) and by 20 months for females (to 6.17 years) (Figure 8.6). In this respect, Wigan has arguably performed better than any of its statistical neighbours. At the same time, in England, improvements in healthy life expectancy have more or less stagnated, having decreased by 2 months for women and increased by only 4 months for men. Other health indicators show that early deaths attributed to cardiovascular disease have reduced by 29 per cent for males and 25 per

Figure 8.6: Healthy life expectancy in Wigan compared with (a) a selection of Chartered Institute of Public Finance and Accounting (CIPFA) statistical neighbours and England, for females (left) and males (right) and (b) CIPFA geographical statistical neighbours

(a)

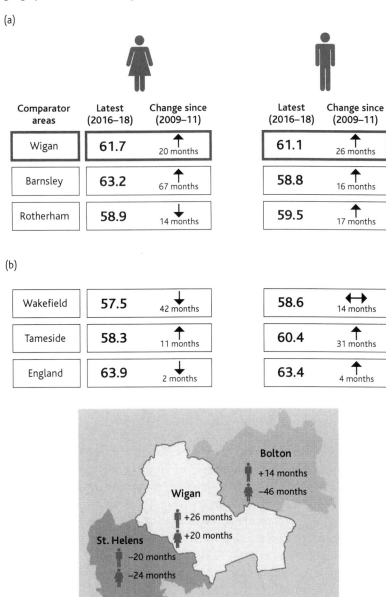

Comparator areas	Latest (2016–18)	Change since (2009–11)	Latest (2016–18)	Change since (2009–11)
Wigan	61.7	↑ 20 months	61.1	↑ 26 months
Barnsley	63.2	↑ 67 months	58.8	↑ 16 months
Rotherham	58.9	↓ 14 months	59.5	↑ 17 months

(b)

Wakefield	57.5	↓ 42 months	58.6	↔ 14 months
Tameside	58.3	↑ 11 months	60.4	↑ 31 months
England	63.9	↓ 2 months	63.4	↑ 4 months

Bolton
+14 months
–46 months

Wigan
+26 months
+20 months

St. Helens
–20 months
–24 months

Source: PHE, 2020

cent for females in the past six years, and the proportion of adults who are physically active has increased from 48 per cent in 2012 to 63.4 per cent in 2017. Smoking rates for routine and manual workers is lower than the England average range, at 22.8 per cent for the first time (England 25.6 per cent). The overall prevalence of smoking is 15.5 per cent (for the fifth year running, this is in the England average range). Smoking rates in pregnant women at the time of delivery has reduced from 16.7 per cent in 2016 to 14.8 per cent in 2017 (this is the greatest improvement for four years, compared with the England average of 10.6 per cent). Hospital stays for alcohol–related harm have reduced from 2,358 in 2014/15 to 2,192 in 2015/16: this is the second year that numbers have decreased, and the gap between Wigan and the England average has reduced significantly since 2013/14. Teenage pregnancy rates are currently at 23.1 per 1,000, which is now in the England average range (20.8 per 1,000). All childhood vaccination programmes achieve 95 per cent herd immunity, including measles, mumps and rubella (MMR) and for children in care (better than England for both these statistics). Over 14,000 children are doing the Daily Mile every day, and this has been extended to two year olds via the Daily Toddle in 20 nurseries. Box 8.5 shows a range of other indicators of improvement, including the Care Quality Commission's assessments of improvements in the quality of social care services.

Box 8.5: Impacts in Wigan

- Wigan's ten programmes across the borough created over 100 Young Health Champions, and Wigan resident Joseph Roberts won the Royal Society for Public Health Young Person Health Champions Hygiea Award (2018).
- A successful video campaign raising awareness of sepsis, toxic shock syndrome and meningitis reached nearly 2,000 people.
- Wigan achieved the third fastest improvement nationally in care home quality.
- Admissions to nursing residential care have reduced by 15 per cent and at a faster rate than the England average.
- For getting people home from hospital, Wigan is best in the North-West and fifth in the country.
- 100 per cent of directly delivered services are rated 'good' or 'outstanding' by the Care Quality Commission.
- 75 per cent of residents who are supported by the reablement service require no further ongoing social care support.
- Wigan is the happiest place to live in Greater Manchester.
- 72 per cent of residents strongly believe that they belong to their local area.

• A balanced budget with growth earmarked 2018/19: £26 million of cashable efficiencies achieved simultaneously with improving services and outcomes.

Challenges in Wigan

There remain some challenges in Wigan. It is a borough that sees more than its fair share of economic hardship. Notably, some of the key challenges lie in the realm of early childhood; for example, only 30 per cent of infants are being breastfed at six to eight weeks. Further, 31 per cent of children in Wigan are not school-ready in time for the reception year, which, although at the England average, is as low as 50 per cent in some localities and among those accessing free school meals. A shocking one in four of the children in one Wigan primary school lives in a house with a reportable incidence of domestic violence in the last two years. In terms of the adult population, when looking at the Live Well cohort, 40 per cent of residents at highest risk of unplanned hospital admission are adults of working age, and these people often have complex dependency on public services. A significant proportion of activity in Wigan's GP practices is socio-economic: debt, domestic abuse, loneliness, access to work and cold homes. Access to quality work for adults of working age needs to be improved as it is a health protective factor. Among older adults, loneliness remains a major determinant of hospital admission.

Conclusion

The National Health Service's Five Year Forward View (NHS, 2014) pointed out that the sustainability of the NHS and the future health of the population relies on a radical upgrade in prevention and public health. It recognises that 'we have not fully harnessed the renewable energy represented by patients and communities, or the potential positive health impacts of employers and national and local governments' (p 9). Wigan has come some way towards harnessing this 'renewable energy'. The King's Fund report found that 'The story of the Wigan Deal can be seen as a case study of effective organisational development and cultural change ... ideas around asset-based working and "different conversations" have become common currency as a result of clear leadership and constancy of purpose over time' (Naylor and Wellings, 2019, p 26).

Reflecting on the lessons that can be learned, it can be seen that a crucial step was the identification of change agents, people with enthusiasm for promoting health and wellbeing, as this was the best way to build society- and system-wide commitment. Wigan has taken every opportunity to appoint the appropriate staff to support transformation, and two of their most important attributes are energy and motivation for change. Innovation is key to future progress, and staff must be given the time and space to try new things, to make mistakes at times and learn from them. Wigan has developed a culture of giving good people the time and space to do great things.

Local transformation is based on the quality and nurturing of relationships and human connection: connecting people back to the humanity of their communities. Wigan's journey has drawn heavily on the asset-based community development approach as proposed by Cormac Russell and others (Kretzmann and McKnight, 1996; Russell, 2011; McKnight and Russell, 2018). The work has been based on Wigan's work as a Nesta creative council. There has been a determined focus on having different conversations between citizens and frontline staff: in keeping with the assets-based approach, this is strengths based, 'co-creation with' as opposed to 'doing to'. The council and partners have used principles of ethnography and anthropology to underpin staff training and transform organisational behaviours and culture. When this work took place in the NHS, it was referred to as 'infecting the NHS with Wellness'. Crucially, the approach embraces the salutogenic paradigm, which focuses on people's and communities' resources and capacity to create health, rather than taking the classic focus on risks, ill-health and disease (Lindström and Eriksson, 2005). However, the Wigan approach goes beyond simply establishing schemes to prescribe non-medical, community or social activities (as in social prescriptions: Husk et al, 2020), although this is part of the response. Rather, the whole society, whole system approach to health and wellbeing was informed by the experiences of North Karelia in cardiovascular disease prevention, Marmot's Fairer Society: Healthy Lives and the 'fully engaged scenario' set out in the Wanless report on the long-term sustainability of a publicly funded health and care system. These principles were underpinned with a 'servant leadership' mentality; that is, an 'expert on tap rather than expert on top' approach. The Deal for Communities investment fund invests in the ideas, talents and passions of local people. In doing so, Wigan has developed citizen-led public health.

In the face of austerity, careful choices for investment were made. Assets-based approaches can be criticised as being an excuse to cut services while relying on communities to look after themselves (Roy, 2017). Conscious of this, the council leadership was careful to base the transformation plans on the premise that community assets are not necessarily free (Naylor and Wellings, 2019). Building upon the principles of 'community wealth building' (CLES, 2019), Wigan Council put in place measures to invest in, and actively stimulate, the community and voluntary sector. In addition, the council shaped the market in a way that promoted ethical employment, social value and community wealth-building.

Figure 8.7 shows reasons to be proud of Wigan. The transfer of public health was a once-in-a-generation opportunity to transform the health and wellbeing of the people of Wigan. The Marmot vision is very clear about what needs to be done: employment, planning, transport, housing, education, leisure and social care are all interlinked

Figure 8.7: Reasons to be proud of Wigan

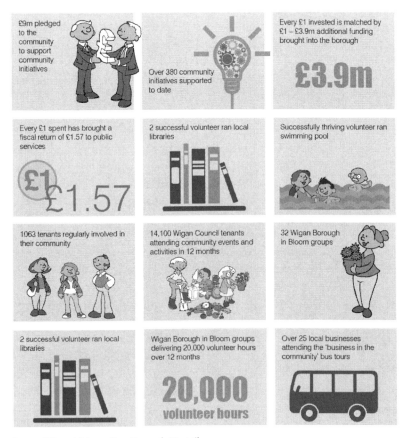

Source: Wigan Metropolitan Borough Council

and have an impact on physical and mental health (Marmot et al, 2010, 2020). Importantly, the achievements in Wigan show that asset-based working should not be seen as a technocratic fix: it is not a tool to be adopted but rather a culture to be grown. It is about rekindling hope in public services and overcoming fatalism about people's capacity to change. Furthermore, the investment in local economies by and for local people, the empowerment of communities and the fostering of a sense of civic pride all, in turn, build the strengths and assets in a virtuous cycle.

References

Antonovsky, A. (1979) *Health, stress, and coping*, San Francisco: Jossey-Bass.

CLES (Centre for Local Economic Strategies) (2019) 'Community wealth building: theory, practice and next steps'. Available from: https://cles.org.uk/publications/community-wealth-building-2019/ [Accessed 1 April 2020].

Cobb, L.A., Baum, R.S., Alvarez H. III and Schaffer, W.A. (1975) 'Resuscitation from out-of-hospital ventricular fibrillation: 4 years follow-up', *Circulation*, 52(Suppl 3): 223–35.

Davis-Hall, M. (2018) 'The Bromley by Bow Centre: harnessing the power of community', *British Journal of General Practice*, 68(672): 333.

Doebbeling, B.N. and Flanagan, M.E. (2011) 'Emerging perspectives on transforming the healthcare system: key conceptual issues', *Medical Care*, 49: S3–S5.

Dougall, D., Lewis, M. and Ross, S. (2018) 'Transformational change in health and care: reports from the field'. London: The King's Fund. Available from: www.kingsfund.org.uk/publications/transformational-change-health-care [Accessed 23 January 2020].

Gray, M. and Barford, A. (2018) 'The depths of the cuts: the uneven geography of local government austerity', *Cambridge Journal of Regions, Economy and Society*, 11(3): 541–63.

Ferry, L., Ahrens, T. and Khalifa, R. (2019) 'Public value, institutional logics and practice variation during austerity localism at Newcastle City Council', *Public Management Review*, 21(1): 96–115.

Harrison, R., Blickem, C., Lamb, J., Kirk, S. and Vassilev, I. (2019) 'Asset-based community development: narratives, practice, and conditions of possibility—a qualitative study with community practitioners', *SAGE Open*, 9(1): 1–11. Available from: https://doi.org/10.1177/2158244018823081 [Accessed 18 May 2020].

Husk, K., Blockley, K., Lovell, R., Bethel, A., Lang, I., Byng, R. and Garside, R. (2020) 'What approaches to social prescribing work, for whom, and in what circumstances? A realist review', *Health and Social Care in the Community*, 28(2): 309–24.

Institute of Public Care (2015) 'Market-shaping toolkit: supporting local authority and SME care provider innovation and collaboration', Oxford Brookes University. Available from: https://ipc.brookes. ac.uk/publications/pdf/Market_Shaping_Toolkit.pdf [Accessed 1 April 2020].

Kretzmann, J. and McKnight, J.P. (1996) 'Assets-based community development', *National Civic Review*, 85(4): 23–9.

Lindström, B. and Eriksson, M. (2005) 'Salutogenesis', *Journal of Epidemiology & Community Health*, 59(6): 440–2.

Marmot, M., Allen, J., Goldblatt, P., Boyce, T., McNeish, D. and Grady, M. (2010) 'Fair society, healthy lives'. The Marmot Review, London: Institute of Health Equity.

Marmot, M., Allen, J., Boyce, T., Goldblatt, P. and Morrison, J. (2020) 'Health equity in England: the Marmot review 10 years on', London: Institute of Health Equity. Available from: https://www.health.org. uk/publications/reports/the-marmot-review-10-years-on [Accessed 1 April 2020].

McKnight, J. and Russell, C. (2018) 'Four essential elements of an asset-based community development process', Chicago: Asset-Based Community Development Institute, DePaul University. Available from: https://www.nurturedevelopment.org/wp-content/ uploads/2018/09/4_Essential_Elements_of_ABCD_Process.pdf [Accessed 1 April 2020].

Naylor, C. and Wellings, D. (2019) 'Citizen-focused public services: lessons from the Wigan deal', London: The King's Fund. Available from: https://www.kingsfund.org.uk/publications/wigan-deal [Accessed 23 January 2020].

NHS (National Health Service) (2014) 'Five year forward view'. Available from: https://www.england.nhs.uk/wp-content/ uploads/2014/10/5yfv-web.pdf [Accessed 1 April 2020].

ONS (Office for National Statistics) (2020) 'Population projections for local authorities: Table 2', Release Date 24 March, London: Office for National Statistics. Available from: https://www.ons. gov.uk/peoplepopulationandcommunity/populationandmigration/ populationprojections/datasets/localauthoritiesinenglandtable2 [Accessed 26 May 2020].

PHE (Public Health England) (2020) 'Public Health Outcomes Framework: statistical commentary', February. Available from: https://www.gov.uk/government/publications/public-health-outcomes-framework-february-2020-data-update/public-health-outcomes-framework-statistical-commentary-february-2020 [Accessed 28 July 2020].

Roy, M.J. (2017) 'The assets-based approach: furthering a neoliberal agenda or rediscovering the old public health? A critical examination of practitioner discourses', *Critical Public Health*, 27(4): 455–64.

Russell, C. (2011) 'Pulling back from the edge: an asset-based approach to ageing well', *Working with Older People*, 15(3): 96–105.

Taylor, M. and Baker, L. (2018) 'The future for communities: perspectives on power', London: Local Trust. Available from: https://localtrust.org.uk/wp-content/uploads/2018/07/local_trust_the_future_for_communities_perspectives_on_power.pdf [Accessed 1 April 2020].

Vartiainen, E. (2018) 'The north Karelia project: cardiovascular disease prevention in Finland', *Global Cardiology Science & Practice*, 2018(2).

Wanless, D. (2002) 'Securing our future health: taking a long-term view'. Final report. London: HM Treasury. Available from: https://www.yearofcare.co.uk/sites/default/files/images/Wanless.pdf [Accessed 1 April 2020].

PART III

Local authority commissioning

Introduction

Mark Cook

The chapters in Part II provide an insight into the impact of austerity on local authority (LA) budgets and LAs' individual responses to protect the wellbeing of their communities. This response is influenced by socio-geopolitical circumstances such as local opportunities for employment (particularly in the North-East, Chapter 7), the extent of devolution (for example, Devo Max in the North-West, Chapters 5 and 8) and the culture of commissioning.

Public services are commissioned and delivered, often on the basis of a hard-line demarcation between the responsibilities of council and contractor, when in fact if wellbeing is to be truly embraced a much more nuanced dynamic has to exist. This is very much an issue of culture and competence on all sides. The connection between Best Value and wellbeing is one that is not well understood in central and local government. However, the 'Wigan Deal' (Chapter 8) provides a consultative approach in which cultural changes in public attitude and behaviour complement financial gains and cost savings in the council budget.

It is important not to conflate 'Best Value' with any understanding of value for money or indeed the best price–quality ratio basis upon which contracts might be awarded in any tender process under the European Union procurement regime. It is clear that for both value for money and best price–quality ratio a range of factors can be taken into account, including socio-economic benefits (for HM Treasury's approach to 'value for money' see, for example, the Green Book (HM Treasury, 2018), which has moved considerably in embracing social value in recent years).

The Best Value Duty as it applies to local authorities in England is enshrined in section 3(1) Local Government Act 1999, which reads as follows:

(1)   A best value authority must make arrangements to secure continuous improvement in the way in which its functions are exercised, having regard to a combination of economy, efficiency and effectiveness.

Much of the complicated apparatus around this duty was repealed by the Conservative/Liberal Democrat Coalition government, including very detailed guidance previously issued by the previous Secretary of State (Hazel Blears), which is now in the shorter form (DCLG, 2015). The sequence of the first two paragraphs of the guidance to which the council must have regard in discharging Best Value Duty is particularly interesting:

1. Best Value authorities are under a general Duty of Best Value to 'make arrangements to secure continuous improvement in the way in which its functions are exercised, having regard to a combination of economy, efficiency and effectiveness'.
2. Under the Duty of Best Value, therefore, authorities should consider overall value, including economic, environmental and social value, when reviewing service provision.

The word 'therefore' is particularly pertinent as it indicates that the United Kingdom (UK) Government regards economic, environmental and social value as intrinsic to the way that a local authority makes arrangements to secure continuous improvement in the way that its functions are exercised. The very act of a council establishing a collaboration or partnering arrangement in itself is an arrangement to secure continuous improvement in the way its functions are exercised. The outcomes follow from that thinking. Both the Scottish and Welsh governments have developed their own approach, which is arguably more committed to wellbeing at the heart of a nation's fabric (see Chapters 20 and 21).

Just gaining this appreciation can make all the difference in establishing relationally based ways of working when the social justice, equalities and the environment are the central theme in public services. This is not an opportunity to be wasted in these times of challenge and conflict in the UK.

The chapters in Part III provide an insight into the culture that is emerging from the changing landscape of LA commissioning (Chapter 9) and the value of relationships (Chapter 10).

In considering the challenges to supporting families and children (Chapter 11) and the care of older people (Chapter 12), clearly the role of relationships and other social determinants adds to the value of resources available via local authorities. The high aspirations of effective partnerships between the public, private and third sectors require a more complex commissioning regime. Commissioning in complexity is the topic of Chapter 13.

References

DCLG (Department for Communities and Local Government) (2015) 'Revised best value statutory guidance'. Available from: https://www.gov.uk/government/publications/revised-best-value-statutory-guidance [Accessed 10 April 2020].

HM Treasury (2018) 'The Green Book. Central government guidance on appraisal and evaluation'. Available from: https://assets.publishing.service.gov.uk/government/uploads/system/uploads/attachment_data/file/685903/The_Green_Book.pdf [Accessed 10 April 2020].

9

The changing landscape of local authority commissioning

Dave Ayre

Introduction

The relationship of public and private sectors in the United Kingdom (UK) and the commissioning, procurement and development of public private partnerships is driven by the prevailing political and economic environment. This chapter explores the history of the relationship between public and private sectors and the extent to which the political and regulatory environment of governments and institutions such as the European Union (EU) can help or hinder the efforts of public bodies in seeking to deliver services that determine the health and quality of life for communities.

The political and regulatory environment

In the mid-19th century, when local government was beginning to develop into a more recognisable form, many urban local authorities began to deliver gas, water and sanitation services (University of Warwick, 2012).

In 1945, Clement Attlee's Labour government was elected at a time of severe post-war austerity. It marked the start of a new social-democratic consensus that was to develop over 30 years under successive governments. By 1973, the top rate of income tax for earned income stood at 75 per cent (Clark and Dilnot, 2002). Key industries such as rail, coal and steel, and all major utilities, water, electricity, gas and telecommunications, were publicly owned.

This post-war consensus was turned on its head with the election of Margaret Thatcher's Conservative government in 1979. Influenced by the free market think tanks of the Adam Smith Institute, the Institute for Economic Affairs and the Centre for Policy Studies, the government embarked on a programme of wholesale privatisation. For councils, the Local Government Acts of 1988 and 1992 introduced and extended compulsory competitive tendering (CCT). Services such as waste collection, construction, grounds maintenance and catering were some of the first to be affected. This was later to be extended to white collar architectural and civil engineering design services towards the end of the John Major Conservative government. Although an enthusiastic proponent of CCT, the Major government was keen to portray a less ideological approach to public services than its predecessor.

In 1992, the Major government introduced the Private Finance Initiative (PFI) and branded it as a new form of public private partnership. The New Labour government of Tony Blair embraced PFI, embarking on an ambitious programme of new hospitals, schools and highways infrastructure. While the Major government signed 21 PFI deals, by the end of Blair's term as prime minister in 2007, 850 had been signed.

PFI was in reality just another form of privatisation. The key principles were the transfer of assets and the consequent risks to the private sector. It was particularly attractive to central government because it also transferred the debt required to fund projects to the private sector, keeping the public sector borrowing requirement lower than it would be otherwise. The debt, private sector profits and ongoing maintenance of the assets for the 25- to 30-year term of the PFI contract is paid for by regular annual payments by the public sector.

By 2011, there was around £300 billion of debt owed by public bodies to PFI companies to deliver new public assets worth just over £50 billion. PFI began to face growing scrutiny and was heavily criticised by the National Audit Office and parliamentary select committees for failing to demonstrate value for money. Even the concept of risk transfer was difficult to sustain as, ultimately, it became clear that the public sector not only carried the liability but also the risk. This is best illustrated by two high-profile examples:

- The London Underground PFI deal at £30 billion over 30 years was the largest in history. Signed in 2003, it began to collapse in 2007. London Underground had to bail out Metronet with a £1.7 billion grant from the Department for Transport. Metronet only managed half of the PFI. The other half was run by Tube Lines, which was finally bought out by the London mayor's Transport for London in 2010, with their contract over cost and behind schedule.
- In south-east London, Lewisham saw the closure of many of its front-line health services as a result of the bankruptcy of the

neighbouring South London Healthcare Trust, brought down by the unaffordable costs of two PFI hospitals.

Despite attempts to revive PFI with the introduction of PFI2, the chancellor in his 2018 budget recognised the shortcomings of PFI and announced that no further PFI or PFI2 projects would be approved. PFI was not universally supported by the private sector owing to prohibitive bidding costs. In the end, only a dwindling number of companies were left participating in the PFI market as investors grew increasingly reluctant to place their funds in what they saw as a declining market with increasing risks.

In 1997, New Labour was elected and set about replacing CCT with Best Value. Although tendering was no longer compulsory, competition was still a fundamental part of the Best Value regime (Ayre, 2016a). The government invited local authorities and private sector-led initiatives to submit applications to be Best Value pilots. The private sector-led initiative was called the Public/Private Partnerships Network (PPN) and provided local authorities who participated with the opportunity to be exempt from the CCT regulations in order to pilot new and innovative forms of partnering between public and private sectors.

Some local authorities made good use of the opportunity, and developed new and innovative approaches to working with the private sector. Dorset County Council was successful in obtaining exemption from the CCT regulations in order to pilot partnering alternatives (Ayre, 1998). The Council carried out a search for a private sector partner with whom it could develop a new form of public–private partnership. Several engineering consultancies were invited to present their approach to public–private partnership to officers of the council and Public Sector Plc (PSP – one of the PPNs). Companies whose overall culture and business model was one of growth through the acquisition of privatised public services were not able to demonstrate a more collaborative approach with the public sector that could add value and contribute to continuous improvement. Buro Happold, on the other hand, had built a worldwide reputation for quality and innovation and saw this collaboration with the county council as mutually beneficial.

Dorset and Buro Happold began exchanging work and best practice and, in the process, developed a non-contractual Memorandum of Understanding that was signed by the then Local Government Minister, Nick Raynsford. This partnership agreement set out:

• shared objectives between the partners;

- a non-adversarial approach to joint working where each partner worked together to address and resolve problems rather than seek to apportion blame;
- two-way work exchange between both partners.

There were significant benefits to the county council and its engineering consultancy. The arrangement helped to maintain the viability of in-house specialist services and to even out peaks and troughs of workload. During times of periodic spare capacity, the in-house workforce were able to carry out work for Buro Happold and its customers, which gave them the opportunity to broaden their skills and work on prestigious projects from across the world. This also generated income for the county council that would not have been available under any conventional contractual arrangement. The arrangement provided a cost-effective and flexible solution able to respond to changes in transport policies. In retaining the in-house service, this acted as a market regulator, reducing the risk of uncontrolled costs in a sector where private consultancy services are generally more expensive than maintaining in-house workforces. The authority applied these partnering principles to a series of procurements, from civil engineering design to highway maintenance and construction. At a time when many councils were continuing to externalise their services, Dorset was procuring service delivery partners to work in collaboration with their in-house workforce. These strategic partnerships served the council particularly well in its preparation for the 2012 Olympic sailing events, which were based at Weymouth. A whole programme of transport infrastructure was constructed on time and within budget.

However, the potential of these Best Value pilots and subsequent initiatives was increasingly constrained by proscriptive procurement regulations introduced to comply with European Directives and a determination by the Treasury that PFI should be the primary partnering model supported by the government.

A further driver of partnering as a concept came from the manufacturing sector. Rather than constantly putting out tenders and choosing different suppliers on the basis of lowest price, assemblers entered into long-term, but relatively informal agreements with a few suppliers. Suppliers worked together with the assembler to deliver continuous improvement in products and processes over time. As a result, all parties delivered lower costs and improved quality without squeezing each other's profit margins. Steady profits then provided the basis for investment in improved products and processes, and a virtuous circle of continuous improvement was established.

In 1994, 'Constructing the Team', the Latham Report (Latham, 1994), the final report of the Government/Industry Review of procurement and contractual arrangements in the UK construction industry was published. The report advocated the transfer of some of the successful practices from manufacturing to construction and indicated partnering as a way forward to improve efficiency and profitability in the UK construction industry. This was followed by 'Rethinking Construction' (Egan, 1998). It identified five key drivers for change: committed leadership; a focus on the customer; integrated processes and teams; a quality-driven agenda; and commitment to people. One of Egan's central recommendations was to replace job-by-job tendering with longer-term strategic alliances between clients and constructors.

Early forms of collaboration took the form of Design and Build contracts that evolved to overcome some of the problems of traditional procurement. This involved collaboration between the construction team along part of the supply chain (for example, the architect, cost consultant and contractor). In this scenario, one party (usually the principal contractor) manages the design and cost consultants on behalf of the client, thus integrating the cost, design and construction processes (CE, 2004).

Demonstration projects extended this early form of collaboration to project partnering. This goes beyond Design and Build by getting more members of the project team together, including client, contractor, sub-contractors and consultants, to work as a team at design stage. Partnering agreements are often entered into with collaborators agreeing to share associated risks as well as the benefits of cost savings. The demonstration projects identified the following benefits:

- Increased collaboration of the supply chain provided more benefits than those resulting from the traditional Design and Build process.
- Improved communication between the team resulted in identifying difficulties earlier than with traditional procurement and in Design and Build contracts.
- Predictability of both cost and time improved as late design changes became less likely with specialist sub-contractors adding to the expertise of the main contractor at design stage.

Some 25 years after the Latham Report, a review of collaborative working in the construction industry noted that the handful of high-profile demonstration projects from the 1990s were still mostly unrepeated and that Latham's 1994 report still described the way things were usually done.

The Project 13 infrastructure initiative (ICE, 2017), launched at the peak of a significant amount of collaboration and alliancing, sets out some notable successes. It notes that governance of procurement and delivery is often based on obtaining the lowest price through a competitive tender and then delivering the construction on time, within budget and to quality. The flaw in this approach is that it assumes that lowest price represents best value and that completion on time, within budget and to quality defines the desired outcome.

As an example, the high-speed rail link between the Channel Tunnel and London's St Pancras Station was delivered within the original budget and schedule but has failed to achieve the revenues forecast from international passengers and property development. Project 13 advocates a new approach to tackle this problem by establishing long-term relationships between the owner, the integrator and their key advisors and suppliers. The relationships should be based on a shared commitment to deliver continuous improvements in performance over periods of several years. Project 13 studies showed that engaging the right suppliers at the right time and integrating them into the team is critical to developing the right infrastructure solutions and to delivering value over the long term. This is more important than extracting the lowest price from suppliers through competition. A few percentage points saved in the price of a supplier's services pale into insignificance when they have a technology that can transform the solution.

They conclude that successful owners understand their suppliers' capabilities and know when to integrate them into their delivery teams to obtain the best results. They invest time in visiting their suppliers' offices and factories and in exploring the products and services they offer. They also commit management time to integrating people from different organisations, professions and backgrounds into a single high-performing team with shared culture, processes and practices.

Effective teams are networks of collaborative relationships that encourage an exchange of knowledge and capabilities to drive improvement and innovation. Owners should take the lead in designing coalitions of suppliers to deliver their programmes and should not allow their supply chains to be the consequence of a series of traditional procurement decisions.

However, this enlightened approach is still far from becoming the norm, especially for building and housing construction where collaboration is more likely to be promoted than actually achieved. Partnering has more often than not stopped at the level of client and principle or management constructor, with the supply chain being procured on a lowest cost basis. Not surprisingly, this has limited the potential for the industry and its customers to deliver the right outcomes for the wider economy and society in general.

These initiatives have clearly demonstrated that longer-term strategic partnerships can deliver real benefits, and some of this learning has been adopted by the public sector in procuring public services. Instead of services being delivered either in-house or by the private sector, many authorities established arrangements whereby in-house services worked with private sector partners who were insourced to top up capacity and skills. The more innovative authorities went further, applying principles of reciprocal working where in-house services used spare capacity to work for their private sector partners, generating income for the authority.

Commissioning and procurement

The securing of health and social care services has followed another commissioning tradition. Commissioning is often confused with procurement, although there are also some similarities, and procurement can often be part of a broader commissioning process. In relation to the delivery of public services, they are both about the introduction of market conditions into the public sector. In environmental and technical services, they spawned the reorganisation of public services into client and consultant or contractor departments, and in health and social care, services were split into commissioners or purchasers and providers.

NHS England defines commissioning as:

> Commissioning is the continual process of planning, agreeing and monitoring services. Commissioning is not one action but many, ranging from the health-needs assessment for a population, through the clinically based design of patient pathways, to service specification and contract negotiation or procurement, with continuous quality assessment. (NHS England, n.d.)

NHS England sees procurement as part of the commissioning process, but what is interesting is that although the two traditions start from different points they are beginning to coalesce. The Project 13 initiative mentioned earlier describes how the high-speed rail link between St Pancras and the Channel Tunnel met its 'procurement' objectives of being constructed on time, to budget and to quality standards but arguably did not meet its 'commissioning' objectives by failing to meet its revenue targets from passenger numbers and property development. Regardless of the terms used, what is really important are the outcomes achieved.

There is one common presumption in both the traditional commissioning and procurement approaches, and that is 'the client or commissioner knows best'. Early Rethinking Construction Demonstration Projects showed the benefits and added value that could be achieved by early constructor engagement in the design build process. The partnering model developed by PSP based upon forging the relationship between public and private sectors first shows what can be achieved when the knowledge and expertise of both sectors can be shared to obtain maximum financial and social value from property projects, before any legal transaction takes place (Smith et al, 2013).

EU law, particularly the EU treaty and the Procurement Directive 2014/24/EU, currently underpins the broad terms under which public procurement and competitive tendering operate in the UK (Crown Commercial Services (CCS, 2016). The rules have been transposed into national law as the Public Contracts Regulations 2015 by the UK's governments, and establish how public authorities, including health and social care commissioners, purchase goods, works and services.

Existing domestic legislation, such as the Health and Social Care Act 2012 and the NHS (Procurement, Patient Choice and Competition) Regulations 2013 in England, currently effectively enshrines the same rules as EU law. These laws, for example, prohibit NHS England or clinical commissioning groups from favouring a single provider and gave powers to the regulator Monitor, and its successor NHS Improvement, to enforce competition rules on NHS trusts. The Procurement Regulations prevent collaboration between commissioners and providers and also between provider trusts. For example, proposals by several hospital trusts to merge in order to create economies of scale, create centres of excellence and focus scarce resources on patient care have been blocked on the grounds of being anti-competitive.

The British Medical Association argues that competition within health systems leads to fragmentation and undermines the NHS's own founding principle of publicly delivered health care. They have advocated that the government must take the opportunity of Brexit to end the application of EU competition and procurement law as soon as possible, reform domestic regulations requiring competitive tendering and not open the NHS up to competition as part of future trade deals (BMA, 2017).

The collapse of giant outsourcer Carillion in January 2018 was one of the highest profile failures of the traditional outsourcing model. Carillion was a major strategic supplier to the UK public sector, its work ranging from building roads and hospitals to providing school meals and defence accommodation. It collapsed in January 2018, when it held some 420 public sector contracts. The Local Government Association estimated that 30 councils and 220 schools were directly affected. It had around 43,000 employees, including 19,000 in the UK, while many more people were employed in its extensive supply chains. Thousands of people lost their jobs. Carillion left a pension liability of around £2.6 billion, and the 27,000 members of its defined benefit pension schemes are now being paid reduced pensions by the Pension Protection Fund, which faces its largest ever hit.

Parliamentary select committees (House of Commons, 2018) and the National Audit Office (NAO, 2018) have called for the government to learn the lessons of the failure of Carillion. The government's response was to set out proposals to strengthen the insolvency framework in cases of major corporate failure by:

- taking forward measures to ensure greater accountability of directors in group companies when selling subsidiaries in distress;
- legislating to enhance existing recovery powers of insolvency practitioners in relation to value extraction schemes;
- legislating to give the Insolvency Service the necessary powers to investigate directors of dissolved companies when they are suspected of having acted in breach of their legal obligations.

They also proposed to create alternative procedures to support business rescue. On corporate governance, the government proposed to:

- strengthen transparency requirements around complex group structures;
- enhance the role of shareholder stewardship;
- strengthen the UK's framework in relation to dividend payments;
- bring forward proposals to improve board-room effectiveness.

They supplemented this by the publication of an Outsourcing Playbook (Government Commercial Function, 2019).

Much of the work of the Parliamentary select committees and the National Audit Office has been understandably focused on addressing issues of corporate governance and the government's capability to procure and manage major outsourcing contracts. The government's response has been mainly technical. This ignores the fact that the failure of Carillion has prompted a much wider rethink of the relationship between public and private sectors. Several local authorities have acted swiftly to bring services back in house that had previously been outsourced. Many more are carrying out a fundamental review of their current outsourcing arrangements. Some progressive local authorities were able to insulate themselves from Carillion's collapse. For example, Carillion was the main contractor on Birmingham City Council's Paradise Birmingham regeneration. The works were being delivered through a limited liability partnership, which was not a contracting authority under the public sector procurement regulations. This allowed the swift appointment of another constructor following the collapse of Carillion. Had it been procured directly by the council, it would have taken nine to twelve months for a replacement constructor to be appointed in compliance with procurement regulations (Jarrett, 2019).

The major outsourcers are under pressure as they go into decline. Capita and Serco are regularly in the media glare. Interserv went into administration and others such as Kier have posted profit warnings. There was a growing reluctance for investors to place their funds in what they see as a declining market with increasing risks. Many traditional outsourcers had consequently been reluctant to fund participation in PFI, PFI2 and Design Build Finance Operate projects as this would continue to add to their debts.

Although Carillion has been perhaps the most high-profile outsourcing failure in recent years, there has been a series of failures in rail franchises, probation and social care, all of which have undermined confidence in outsourcing.

Public and private sectors and the social determinants of health

The social determinants of health rainbow model (Dahlgren and Whitehead, 1991) sets out a hierarchy of determinants with the general socio-economic, cultural and environmental conditions at the top. We have touched on some of these in the historic changes in the relationship between public and private sectors and the political ideologies and culture that drive these changes. We have not yet dealt with the economic context.

The recent problems for the economy started with Northern Rock in the autumn of 2007. More banks with exposure to the sub-prime mortgage market in the United States were having difficulties, leading to bailouts by the government. The costs of the bank bailouts and the reduction in tax income due to the recession that followed created a public sector funding deficit for the government. In 2010, the Conservative/Liberal Democrat Coalition government was elected, and together with subsequent Conservative majority governments followed a policy of public sector austerity to seek to bridge the public sector deficit.

The NHS, schools, overseas development and defence budgets had all initially been protected, although demographic pressures from a growing pupil population and increases in life expectancy continued to bring challenges to these services. NHS plans also assumed a hitherto unachievable scale of efficiency savings, and cuts in councils' unprotected social care budgets have contributed to the growing pressures on accident and emergency services (Crawford et al, 2018).

Local government has been particularly badly hit, and this has resulted in consequential pressures on services that were ostensibly 'protected'. Studies have shown a correlation between cuts in youth and community services and the rise in knife crime (BBC, 2019). Special educational needs services have come under scrutiny. Since 2015, government funding through the 'high needs block' has increased by 11 per cent across England, but demand has increased by 47 per cent (CCN, 2019). Public health services have a specific remit to address the poor health prevention agenda, yet they have seen annual cuts up to £700 million per year over the last four years since responsibility was returned to local government (LGA, 2019). Consequently, local authorities have significantly reduced spending on a range of public health activities, including substantial cuts to sexual health promotion and smoking cessation budgets. The Local Government Association considers that further reductions to the public health budget reinforce the view that central government sees prevention services as 'nice to do', but non-essential.

While the austerity agenda has undoubtedly impacted on the capacity of local government and other agencies to tackle some of the key social determinants of health, failures in the wider economy have also contributed to poorer health outcomes. There were 4,359 deaths related to drug poisoning in England and Wales in 2018, the highest number and the highest annual increase (16 per cent) since the time series began in 1993. The North-East had a significantly higher rate of deaths relating to drug misuse than all other English regions; London had the lowest rate (ONS, 2019). While the explanations offered by many commentators were many and varied, some factors related to cuts in public health budgets, which have resulted in the closure and underfunding of drug prevention and rehabilitation programmes. One factor is undeniable, and it is that the variation in death rates across the country is closely related to imbalances in the economy. The North-East has seen some of the worst ravages of economic decline over decades. The traditional industries of shipbuilding, mining and steel production have all but disappeared, leaving a legacy of unemployment and ill health. If evidence was needed that work environment and unemployment are two key social determinants of health, the higher rates of drug deaths in the North-East are compelling.

Work-related ill health and accidents at work are two other social determinants of health. There were 2,595 deaths due to mesothelioma and a similar rate of lung cancer in 2016 due to previous exposure to asbestos. Many victims worked in construction (HSE, 2018), where accident rates have not been helped by a history of blacklisting of safety and trade union representatives exposed by an investigation by the Information Commissioners Office (Smith and Chamberlain, 2015). Commissioning and procurement of construction by the public sector can address some of these endemic problems by including safety as part of the quality criteria for selection and regular monitoring of construction industry key performance indicators (Glenigan, 2018).

Housing is another key determinant of health. Successive governments have been committed to increasing housing supply, with a particular emphasis on expanding home ownership. The 1979 Thatcher government was the first to make it mandatory for council tenants to have the Right to Buy at a discount, although some Labour councils such as South Tyneside had already introduced a similar policy. The evidence suggests that this policy approach contributed to a reduction in long-term home ownership (DHCLG, 2016).

The proportion of households in the social rented sector fell from 31 per cent in 1980 to 19 per cent in 2000. It was standing at 17 per cent in 2013/14, where it remained in 2019. The proportion of all households in owner occupation increased steadily from the 1980s to 2003, when it reached a peak of 71 per cent. Since then, there has been a gradual decline in owner occupation to 63 per cent in 2013/14. In 2015/16, 4.5 million households were renting in the private sector. This represents 20 per cent of all households in England. Throughout the 1980s and 1990s, the proportion of private renters was steady at around 10 per cent. However, the sector has more than doubled in size since then, and there are now 2.5 million more households in the private renting sector than there were in 2000. This has been driven by a number of factors. In the late 1990s, rent controls were removed and assured short tenancies became standard. Lenders also introduced the buy-to-let mortgage at around the same time. Paradoxically, the Right to Buy has also been a major driver. By 2013, one-third of all council homes sold in the 1980s were owned by private landlords (Fisher, 2014). Shelter now estimates that over 40 per cent of homes bought under the Right to Buy are now in the private rented sector, and on current trends it is set to increase to more than 50 per cent by 2026. Selling off social housing and not replacing it has inflated house prices and created the conditions in which home ownership has become unaffordable for a growing proportion of the population.

So how do the historic decline of social housing, the shifts from home ownership and the growth of the private rented sector impact on health outcomes? One way of measuring housing quality is to use the Housing Health and Safety Rating System (HHSRS) (Barton, 2018). The HHSRS lets an assessor judge whether housing conditions are poor enough that there is a risk to health and safety. It can be applied to all tenure groups and is one of the main tools local authorities have in order to act against poor housing conditions in the private rented sector. Problems identified by HHSRS that are likely to have a serious impact on a tenant's health are termed 'Category 1 hazards'.

In 2015, 17 per cent of private rented homes had a Category 1 hazard. This compared with 13 per cent of owner-occupied homes and 6 per cent of the social rented sector. Of the two most common Category 1 hazards, excess cold and falls, 6 per cent of private rented homes were found to have excess cold compared with just 1 per cent for social rented, and 10 per cent of private rented homes were a fall hazard, compared with 4 per cent for social rented.

Energy efficiency and quality of the private rented sector have improved, but standards lag behind the social rented sector. Over a quarter (28 per cent) of private rented homes failed to meet the Decent Homes standard in 2015. The comparative figure for the social rented sector was 13 per cent. Although the private rented sector has always performed less well than other tenures using this measure of housing quality, there was a marked improvement in the proportion of non-decent private rented homes over the 2006 to 2013 period from 47 per cent to 30 per cent. Since then, the proportion of non-decent homes in the sector has remained virtually unchanged.

Within the private rented sector, households on low incomes and those supported by housing benefit are more likely to have a Category 1 hazard in their home. The same is true of households with a disabled or long-term ill person, or households with someone over 60 living in them (DHCLG, 2016). Housing policy over the last 40 years has, therefore, contributed to housing being a greater determinant of poor health than it needs to be. There has been a significant growth in the private rented sector and consequential reductions in the social rented sector. Private rented homes have the greatest risk to health and safety and have the highest proportion of poor and disabled residents. Homes for social rent are the safest.

Social and community isolation has also been identified as one of the determinants of poor health. Local authorities deliver or provide support to community groups to provide social care and community services. Facilities for community groups such as community centres, parks and gardens are often provided, although many have been closed because of their non-statutory nature. Subsidised public transport can be an essential lifeline for communities suffering from rural isolation (Transport Select Committee, 2019). According to the Campaign for Better Transport, council funding for public transport has been cut by almost 50 per cent over the last ten years (Topham, 2018).

Many local authorities have tried to implement innovative rural transport solutions, with some success, but have been hampered by a combination of a more adversarial marketplace following deregulation and the constraints of the procurement regime. Dorset County Council sought to build on a successful tradition of collaborative public private partnerships in civil engineering design and construction by seeking to procure transport partners in a major reprocurement exercise in 2010 (Ayre, 2016b).

Dorset sought to procure arrangements that incentivised a collaborative approach with its transport operators, but when portfolios of routes were awarded, anti-competitive activity was prompted. Previously subsidised routes were suddenly declared profitable by incumbent operators to keep out the competition. The council had anticipated this in part, and included a variation clause in the contract to enable it to respond by the flexible reallocation of routes to successful partners. Unfortunately, when it came to the application of this clause, EU regulations were quoted as the obstacle, even though it was in response to anti-competitive activity by the market and supported by the Competition Commission (now the Competition and Markets Authority). There followed a period of market turbulence as successful operators were excluded from some public transport routes, causing them to withdraw from complementary home to school transport routes. This contributed in part to major service failures at the beginning of the new school term. Once the competition had withdrawn, public transport operators gave notice that the routes were no longer profitable and needed subsidy to be reintroduced or they would cease operations. This put increased pressure on the council's transport budgets.

The stated intention of EU procurement regulations is to encourage competition, but like many regulations, the law of unintended consequences ends up taking precedence. In Dorset's case, instead of providing the council with the tools it needed to confront anti-competitive activity by the market, it became an obstacle to any effective response. Instead of rewarding collaborative behaviour and supporting the council's attempts to change the culture of the market, adversarial behaviour proved to be a successful strategy for the operators. Those operators who had bought into the collaborative vision of the council felt let down and lost faith in the council's abilities to incentivise innovation. Effort and resources of public and private sectors became deployed on non-productive activities, and service failures prompted a blame game instead of joint problem-solving and innovation to improve transport services for the people of Dorset.

Although much was done to recover the situation, thanks to the hard work of the council's staff and operators, a major opportunity was missed to transform the transport market to one focused on the needs of isolated communities.

Conclusion

The way that governments, businesses and wider society interrelate at local, national and international level can determine the success or failure of economies and the health, wellbeing and quality of life of communities. The case needs to made for greater partnership working between nations, public and private sectors, different public bodies and between private sector organisations. Evidence needs to be gathered to show that partnerships can make a positive contribution to the health, wellbeing and quality of life of communities.

Health inequalities and the social determinants of health are major societal challenges. Can public and third-sector organisations form successful partnerships to address some or all of the social determinants, or should this be left to the market? It is clear that market forces alone cannot address the social determinants of health. The provision of affordable housing is a case in point. It is self-evident that the market alone cannot build viable homes that are affordable for the poorest in society who cannot afford to buy or rent them. Without some form of social intervention, either through the planning system or the building of homes for social rent, the market cannot tackle homelessness or deliver homes that are safe and healthy for some of society's most vulnerable citizens. Having said this, the UK cannot build sufficient homes for its needs without the housebuilding and construction industry, and it is only through greater collaboration between public and private sectors that high quality, sustainable housing can be delivered which meets the diverse needs of communities.

Rigorous academic research on the benefits of partnering to organisations, societies and between countries is limited. That is why several contributors to this publication, together with a group of academic institutions, are working to establish the Centre for Partnering (see Chapter 10). The partners are committed to building a consortium of academic institutions that will design and deliver a comprehensive research programme to compile the evidence necessary in order to deliver innovative and successful approaches to partnering.

Evidence is needed to fill the policy vacuum. Responses to the failure of Carillion and the crisis in outsourcing have been largely technical. A bolder approach is necessary to work with public and private sectors to develop and implement successful partnering alternatives to the outsourcing of public services. The growing catalogue of outsourcing failures in construction, probation, rail franchising, health and social care is creating an appetite for change, and the exit of the UK from the EU provides the opportunity. It is for local and central government working with academic institutions to grasp this opportunity to pilot new and more innovative approaches to the delivery of public services through collaborative partnerships between public, private and third-sector organisations.

References

Ayre, D.N. (1998) 'Environmental services best value proposal'. Dorset County Council.

Ayre, D.N. (2016a) 'The political environment', in R. Smith and A. Sparke (eds), *Engaging with Success*, pp 7–18, London: PSP Publishing.

Ayre, D.N. (2016b) 'PSP Dorset LLP', in R. Smith and A. Sparke (eds), *Engaging with Success*, pp 53–61, London: PSP Publishing.

Barton, C. (2018) 'Private rented housing: what are conditions like?' House of Commons Library. Available from: https://commonslibrary. parliament.uk/social-policy/housing/private-rented-housing-what-are-conditions-like [Accessed 14 May 2020].

BBC (2019) 'Rising knife crime linked to council cuts study suggests'. Available from: https://www.bbc.co.uk/news/uk-48176397 [Accessed 14 May 2020].

BMA (British Medical Association) (2017). 'Brexit briefing – competition and procurement in the healthcare system'. Available from: https://archive.bma.org.uk/collective-voice/influence/europe/brexit/bma-brexit-briefings/competition-and-procurement [Accessed 10 April 2020].

CCN (County Councils Network) (2019) 'Special educational needs and disabilities: the challenge facing county authorities'. Available from: http://www.countycouncilsnetwork.org.uk/download/2314 [Accessed 14 May 2020].

CCS (Crown Commercial Services) (2016) 'A brief guide to the 2014 EU public procurement directives'. Available from: https://assets.publishing.service.gov.uk/government/uploads/system/uploads/attachment_data/file/560261/Brief_Guide_to_the_2014_Directives_Oct_16.pdf [Accessed 14 May 2020].

Clark, T. and Dilnot, A. (2002) 'Long term trends in British taxation and spending', Institute for Fiscal Studies (IFS). Available from: https://election2017.ifs.org.uk/bns/bn25.pdf [Accessed 14 May 2020].

CE (Constructing Excellence) (2004) 'Demonstrating excellence'. Available from: https://constructingexcellence.org.uk/wp-content/uploads/2015/03/demonstrating_exc.pdf [Accessed 14 May 2020].

Crawford, R., Stoye, G. and Zaranko, B. (2018) 'The impact of cuts to social care spending on the use of accident and emergency services in England', Institute for Fiscal Studies (IFS). Available from: https://www.ifs.org.uk/publications/13071 [Accessed 14 May 2020].

Dahlgren, G. and Whitehead, M. (1991) 'The social determinants of health model' Available from: https://www.researchgate.net/figure/Dahlgren-and-Whitehead-1991-model-of-the-determinants-of-health_fig1_303321662 [Accessed 14 May 2020].

DHCLG (Department for Housing, Communities and Local Government) (2016) 'English housing survey 2015 to 2016 – private rented sector'. Available from: https://www.gov.uk/government/statistics/english-housing-survey-2015-to-2016-private-rented-sector [Accessed 14 May 2020].

Egan, J. (1998) 'Rethinking construction: the report of the construction task force'. Available from: https://constructingexcellence.org.uk/wp-content/uploads/2014/10/rethinking_construction_report.pdf [Accessed 14 May 2020].

Fisher, A. (2014) *The failed experiment: and how to build an economy that works*, West Wickham: Comerford & Miller.

Glenigan (2018) 'UK industry performance report: based on the UK construction industry key performance indicators'. Available from: https://www.glenigan.com/wp-content/uploads/2018/11/UK_Industry_Performance_Report_2018_4456.pdf [Accessed 14 May 2020].

Government Commercial Function (2019) 'The outsourcing playbook: central government guidance on outsourcing decisions and contracting', London: Cabinet Office. Available from: https://assets.publishing.service.gov.uk/government/uploads/system/uploads/attachment_data/file/816633/Outsourcing_Playbook.pdf [Accessed 14 May 2020].

House of Commons (2018) 'Carillion', Business, energy and industrial strategy, and work and pensions committees. Available from: https://publications.parliament.uk/pa/cm201719/cmselect/cmworpen/769/769.pdf [Accessed 14 May 2020].

HSE (Health and Safety Executive) (2018) 'Health and safety at work summary statistics for Great Britain 2018' Available from: https://www.hse.gov.uk/statistics/overall/hssh1718.pdf [Accessed 14 May 2020].

ICE (Institution of Civil Engineers) (2017) 'From transactions to enterprises: a new approach to delivering high performing infrastructure', London: Project 13. Available from: http://www.p13.org.uk/wp-content/uploads/2018/04/From-Transactions-to-Enterprises.pdf [Accessed 14 May 2020].

Jarrett, A. (2019) 'Presentation to the CIPFA property conference – regeneration 2019', speech. 10 July, International Convention Centre, Birmingham.

Latham, M. (1994) 'Constructing the team: final report of the government/industry review of procurement and contractual arrangements in the UK construction industry'. London: Her Majesty's Stationery Office. Available from: https://constructingexcellence.org.uk/wp-content/uploads/2014/10/Constructing-the-team-The-Latham-Report.pdf [Accessed 14 May 2020].

LGA (Local Government Association) (2019) 'Health and local public health cuts', House of Commons briefings and responses, 14 May. Available from: https://www.local.gov.uk/parliament/briefings-and-responses/health-and-local-public-health-cuts-house-commons-14-may-2019 [Accessed 14 May 2020].

NAO (National Audit Office) (2018) 'Investigation into the government's handling of the collapse of Carillion', London: NAO. Available from: https://www.nao.org.uk/wp-content/uploads/2018/06/Investigation-into-the-governments-handling-of-the-collapse-of-Carillion.pdf [Accessed 14 May 2020].

NHS England (n.d.) 'What is commissioning?'. Available at: https://www.england.nhs.uk/commissioning/what-is-commissioning [Accessed 14 May 2020].

ONS (Office for National Statistics) (2019) 'Deaths related to drug poisoning in England and Wales: 2018 registrations' Available from: https://www.ons.gov.uk/peoplepopulationandcommunity/births deathsandmarriages/deaths/bulletins/deathsrelatedtodrugpoisoning inenglandandwales/2018registrations [Accessed 14 May 2020].

Smith, D. and Chamberlain, P. (2015) *Blacklisted: The Secret War between Big Business and Union Activists*, Oxford: New Internationalist.

Smith, R., Hammersley, M. and Davis, H. (eds) (2013) *Relational Partnering*, London: PSP Publishing.

Topham, G. (2018) 'Bus services in "crisis" as councils cut funding, campaigners war', *The Guardian*, 2 July. Available from: https://www.theguardian.com/uk-news/2018/jul/02/bus-services-in-crisis-as-councils-cut-funding-campaigners-warn [Accessed 14 May 2020].

Transport Select Committee (2019) 'Bus services in England outside London' Available from: https://publications.parliament.uk/pa/cm201719/cmselect/cmtrans/1425/1425.pdf [Accessed 14 May 2020].

University of Warwick (2012) 'Elected mayors and city leadership', Coventry: University of Warwick. Available from: https://warwick.ac.uk/research/warwickcommission/electedmayors/summaryreport/the_warwick_commission_on_elected_mayors_and_city_leadership_summary_report.pdf [Accessed 14 May 2020].

10

The power and value of relationships in local authorities' and central government funding encouraging culture change

Richard Smith

Introduction

This chapter describes the emergence and development of the Centre for Partnering (CfP), a think tank that has been formed to explore the role and effect of partnering between different kinds of organisations from within the public, private and voluntary sectors. The research projects that the CfP will undertake include an examination of the role that procurement and commissioning of services has played and could play in the future of partnering. The research agenda is also focused on the value of partnering as it could impact on large scale infrastructure projects where social and other community (local and national) issues are addressed. The CfP agenda also addresses 'wicked issues', as identified as part of the consideration of the social determinants of health. The focus of this research is upon the value of establishing a legal framework through which prospective partners can enter into a dialogue to build trust and a relationship ahead of formal contract relationships.

Procurement, a city council perspective

The author's history and experiences over the past 40 years in the field of partnering have been many and varied. The author was called to the Bar in 1978 and initially worked with GEC Marconi in the field of contracts tendering and monitoring for the Ministry of Defence. In 1988, he was appointed as Director of Contract Services to Portsmouth City Council, and in 1991, he was appointed the council's Head of Businesses. From 1995 to 2019, he established a new-form Public

Sector Plc (PSP). This chapter considers the various events that led to the formation of the CfP, its aim being to create a centre for excellence in research, development and implementation of innovative approaches to partnership working.

Beginning first in Marconi and then at Portsmouth City Council, over a period of seven years from 1998 to 1995, it became possible to evolve what came to be known as the Portsmouth City Business Group (PCBG). It was the culture that predominantly dictated this turn of events; indeed, the council's strapline at this time was 'Portsmouth City Council means Business'.

In 1988, the council, in response to the Local Government Act and the introduction of compulsory competitive tendering (CCT), placed an advertisement for the recruitment of a Director of Contract Services. This followed a report by the council's consultants, who had recommended the establishment of an in-house organisation to compete openly with the private arena for the retention of the manual services that were run by the Direct Services Organisation (DSO).

The consultants recommended the appointment of a director and a new management team, perhaps drawing on a combination of experienced private sector and public individuals. However, with the establishment of this new organisation came a cultural divide, with the contractor on one side and the client on the other. There was a clear division of roles and responsibilities within the council – to the point where council officers who used to work together, take holidays together and share common experiences in the delivery of public services now stood facing each other from opposite positions, the one at risk of losing their job, the other making judgements as to whether they should keep it or not.

The author, as Director of Contract Services, had to reconcile his contracted role with that of his corporate responsibility as a senior employee. This was achieved through securing six of the seven tendered services and demonstrating the savings to the council's budget that could be achieved. More than this, he demonstrated the need for a corporate strategic director – the Head of Business – who was given responsibilities for extending the remit of the contractor side of the council to areas that were not affected by CCT. In addition, it gave rise to the establishment of an internal market, which was used to refocus the council's budget setting process. It is an irony that the contract that at first was subject to the demands of the client became the strategic influencer of the client side.

In 1995, there was no private sector marketplace sophisticated enough to recognise this public sector achievement. The private sector failed to understand the differences between a form of public–private partnering where investment in resources dictated the form of legal arrangement as opposed to a contract for service based on a number of transactions. They recognised, of course, that because of CCT there was an opportunity to take over and run public services, but not that their skills and expertise could be applied more positively and strengthen the public sector's use of its own resources (HMG, 1988). It was not until this externalisation process, 1994–5, that the inadequacy of the market came to be fully recognised. Indeed, what had started as a search for a private sector long-term partner to the PCBG ended with the outsourcing of the majority of PCBG services to the market.

Ironically, the establishment of the PSP initiative led, in the author's view, to the establishment of the very organisation (PCBG) that had been sought as a private sector partner to the council's internal business group. The history of the development of PSP has been fraught with difficulties. The political environment leading up to 1997, when PSP published its first volume (PSP, 1997), was fixated upon the question of which public service better belonged in the public or private sectors.

In 2019, 15 years after the attempted partnering of the PCBG, there is still a lack of understanding of how to resolve the cultural obstacles that impede the true sense of partnering, owing to the suspicions, mistrust and lack of transparency in public–private partnership contracting regimes. Recent experiences of Carillion, and doubt over the financial competence of other major private sector companies, continues to pervade the thinking processes of both sectors (see Chapter 9). This loss of confidence in outsourcing has now caused local government to insource services that had previously been put out to tender, bringing them back under its management control.

In the author's opinion, the cultural obstacles of outsourcing are more easily dealt with prior to contract award. It does not seem helpful to place a procurement regime ahead of the need to develop relationships first – to develop a form of trust between the organisations wishing to do business with each other. PSP volumes 1–3 (Smith and Hollsworth, 2013; Smith et al, 2013; Smith and Sparke, 2016) promoted a fundamental change in thinking to the extent that a new organisational structure and process was demanded, through which blue sky thinking could progressively evolve into firm contract commitments.

Public Sector Plc (PSP)

PSP initially received government backing in 1998, when Hilary Armstrong MP, then Local Government Minister and Secretary of

State, established it as one of six new Pilot Partnership Networks (PPNs) to explore how new ideas around public–private partnering could develop under the new government 'best value' regime. With government backing for new ideas, PSP was given a boost. Even more significant, in the author's view, was the opportunity to present an alternative to outsourcing – in those days referred to by PSP as insourcing – to the select committee meeting in the House of Commons in 1998. The committee considered the differences in the two partnering regimes.

So why has all this change to partnering culture taken so long? The idea of relational partnering, as this idea of putting relationships first and contracts second came to be known, has consumed an inordinate amount of time, resources and long-standing commitment. The idea has been promoted from within the private sector and has therefore taken its place in the long list of private-sector initiatives that have been advanced over the years to improve the relationships between public and private sectors. However, the profound nature of the change being advocated through a form of relational partnering has lacked formal government backing over the years since 1998.

The Local Government Council Consortium Group

To support the development of relationships between public and private sectors, it became crucial to evolve the Local Government Council Consortium Group (LG-CCG). Initially, this began in Dudley, Dorset and Bolton. From 2011 to 2018, the LG-CCG has grown to over 20 councils. There have also been significant contributions from Cheshire West, Gateshead, Southend and Warwick. The LG-CCG, through its annual meeting, exchanged information on the individual experiences of the use of this new form of partnering. This work culminated in a proposal to develop a Commission Report (CCG, 2018) that would incorporate recommendations as to the benefits of local government making use of a new partnering alternative. It recommended that local government could develop a fourth option when considering partnering, particularly in relation to its property estate. The other three alternatives would of course continue to be available, namely adopting the status quo, utilising its own public sector funds or making use of a traditional European Union (EU) procurement process.

It is time that these cumulative experiences be promoted on a different level. The contributors to this book have all raised issues in relation to the social determinants of health and wellbeing. This chapter advocates the crucial role that the use of partnering or different organisations working more effectively together can play, providing that the cultural obstacles are overcome. In this regard, there should be more of a national debate concerning what new ideas are necessary, which structures and processes, to foster a cultural environment built upon greater trust.

If the objectives set by this book are to be recognised and acted upon, then the national debate must be properly researched and evidenced. The CfP has been established as an entity seeking to work with a number of universities across the United Kingdom (UK). The author hopes that the issues raised within this book can form part of the research programme established by the CfP in relation to improving the value of partnering. The CfP's broad aims are to examine the benefits of partnering in the context of the public and private sectors, but also to consider the workings of the public sector within itself. The workings of local government with the National Health Service (NHS), education, police and the third sectors (see Part IV of this book) must be improved. This is particularly important in dealing with the 'wicked issues' identified in Chapters 4, 10, 16 and 19.

When the author worked with GEC Marconi, much of his work related to an examination of the contract specification as compared with ongoing contractor performance. Where there were deviations from the contract specification, the company would seek variation orders. The success of this largely depended on the quality of the original Request for Quotation and its specification, linked to the company's form of tender and contact agreements. The culture was largely adversarial as far as the client and contractor were concerned.

In 1988, the author was appointed Director of Contract Services for Portsmouth City Council with responsibility for a large blue-collar manual workforce (about 1,000 employees), who were subject to the Local Government Act 1988 and required to tender in open competition with the private sector in order to retain their jobs. Experience of a contract tendering environment was essential for this post.

Over the next three years, intense negotiations followed with respect to changes to working practices and to the culture of the council organisation. A cultural division arose within the council as groups of employees came to be client or contractor. So, while one group of employees had job security in a client role, the others – those in a contractor role who were subject to the legislation – did not.

By 1991, the cultural transformation within the DSO had largely been agreed with the trades unions in the form of a number of collective agreements, albeit that the cost of securing jobs for the workforce had been the partial loss of two of the services. The result and cost savings that accrued to Portsmouth Council were welcomed, and, in 1991, the council took a further step forward in what today we would understand to be commercialisation. An organisational change resulted in the establishment of the post of Head of Businesses, who had responsibility for all the services that were provided directly to the community. The significance of this appointment was that the post holder would carry corporate and strategic responsibilities, ranking as one of the top three officers of the council.

Aside from this structural change to the organisation, following the author's appointment to the post, an additional responsibility arose to introduce a further cultural change to processes within the council; this came to be known as the internal market.

The internal market was an evolution of the idea of separation of roles into those who specified services and/or commissioned them as distinct from those who were the service deliverers. It was a cultural change that required all employees, depending upon their different roles, to question what they were doing, why they were doing it and for whom.

Compulsory competitive tendering

The advent of CCT and the Local Government Act in 1988 (see Chapter 9) forced a substantial cultural change, while the adoption of the internal market some years later was an optional strategy for the council but consolidated the change processes that had grown up with the organisation. This was particularly true when it came to defining people's roles and making them more responsive to budget-setting activities.

The Portsmouth experience (Portsmouth City Council reports to Contract Services Board 1988–95) demonstrated what was achievable through the imposition of a regime change and a more pragmatic and realistic approach to the subject of council service delivery and financial costs. It was a successful experiment in Portsmouth, but the adoption of the internal market, although much talked about in other councils, largely failed to materialise elsewhere owing to a change in government in 1997 and their new focus upon best value (see Part III introduction by Mark Cook). It was perfectly possible for different skill sets and talents to come together with a common aim of delivering more successful service outcomes for local communities. The trick was to ensure that adequate processes were in place within an integrated organisational structure.

The cultural obstacles were no more self-evident than when the PCBG sought to engage with the private sector on a different partnering baseline. The council invited the private sector to invest in the resources of the PCBG as opposed to taking over the management and delivery of the services that were undertaken by the group. This was a subtle difference but had enormous implications. The market was clearly not used to an investment-type opportunity when it came to public–private partnerships within local government. What started with good intention rapidly became beset with cultural and legal problems, with the council gradually falling back to a traditional partnering approach. In other words, the process evolved into an outsourcing of services rather than an insourcing of private sector skills and expertise to strengthen its own businesses organisation.

Despite the council organising a management and employee buyout on behalf of its workforce and an innovate investment partnership deal with Générale des Eaux in the bidding process, it did not prove possible to secure this outcome, since the evaluation criteria utilised at that time were still largely based upon cost with less focus upon future sharing of financial benefits.

The Head of Business (the author of this chapter), who had largely introduced the idea of market insourcing, using its skills and resources to strengthen the public sector, not replace it, was required to resign from the council's corporate strategic decision-making role and focus upon developing a business group proposal to the council. This resulted in the development of a management/employee buyout. This was because it was not possible to carry out two roles, one representing the council's client function and the other representing the interests of the council's contractor, as this would have led to a conflict of interest. Perhaps this was a fault within the tendering process, since it led to the exclusion of one of the council's officers who had the knowledge and skill to successfully deliver a business group that could have been invested in by the private sector.

In 1997, having recognised the inability of the private sector to offer adequate investment proposals to support a council's resources where they were labelled 'contractor'. Three publications were produced: Smith (1997), Smith et al (2013), and Smith and Hollsworth (2013). These volumes contributed to the establishment of the Public Sector Plc organisation, known as PSP. This discussion volume, involving a number of local government experts from both public and private sectors, considered issues that might arise if CCT was replaced with a new political objective. In the event, and after publication of the book, CCT was replaced by the incoming New Labour government and their introduction of the best value regime. Many of the factors that led to the unsuccessful attempt by the PCBG to establish an early form of public enterprise, blending the best of public and private sectors, were at last reconsidered within the best value initiative – albeit late in the day.

Changes in the procurement legislation

PSP was supported by New Labour in 1997 when it became one of six PPNs established by the Local Government Minister, Hilary Armstrong MP. PSP was also invited to provide evidence about the nature of 'insourcing' when compared with 'outsourcing'. This evidence was provided to the Select Committee which was meeting in 1998 to consider new options for public–private partnering. There was some political support to the idea of a market strengthening the skills and capacity within the public sector, as compared with the introduction of the market to run public services.

One of the big political issues behind 'best value' was the whole problem of employment protection and employee rights following the transfer of workforces from the public sector to the private sector, following unsuccessful tendering by local government to retain the right to continue delivering local community services. Transfer of Undertakings (Protection of Employment) Regulations were introduced in 2006 to alleviate the change process, but this in no way dealt with the disruptive impact that such a transfer of people involved. It would surely have been preferable for public workforces to remain within the public sector, as was advocated within the 'insourcing' regime upon which PSP was based.

From 1997 to 2007, the best value debate ensued. It was a time for new ideas affecting the partnering culture of organisations – be they public or private sector, or even public and private partnering with the voluntary and/or not-for-profit sectors. However, the continuing application of an EU procurement regime, together with a natural inbuilt tendency towards maintaining the status quo, impeded progress in making any fundamental change. This was further complicated by the theoretical debate that, when contemplating substantial change, there is a question over the prominence that is attached to changes to organisational structure as opposed to changes that are made to process upon which best value is based. It would have been more advantageous if, at the time of best value introduction, there had been more emphasis upon the need to make changes within organisational structures and among individuals' attitudes. How to avoid the cultural divide that was born within local government during the time of CCT, when the notion of client and contractor was first conceived, has proved a major obstacle over the years to the promotion of more strategic out-of-box thinking .

The overwhelming prominence of the best value approach to process manifested itself in four words: challenge, consult, compete and compare. PSP took a different path in 1998, advocating more change to organisational structures so the focus was much more on an organisation's ability to overcome cultural differences with other organisations through their mission statements. This applied both to public and private sectors, and focused upon a more flexible contract and legal framework that strengthened the possibility of evolving relationships ahead of contract commitments.

The structural strategy led to the establishment of PSP as an entity in its own right in 2006. This new organisation was founded upon the principles enunciated through the origins and development of the PCBG from 1991 to 1995. The company advocated a new approach to the delivery of commercial outcomes within local government. This involved discussions and negotiations with a number of 'pathfinder' councils, where the focus of partnering was based upon the establishment of a relationship between the contracting parties before legal commitments were entered into. The organisation reflected the principles raised in PSP volumes 1–3.

Relational partnering

After the publication of the first volume of PSP, there followed two further PSP publications. The second of these introduced the new concept of relational partnering. This was intended to be an alternative partnering model to that traditionally required, with the issue of a service specification and selection of potential tenderers including a 'beauty parade' before formal award of contracts and legally binding commitments. It was far better (according to PSP's argument) that where medium- to long-term business relationships were to be forged, a culture of trust and transparency of transactions should be promoted. The focus of this quasi-commercial business approach was much more focused upon both contracting parties compromising their ambitions to deliver successful community outcomes, alongside adequate profit returns. More significantly, such a partnership focused upon strengthening the overall capacity of a local authority's resources as a partner organisation, as distinct from a contractor running council services or delivering council service requirements. It is important to emphasise that this form of discussion ultimately led to a discussion about the different forms of resources, be they people, finance, property or know-how. PSP's ultimate evolution became progressively more focused on property.

Progress towards the establishment of these new forms of partnership from 2006 onwards was slow. This was primarily because of the lack of working examples of the success of the relational partnering philosophy. It proved extremely difficult for the first council to take the first step so as to give confidence to other councils to follow likewise. In 2013, PSP vol 2 focused upon six councils that had taken the first steps to applying the new relational partnering approach. Those six councils became significant pathfinders in developing the government's framework that was appropriate to this form of partnering. They were Dudley, Dorset, Bolton, Cheshire West, Southend and Warwick.

It followed from these early pioneering days that there was a mutual need to share experiences in relation to the development of the new relational partnering governance and legal framework. The six early councils met in 2013 to form the LG-CCG. The six councils were all different in terms of political complexion, size and demography, and had substantially different political aims. The linking factor with all of these authorities was that they shared a common ambition to evolve a new form of partnering and wished to share their experiences amongst each other.

The LG-CCG was a unique opportunity to study the impact of developing a new relational partnering governance framework. PSP's evolution had increasingly focused upon local government's property resource. Through the LG-CCG, it was now possible to gain an understanding of what worked and what did not. The pooling of these experiences dramatically affected the learning curve, making it easier for other councils to join the initiative.

Between 2013 and 2017, the LG-CCG met annually to consider the contribution that a more efficient and effective use of property resources could make to mitigating the impact of the government's austerity programme. During this time, the group of councils grew from six to 22.

The impact of the government's austerity programme was reflected in the following two figures. The 'Graphs of Doom' (Figures 10.1, 10.2) reflected the gap between money received by the council and likely costs of services to be provided. This heightened the importance of the debate within the LG-CCG insofar as they were seeking additional financial benefits that could be achieved from a council's property estate.

Figure 10.1: The Barnet Council 'Graph of Doom'

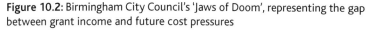

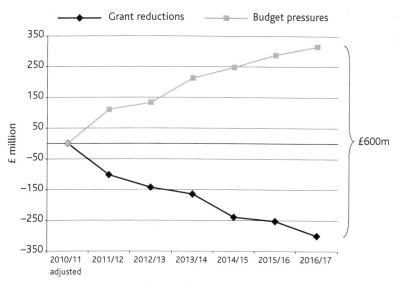

Source: Brindle, 2012

Figure 10.2: Birmingham City Council's 'Jaws of Doom', representing the gap between grant income and future cost pressures

Source: Image from Birmingham City Council

The impact of austerity had far-reaching consequences and led to a new focus on resources. Whereas previously the CCT public–private partnership was all about the transfer of public services to the market, substituting the private sector for the public sector, austerity was much more about the council's use of its resources; ironically, the PCBG externalisation process should have been about this same resources issue. It should have been how the PCBG merged its use of resources with the market, rather than giving up all its contracts and ceasing to exist.

The group meeting each year was preceded by an advisory group of senior officers who considered their council's use of the new framework in the context of its political aims and ambitions. Issues considered by the LG-CCG included the introduction of new management monitoring arrangements designed to enable members of the councils to have earlier information about the performance of their projects and the likely delivery of outcomes originally contemplated. Such a change to process was also considered alongside the change in culture within the council organisation itself. That is to say, consideration was given as to the role and value of the new legal entities (limited liability partnerships) in the council's organisational structure. The aim was to regard the partnership vehicle as a part of the council's capacity to deliver more effective resource outcomes. This objective proved extremely difficult to deliver given the necessary change to culture that was required. The initiative was hampered by a procurement culture that before the making of new contract commitments always sought a market appraisal of other private sector options, only then committing to the idea of a joint working arrangement that was designed to explore new possibilities within an informal working arrangement.

While the second PSP publication had contemplated the cultural change of placing relationships first and contracts second, the third PSP publication contemplated the establishment of the LG-CCG in a broader national perspective. This intent became manifest in 2016 when the LG-CCG and its growing number of councils proposed the establishment of a commission report to formulate recommendations for use by the rest of local government and elsewhere in the public sector.

This report was published in 2017 (CCG, 2018). It followed a consultation process involving over 100 individuals with varying experience in public–private partnering. The report recognised that all councils had three property alternatives when it came to unlocking their value. These were first, to adopt the status quo; secondly, to undertake changes to their property opportunities with their own resources, which could include prudential borrowing; or thirdly, utilise a traditional procurement route, including competitive tendering and dialogue.

The report recommended use of a fourth alternative, which had been pioneered as the relational partnering option by the LG-CCG. It contained 11 recommendations that, if accepted, would deliver additional substantial financial returns within local authorities. If the idea of relational partnering was to be promoted at this point, it was important to move beyond the realm of property alone. The original notion that lay behind the PCBG was a redefinition of structure and process that would lead to a different form of relationship between the private and public sectors. It was the importance of the value of *partnering* that should be considered, particularly in the cultural context. It became increasingly important to identify what had worked and what had not worked when it came to understanding the value of public–private partnerships. This was significantly apparent following the demise of Carillion, with all the outsourcing issues that arose when the public sector contracted out work opportunities.

It was also apparent that an exclusive focus upon resource and service financial improvements missed out on the considerable value that such partnering could bring in terms of socio-economic benefits. These benefits should be seen as important as, if not more important than, purely delivering financial outcomes. Because the Commission Report largely dealt with property benefits and its recommendations were focused on economic regeneration activities, most councils outside the LG-CCG maintained that they had their own strategies and were delivering their own satisfactory outcomes within the three property strategy alternatives already available to them, and therefore they did not see any benefit from the use of this new fourth option. It was apparent that if relational partnering could be seen to apply both to economic regeneration and to socio-economic regeneration, then recommendations in relation to it would have a wider appeal. In 2018, Professor Adrian Bonner published the predecessor to this book in which the social determinants of health (Bonner, 2018) were examined from an international perspective. The current volume is intended to develop and consider the issues raised, particularly in the context of local government and elsewhere in the public sector.

These two books raise many 'wicked issues' – those issues that are difficult to confront and give rise to difficulties that different kinds of organisation to deal with. In this context, it is apparent that the role of partnering has much to offer. This is not only the case where public and private sectors are concerned, but also in the wider realm of public sector entities working with each other and with the not-for-profit sector.

Partnering therefore has a key role to play in the delivery of socioeconomics, particularly if the social determinants of health and wellbeing are to be fully recognised and acted upon. If this is to be the case, a new form of culture that blends the best of different sector interests through an open and transparent model is required, pointing the way to an opportunity to consolidate the work of the LG-CCG and establish the relational partnering option.

The Centre for Partnering

The CfP has been formed with the aim of examining the role of partnering and how it can, in different circumstances, deliver effective community outcomes (CfP, 2018).

There are four pillars upon which the CfP has been created. The first is an examination of the current evidence base for successful or unsuccessful partnering – that is, public–private sectors and, crucially, the public sector working within itself through different public agencies, such as the NHS, law enforcement, education and local government. The CfP will also examine the working relationship of all sectors with not-for-profit organisations and other third-sector organisations.

The work of the CfP is therefore clearly conducive to supporting the work of Bonner (2018, 2020) and the team of authors who have contributed to the publications. To this extent, the CfP's terms of reference have included research into those 'wicked issues' identified as having a major impact on delivering socio-economic benefits to local communities.

The work of the LG-CCG in the bringing together and partnering of the different local councils will be crucial to the CfP, particularly since one of the aims is to explore the value that can be added by the academic sector. The CfP therefore comprises a network of universities of different types, based in different regions of the country and with different academic skill sets. Discussions in relation to the setting up of the CfP have so far involved Stirling, Manchester Metropolitan, Northumbria, Oxford (the Blavatnik School of Government) and Cardiff universities, although these are early days for the development of such an academic network. All these universities have contributed chapters to this book.

Perhaps one of the most important elements of the work of the CfP (as with the LG-CCG) is to agree a common research aim based upon examining the cultural obstacles that impact on partnering. When it comes to public–private partnering, and in the wake of the Carillion experience, it is important that the CfP carefully selects private sector partners who share the same socio-economic agenda. In this regard, the CfP working with universities is determining the selection criteria for private sector companies – particularly the first half-dozen companies that are likely to represent different market sectors. A likely focus for the CfP will be a selection of private sector interests that are prepared to work with and strengthen the capacity of the public sector.

In summary, it is interesting to note how the evolution of relational partnering as an idea has come about. It is unfortunate that in the days of the PCBG, the private sector found the idea of insourcing their skills and resources as a form of investment proposal, hard to understand. It was even more apparent that the legal framework around which the Portsmouth externalisation program was largely based, was rigid and inflexible. It involved a competitive commercial tendering process which was more focused on cost efficiencies and public services undertaken by the private sector than on an investment-style proposal that would maintain the need for the council's own business group.

Since 1995 and the evolution of a new form of partnering model that does not always require competitive tendering it has been possible to prove that different organisations and individuals can sit together to resolve ideological and cultural issues first. Most importantly, to gain trust in each other's partnering approach.

There is clearly however a need to address the procurement question which so often impacts on the ability of the private sector, and elsewhere in the public sector, to make flexible choices about the use of public sector funds and investment options.

The author recalls a conversation over 20 years ago with a local authority chief executive who was most interested in the offering of the private sector, but felt unable to accept it, given that it had been advanced by the private sector and had not arisen as part of a procurement and tendering process. In terms of difficulties in changing culture this issue still exists, with the public sector finding it hard to accept an unsolicited proposal from the market. There is too much of 'How do they know the proposition is best value without a market appraisal?' Surely the question should be why such a competitive appraisal is necessary if the unsolicited proposal can demonstrably deliver best value.

On 5 September 2019, in the House of Lords, a group of academics, professionals and business leaders came together to begin the process of investigating the benefits to the health, economic and social wellbeing of communities that can be achieved by partnering between public, private and third-sector organisations. The event heralded the setting up of a new think tank, the CfP. This involves the cooperation of a number of universities that represent different regions of the UK.

This CfP Group currently exchanges information and is involved in the establishment of the research projects. The CfP Group is currently planning an Economic and Social Research Council proposal for submission at the end of the year.

Conclusion

In order to ensure that market issues are properly addressed, the CfP Group is embarking upon a private sector selection process. It is an aim of the CfP to find longer-term business partners, of different sizes and cultural experiences, representing different market sectors. As part of this process, a 'debate' day is being organised to explore the various public–private sector experiences and the obvious improvements that could be made to the procurement regulatory and project design and implementation priorities. A long list of organisations to be invited is currently being compiled.

The very important issue of cultural differences needs to be recognised. There are cultural obstacles within all sectors and between them. This is true within public-to-public sector activity (local government and the NHS in the field of care, for example) and within and in conjunction with the private sector, where the profit motive sometimes conflicts with a social and more community-driven ambition.

The CfP has at its core the need to address the forming of productive and trustworthy relationships before business is transacted. The research projects address this point in particular. Organisations and individuals are often too steeped in their own cultural environments to consider stepping out of the box. One example with which to conclude concerns the need for the elderly to have proper heating within their homes, which the author recalls from a discussion in relation to public sector budgeting. The budget to provide heating in council houses would need to come from a local authority, yet the benefits to the NHS in terms of the elderly population not falling ill are obvious. There should be more focus on the partnering objectives of both these organisations when it comes to simple proposals that would improve social wellbeing within local communities.

References

Bonner, A. (ed) (2018) *Social Determinants of Health: An Interdisciplinary Approach to Social Inequality and Wellbeing*, Bristol: Policy Press.

Bonner, A. (ed) (2020) *Local authorities and Social Determinants of Health*. Bristol: Policy Press.

Brindle, D. (2012) 'Graph of doom: a bleak future for social care services', *The Guardian*, 15 May. Available from: https://www.theguardian.com/society/2012/may/15/graph-doom-social-care-services-barnet [Accessed 15 May 2020].

CfP (Centre for Partnering) (2018) Report. October (v37).

CCG (Council Consortium Group Report) (2018) 'Putting relationships first … an exploration into the benefits of the relational partnering model', PSP report for local government. London: CCG.

HMG (1988) 'Local Government Act'. Available from: http://www.legislation.gov.uk/ukpga/1988/9/contents [Accessed 20 April 2020].

Smith, R. (ed) (1997) 'A discussion paper exploring a new form of public services company', vol. 1, Public Sector PLC. London: Local Government Communications.

Smith, R., Hammersley, M. and Davis, H. (eds) (2013) *Relational Partnering*, vol. 2, London: PSP Publishing.

Smith, R. and Hollsworth, A. (eds) (2013) 'A synopsis of PSPS volume 1 – a discussion paper exploring a new form of public services company', London: PSP Publishing.

Smith, R. and Sparke, A. (2016) *Engaging with Success*, vol. 3. London: PSP Publishing.

11

The challenges facing local authorities in supporting children and families

Gayle Munro and Keith Clements

Introduction

Younger members of our communities and their families have been particularly affected by austerity measures and the associated impact upon the provision of services by local government. There is significant variation across the country in terms of thresholds for accessing social care and support provided by local authorities, with increasing expectations on the voluntary sector to fill any gaps, against a backdrop of cuts to commissioned statutory services and a heightened call upon the availability of funding via trusts and foundations. This chapter discusses some of the challenges for local authorities providing services to children, young people and their families within such a context, the impact upon the health of those young people seeking support and the intersection with the work of the voluntary sector.

This discussion draws upon the research and policy work of the National Children's Bureau (NCB), which works with children, young people and their families through research, advocacy, the delivery of training and the facilitation of learning and development across a range of child-focused programmes. The overall aim of the body of work across the fields of early years, education, health and participation is to support those who work with children and young people to achieve better outcomes and a better childhood for all children. This chapter provides a brief outline of some of the background to the financial pressures under which services find themselves working before focusing on some of the implications for social care and health outcomes for children and young people. (The authors are writing in a personal capacity and, while drawing on the work of NCB, the discussion in this chapter does not represent the official position of the NCB.)

Funding of services

The relationship between the provision of statutory and non-statutory services in the United Kingdom (UK) is complex and the voluntary sector is not always as 'non-governmental' as the name would suggest. Many large non-governmental organisations (NGOs) that have national reach are able to carry out their work because they have been awarded contracts via different central government departments to run programmes aimed at separate sets of beneficiaries or service users, usually categorised by support need. The demarcation between statutory and non-statutory services is therefore not always as unambiguous as might immediately appear to a member of the general public, who may not expect such a blurred relationship between a charity that he/she has chosen to support and the government of the day. A review of the financial returns to the Charity Commission (the regulator of charities across England and Wales) also illustrates a degree of opacity around the detail of the funding of individual charities. For example, some returns include a reference to government grants in their official returns, but they do not always provide any more detail around the type of funding and area allocated; others simply make a distinction between 'restricted' and 'unrestricted' funds (the distinction being funds that come with stipulations around how the money is to be spent, versus money that can be spent more freely), without indicating the exact source of income.

The extent to which the voluntary sector relies on governmental sources of funding becomes a particularly relevant issue for the sustainability of an NGO (and is ultimately of importance to the recipients of services run by a charity) at two key junctures. The first of these is when the relationship between the charitable organisation and the government of the day is wedded to the particular political party in power. A change in government can have a disastrous impact upon a charity that has heavily relied upon its relationship with a particular political party to fund its services. Support providers become particularly at risk when they might be considered as a 'nice to have' service rather than one that the government has a statutory duty of care to provide. The second point at which the government-funded elements of non-statutory services are at significant risk are in times of state-mandated austerity programmes.

In 2009, the British government announced a series of austerity measures aimed at curbing spending across the welfare state, ostensibly with the ultimate goal of reducing the national debt. Across 2017 and 2018 the Local Government Association and a number of children's charities have produced reports and briefings aimed at highlighting and drawing attention to the impact of funding cuts to frontline services on vulnerable children, young people and their families. In 2016, Action for Children, NCB and the Children's Society published 'Turning the Tide' (Action for Children et al, 2016), which illustrated how local authority children's services had been driven by cuts in funding to 'crisis-driven firefighting'.

Particular casualties of the cuts have been early intervention support services for families in need of help, with a subsequent knock-on effect upon increased levels of demand in crisis care further up the spectrum of support needs.

Accessing social care services

In 2017, the NCB, via its work with the All-Party Parliamentary Group for Children (a group of Members of Parliament representing different political parties and members of the House of Lords who have made a commitment to taking action on improving policy affecting children and young people), carried out an inquiry into the resourcing of children's social services, bringing together evidence about changes in the nature and level of demand, with the aim of improving understandings of the challenges facing under-performing children's services and how to address them. The inquiry, which resulted in the publication of the 'No Good Options' report (NCB, 2017), highlighted the reduction in local authority resource allocation towards children and families in need of early intervention support. The evidence showed that support was more heavily weighted towards services that provide crisis interventions where needs have often escalated significantly.

A survey of directors of children's services carried out by the inquiry found that 89 per cent reported finding it increasingly challenging to fulfil their statutory duties under Section 17 of the Children's Act in the five years leading up to the inquiry. Where children were in touch with services, interventions were focused more on child protection concerns, rather than on identifying and responding to a broad range of needs.

The report of the inquiry highlighted how local authorities were facing a 'perfect storm' of increased demand set against reduced resources. The inquiry heard a wide range of possible explanations for increases in demand. These included increasing numbers of children who were vulnerable or at risk from female genital mutilation, gang violence, child sexual exploitation and radicalisation, and increasing numbers of unaccompanied children seeking asylum. It also included concerns that perceived increases in child poverty and cuts to early intervention services were leading to more children being at risk from mental illness, substance abuse and domestic violence. Other submissions suggested the data could be explained by better identification, rather than an actual increase in the number of children at risk.

'No Good Options' included a number of case studies that illustrated the challenges facing families trying to access appropriate mental health support for their children and the difficulties experienced by families of children with disabilities who were struggling to access respite and other local authority help. One mother shared her experience of how the services her family received had changed over time:

> The catastrophic cuts to funding leave us families with less and less support. They leave families struggling to get even a minimum of intervention that might help secure them greater independence and wellbeing later in life.

As a follow-up to the 'No Good Options' inquiry, NCB carried out a second inquiry in 2018, this time with a focus on whether thresholds for accessing social care support varied across the country and the extent to which thresholds for support are linked to available resources. The findings of this inquiry were detailed in 'Storing up Trouble: a postcode lottery of children's social care' (NCB, 2018a). The methods adopted across the inquiry included the facilitation of parliamentary evidence sessions, which took oral evidence from local children's service leaders, children and young people, social workers, teachers, academics, the Children's Commissioner and the Parliamentary Under-Secretary of State for Children and Families; a survey of Directors of Children's Services (DCSs) in England; a survey of social workers in England; and an analysis of a sample of Local Safeguarding Children Boards' threshold documents, which outline the criteria for referring a child to a local authority for assessment and provision of services.

Elements of the inquiry were structured around and reflected the levels of support available via children's social care. The analysis of local authority threshold documents describes four levels of intervention, depending on the intensity of support required. Level A is where early help is recommended but this is to be led by universal services without support from children's social care. The next level up (Level B) is also classed as early help, but this involves some kind of advice, coordination or additional service from children's social care. Level C is when a child is considered potentially a 'child in need' and should be referred to children's social care for assessment and support under Section 17 of the Children Act. Level D is the highest level of support available, which involves an urgent referral to children's social care, so that Section 47 inquiries, child protection plans and/or emergency accommodation (Section 20) orders can be considered. The findings of the inquiry highlighted the confusion around the language and terminology associated with 'early help', sometimes even within a single local authority's children's services department. Again, this confusion around what exactly is meant by 'early help' can be read against a backdrop of a reduction in spending associated with early intervention services of 40 per cent between 2010/11 and 2015/16, while spending on acute statutory services increased by 7 per cent over the same period (Action for Children et al, 2016). The inquiry also heard that there have been cuts to the government's Early Intervention Grant of almost £500 million since 2013, with projections for funding to fall by a further £183 million by 2020.

'Storing Up Trouble' highlights how the number of children subject to a child protection plan had increased by 29.2 per cent between 2010/11 and 2015/16, compared with a backdrop of a cut in local authorities' spending power across the same time period by more than 20 per cent. The majority of social workers consulted as part of the Inquiry reported that thresholds for accessing early help and for qualifying as a 'child in need' had risen in the three years prior to the inquiry. One social worker explained how limited resources have meant that families no longer receive the support they need at an early stage, but that those families are being referred for support much later, when support needs have become more complex.

As part of the inquiry, a survey of DCSs was carried out to elicit their views on the level of need a child has to reach before he/she can access support. Through the survey responses, more than 80 per cent of DCSs said there were variations in accessing early help; almost three-quarters of respondents reported variable thresholds for 'children in need' support and almost two-thirds indicated variations for making a child subject to a child protection plan. The analysis of threshold documents found that children and young people with very similar needs or facing similar levels of risk receive different levels of intervention, depending on the local authority through which they access care. Particular variations were found to be prevalent across accessing social care support connected to domestic violence, self-harm, housing and bullying.

More than 90 per cent of DCSs surveyed reported that it had become more difficult for children's social care teams to fulfil their duties and responsibilities to 'children in need' in the three years before the inquiry. Reasons attributed to these challenges included a 'rising demand in services' (91 per cent), 'more complex cases involving vulnerable children and families' (90 per cent), 'availability of appropriate services' (73 per cent) and 'reduction in resource' (69 per cent). Crucially, 66 per cent of lead members for children's services did not think their local authority had sufficient funding to provide universal services for children and families. One DCS commented on the impact that austerity has had on outcomes for children, as the sector as a whole struggles to meet the demand for support:

> The impact of austerity on other partners as well as the local authority – schools, health services, police and others means that every service is stretched beyond their full capacity; while demand has risen in our area this is not at the level it was three years ago but the complexity of the needs is increasing. The ability of all to intervene early and provided a comprehensive range of support and services is compromised and is one of the reasons behind an increase in numbers of children in care. (Director of Children's Services)

Variations and finance

One of the aims of the inquiry was to investigate whether inconsistent and rising thresholds could in part be explained by differences in the availability of resources across local authorities. The inquiry received evidence that 60 per cent of front-line practitioners reported that financial worries and availability of resources were influencing decisions to intervene in supporting children and families who need help. The evidence was particularly compelling in relation to the provision of early help and support for 'children in need' under Section 17.

The inquiry was told by 40 per cent of councillors who are lead members for children's services that a lack of resources prevented them from meeting at least one of their statutory duties for children. One of the academics whose work fed into the inquiry, Professor Paul Bywaters, highlighted how deprivation factors at a smaller level than at the local authority can also have an impact. Deprivation across areas is measured at different regional scales and captured via the Indices of Multiple Deprivation (the method used by the government to measure deprivation by collecting data on small areas on a range of different indicators, including housing, education, crime and health).

Bywaters referred to the 'inverse intervention law' that he saw in his work comparing children in similarly deprived neighbourhoods in local authorities from both ends of the 'high–low' spectrum. Local authorities where there are overall lower levels of deprivation are intervening more than 50 per cent more often than local authorities with high levels of deprivation.

Those frontline practitioners who responded to the survey of social workers carried out as part of the inquiry clearly articulated how the variations in thresholds between local authorities can be attributed to financial decisions. The following citations were all made by social workers of varying degrees of experience as responses to the NCB survey carried out as part of the inquiry:

> it varies dramatically from borough to borough in London and means some children are supported while others are not. It seems this can be due to costs and finances.

> [The] opinion of skilled social workers with knowledge of the family is considered less important than financial implication for authority.

The widening gap between the demand for support and the ability of those services to respond was highlighted by a number of respondents, with high caseloads referred to by many:

> Children's services are in crisis in my view. The budget does not reflect the level of need.

> If I do not make our quotas set forth by the senior management, I/we receive reprimands. I am caught in an unethical situation pushing profit over the child's true requirements.

> The system and the people are cracking.

Several respondents referred to the impact that higher thresholds are having on voluntary sector agencies, which are being asked to step into the gap in services for those children and young people whose circumstances don't meet the increasingly high thresholds for support. The pressure placed upon charitable organisations when statutory agencies struggle to meet the demand has also been illustrated in other research. In 2018, NCB was commissioned by Hospice UK and

Together for Short Lives to carry out research into hospice provision and palliative care services for children and young people across the UK (NCB, 2018b). This research highlighted the pressure placed upon voluntary sector organisations as a result of funding cuts within the National Health Service (NHS). A number of participants in that research also emphasised the greater demand placed on non-statutory services when staffing recruitment and retention rates within the NHS impact upon front-line service delivery. One survey respondent who participated in the research said:

> The voluntary sector to date has not been included effectively in overarching long tern health service work force planning. It is imperative that this changes going forward as a significant amount of health care is provided by the voluntary and other third sector providers and this sector will struggle to compete with an equally challenged NHS for a shrinking nursing workforce. As a children's hospice we cannot compete fully with the full range of the NHS pay bands and unsocial hours payments and over the last two years this has significantly affected our ability to recruit and retain experienced nurses. (Hospice worker and survey respondent)

Regarding the social care inquiry and 'Storing up Trouble', the effect of rising thresholds on early intervention services was a theme that ran across much of the evidence gathered:

> The thresholds have increased to such a degree that social work is now effectively crisis management, preventative work and 'early help' still remains extremely limited, very difficult to access and the referral process is confusing and acceptance very selective.

> 'Child In Need' services have been significantly impacted on by the reduction in funding and provisions. There are next to no services now available to help support families in the community in order to help them avoid escalating. For example there are currently no perpetrator courses for [domestic violence] in the locality.

> We have increasingly found that there is no longer a 'child in need'. Rather there are cases that have to close or that

they go to court/child protection. We do not have the resources or finances. We our heavily stretched and there is a serious crisis, despite great work by all.

The ways in which services across local authorities and the children's sector as a whole are often segregated by support need is not always helpful in taking a holistic view of the needs of children, young people and their families. However, the intersection between health outcomes (both physical and mental health) and supporting children in need of protection was highlighted across the breadth of evidence heard by the inquiry. One social worker commented on the intersectionality of child protection at different stages, wellbeing and the transition from childhood into adolescence:

we find children stepped down [from Children in Need] to Early Help will later 'bounce back' as Child Protection cases in their teens when they become beyond parental control, engage in criminality or suffer mental and emotional ill-health as a result of persistent and chronic relationship difficulties within their families.

And as these young people transition into adulthood, crisis services within adult social care will also be impacted by a lack of early intervention support for younger people.

Disparities in health outcomes

In 2014, along with the Royal College of Paediatrics and Child Health and the British Association for Child and Adolescent Public Health, NCB published 'Why Children Die' (Wolfe et al, 2014). The report highlighted the progress that had been made in reducing child mortality in the decades prior to the release of the report. However, it also showed that children from poorer families are more likely to die before their 18th birthday than their wealthier peers, and that mortality rates are significantly higher in the UK than across some areas in Europe. The report highlighted, for instance, that if the UK had the same all-cause mortality rate for children under 14 years as Sweden, there would be nearly 2,000 fewer deaths among children in that age group per year – five fewer deaths per day. Many of these preventable deaths would be in the pre-school years – at the time the report was published, 1,500 children between one month and four years old died every year in the UK.

NCB's 'Poor Beginnings' study (NCB, 2015) was published at a time when responsibility for public health outcomes was moving to the remit of local authorities and aimed to explore some of the variations in health outcomes across the country. The study's overall finding was that 'simply by growing up in a certain part of England a child under five is more likely to have poor health that will impact the rest of their lives'. 'Poor Beginnings' focused on four key areas of young children's health and wellbeing: obesity, tooth decay, injury and 'school readiness', and illustrated some of the stark differences in outcomes across these areas, depending on where in the country the child was living.

The study found that some regions performed very differently across the four health-related outcomes. However, the North-West region reported consistently poor outcomes across the four categories. Overall, the South-East had the best outcomes for early childhood obesity, tooth decay, injury and development, while the North-West had consistently poor results. If the North-West had the same early childhood outcomes as the South-East, then the North-West region would have 19 per cent fewer obese four- to five-year-olds, equating to more than 1,600 fewer children; 43 per cent fewer five-year-olds with tooth decay, equivalent to 11,000 fewer children; 31 per cent fewer children under the age of five admitted to hospital with an injury (2,500 children a year) and 11 per cent more children with a 'good' level of development by the end of reception class (5,500 more children).

There were even greater levels of variation in children's outcomes across local authorities. A five-year-old in Leicester, for example, is five times more likely to have tooth decay than a five-year-old growing up in West Sussex. The proportion of young children who are obese ranges from 5.5 per cent in Richmond upon Thames (west London) to 14.2 per cent in Barking and Dagenham (east London). The proportion of young children with tooth decay ranges from 9.5 per cent in West Sussex to 51 per cent in Leicester. The proportion of young children who suffer an injury serious enough to be admitted to hospital ranges from 67.6 per 10,000 in Westminster to 316.4 per 10,000 on the Isle of Wight. A young child on the Isle of Wight is therefore over four times more likely to be admitted to hospital with an injury than one of their peers in Westminster. The proportion of children who are developing well and ready for school by the age of five ranges from 75.3 per cent in Lewisham to 41.2 per cent in Leicester.

Data reviewed as part of the research for 'Poor Beginnings' illustrated how young children growing up in deprived areas are more likely than those living in more affluent areas to suffer from poor health and development. However, poor outcomes in deprived areas are not inevitable. Some local authorities with high levels of deprivation buck the trend, with average or better outcomes for young children.

Overall, the data illustrated the potential impact on children and young people that could be achieved through less disparity in health outcomes across local authorities. If all local authority areas had the same outcomes as the least deprived fifth, across England there would be a 16 per cent reduction in cases of obesity in reception class, equivalent to 10,000 fewer obese children; an 11 per cent reduction in the number of children under five admitted to hospital with an injury, equating to 5,000 fewer cases of early childhood injury; and 26 per cent reduction in the number of five-year-olds with tooth decay (35,000 fewer children with poor dental health). However, the difference in outcomes related to school readiness are not so stark. The difference between the local authorities on either end of the spectrum of deprivation amount to a 3 per cent difference in children achieving a good level of development, amounting to nearly 12,000 more children better prepared for school.

Current (and future) political climate

The United Nations' Special Rapporteur on extreme poverty and human rights, Professor Philip Alston, reported on his visit to the UK on 18 November 2019 with a searing assessment of the circumstances for those living in poverty, destitution and unable to afford basic essentials. The report attributes the growth in food banks and increasing levels of rough-sleeping and homelessness directly to the 'gutting' of local authority services by a series of central government policies rooted within austerity measures. The situation for children vis-à-vis poverty is highlighted through his citing of the Institute for Fiscal Studies, which predicts a rise in child poverty of 7 per cent by 2022, and reference to 'other sources' that predict child poverty rates as high as 40 per cent. He concludes: 'for almost one in every two children to be poor in twenty-first century Britain is not just a disgrace, but a social calamity and an economic disaster, all rolled into one' (Alston, 2018).

Alston describes what he and his team witnessed as part of his visit across the UK: 'great misery has also been inflicted unnecessarily, especially on the working poor, on single mothers struggling against mighty odds, on people with disabilities who are already marginalized, and on millions of children who are being locked into a cycle of poverty from which most will have great difficulty escaping.' The response from the British government is described in the report as being an actor that has 'stubbornly resisted seeing the situation for what it is' and has 'remained determinedly in a state of denial'.

The backdrop to the austerity measures and cuts in local authority funding has been a period of significant political uncertainty, following repeated failed attempts by the British government to negotiate its way through Brexit and the machinations of Britain leaving the European Union (EU). At the time of writing, there was still considerable uncertainty as to the practical impacts of Brexit on children and families. However, there is little doubt that domestic policies (which may, at first glance, seem not to be directly related to Brexit) have been subject to delays and diversion since the vote to leave the EU in June 2016. Government resources have been redeployed to dealing with Brexit-related issues at the expense of other work, and policy development has been subject to periods of limbo and delay while Brexit-related decisions are being negotiated.

Researchers have been documenting the impact that Brexit is having and is likely to have on families in Britain – with a focus on those where one or more parent is an EU national. The University of Birmingham's 'EU families and Eurochildren in Brexiting Britain' project highlights how the Brexit process has produced a 'stark "us and them" narrative', and through the study aims to 'portrait the emergence of a new politics of belonging which reconfigures discursively and legally who belongs to a post-EU Britain'.[1] Many of the families whose experiences are documented as part of the project refer to the impact of such an enforced period of limbo and uncertainty on their plans for the future, their careers, their children's education, their family dynamics and their mental health. The Children's Legal Centre, run by children's charity Coram, has produced a series of briefings documenting the likely impact of Brexit on children's rights in Britain. These briefings have particularly highlighted the complexity faced by some families in seeking settlement rights, the risks faced by those children who may find themselves 'undocumented' in a post-EU Britain and the effects of such an uncertain future on those children and young people who are required to prove that they have the right to remain in the UK.[2]

Alston's report comments on the links between Brexit and poverty: 'anyone concerned with poverty in the UK has reason to be very deeply concerned' (Alston, 2018). The prolonged period of uncertainty related to the Brexit process is likely to have a profound impact upon rates of economic growth, and Alston predicts that the impacts will be disproportionately felt in deprived areas and by the most vulnerable and marginalised, including children and young people.

Conclusion

The weight of evidence from those working at the service delivery end of children's support suggests that vulnerable children, young people, their families and those who work with them are increasingly battling against a 'perfect storm' of cuts in services and increased pressures. The analogy of a 'battle', 'fight' or a 'struggle' is one that has run as a thread throughout much of the research and policy work carried out with those involved in the children's support sector in the UK. Families are in the position of having to battle to gain the support they need for their children against increasingly pared down services; and service providers are having to fight to gain the resources they need to meet the demand for their support. The cuts to early intervention services are already having a significant impact on families who are only able to access support when they reach crisis point. But as the young people in those families transition into adulthood (and may have families themselves), this fight will intensify and the fires will be increasingly difficult to battle against. A longer-term view on the funding of children's services now along with greater investment in the future would help to alleviate some of the burden on both support providers and those who need them throughout the life course.

Notes

[1] University of Birmingham, 'EU families and Eurochildren in Brexiting Britain', project information. Available from: https://eurochildren.info/ [Accessed August 2019].

[2] Coram Children's Legal Centre, 'Brexit and children's rights'. Available from: https://www.childrenslegalcentre.com/promoting-childrens-rights/policy/brexit-childrens-rights/ [Accessed August 2019].

References

Action for Children, National Children's Bureau and The Children's Society (2016) 'Turning the tide: reversing the move to late intervention spending in children and young people's services', London.

Alston, P. (2018) 'Statement on visit to the United Kingdom by Professor Philip Alston, United Nations special rapporteur on extreme poverty and human rights'. Available from: https://www.ohchr.org/EN/NewsEvents/Pages/DisplayNews.aspx?NewsID=23881&LangID=E [Accessed August 2019].

NCB (National Children's Bureau) (2015) 'Poor beginnings: health inequalities among young children across England', London.

NCB (National Children's Bureau) (2017) 'No good options: report of the inquiry into children's social care in England', National Children's Bureau and the All-Party Parliamentary Group for Children, London.

NCB (National Children's Bureau) (2018a) 'Storing up trouble: a postcode lottery of children's social care', National Children's Bureau and the All-Party Parliamentary Group for Children, London.

NCB (National Children's Bureau) (2018b) 'Children's palliative care and children's hospice provision in the UK', Hospice UK and Together for Short Lives.

Wolfe, I., Macfarlane, A., Donkin, A., Marmot, M. and Viner, R. (2014) 'Why children die: death in infants, children and young people in the UK', Royal College of Paediatrics and Child Health, National Children's Bureau, British Association for Child and Adolescent Public Health.

12

The cost of care if you don't own your home

Glenda Roberts

Introduction

A major theme throughout this book is the range of issues that local councils are faced with at a time of austerity and socio-economic drivers, such as the cost of housing and the demographic changes relating to people living longer. Although advancements in health care have increased longevity, a long life can add more years of disabilities and poor wellbeing. The social gradient described by Marmot (2010) emphasises that those who are most socially deprived have poor health, not only as a result of lack of resources (for example, accommodation, heat and food) but also because of feelings of worthlessness and low self-esteem.

Accommodation in the later years of life can be problematic for some, particularly for those without a supportive family and social network. In Chapter 7, we read that a major concern for councils in the North-East is the increasing health costs of people who, in retirement, move into low-cost housing areas where they can be mortgage free. The aggregation of increasing numbers of people with health needs relating to ageing and poor lifestyle choices is placing significant health costs in those localities already challenged by poor economic growth.

Successful ageing is good for individuals and their communities; however, the cost of care in old age can be profoundly influenced by housing provision. This chapter addresses the complex set of issues when a person does not own their home.

It has been acknowledged and debated for a long time that the social care funding system is not fit for purpose (Blake, 2011), and in its current form is untenable both monetarily and politically (Green, 2019). At the Labour Party conference in 1997, Tony Blair said 'I don't want [our children] brought up in a country where the only way pensioners can get long-term care is by selling their home' (Bottery et al, 2018, p 7). The focus of the funding debate continues to be on these individuals who do own their own home and how they make a valuable contribution to maintaining the current system (Blake 2011; Bottery et al, 2018). There is consideration that this system is unfair on individuals who are deemed to have provided for their future (CFCS, 2011; Green, 2019), but little consideration of the implications for individuals who, whether through choice or circumstance, have no assets to use towards the cost of their care (TSA, 2018). Despite one in four people over the age of 75 not owning their own home (TSA, 2018), they have been largely ignored as part of the deliberations. Disappointingly, the interpretation of what is fair seems based on what can be contributed in financial terms. Unfairness should also be measured morally and ethically: people who do not own their own home also face an unfair system, one of limited choice and delayed access to care (TSA, 2018).

Older age renters

The largest group of people who own their home outright are in the older age group (MHCLG, 2018). However, the growth in house prices now puts homeownership out of the reach of many typical wage earners (Melican, 2018); therefore the number of people who privately rent property has steadily climbed over the last 20 years (Shelter, 2018) and has doubled since 2002 (MHCLG, 2018), with no indication this trend will change. The increase is slower in the over 65 age group (Shelter, 2018), but, owing to the ageing population, there is a rising tide of older people renting, with one in four of the over 75s not owning a home (TSA, 2018). Social renting, as opposed to private renting, has stabilised over the last decade (MHCLG, 2018), and over 65s are the most prevalent in this group, making up 27 per cent of the market (MHCLG, 2018). The increase in renting among older people further threatens the precarious balance of the current funding model (Blake, 2011), which sees self-funding individuals accounting for 52 per cent of care home residents (LaingBuisson, 2018).

To clarify, a large proportion of older people rent property and therefore do not have assets to pay for their own care. That proportion is set to increase with an ageing population, making it incomprehensible why they are not being included as part of the debates on funding for the future. Additionally, it is difficult to understand why there has been little exploration of whether the number of people who can afford to pay for their own care, and currently subsidise the market, will fall in line with this increase in older renters.

Choice and quality

The ongoing debates about this two-tier system of funding appear to empower and give voice to people paying for care, but what, if any, are the differences in the day-to-day access to and experience of care? As discussed here, it appears this system favours those who pay for their own care and puts those who do not at a disadvantage.

First, the cost of care should be considered to understand how and why we have two levels of funding. While the cost is dependent on the type of care that is required and the location (PayingForCare, 2019), some averages can be assumed to help understand the shortfall in funding and the business implications to private care providers. It should also be noted that for ease of understanding, the chapter does not discuss National Health Service (NHS) continuing care funded placements or Free Nursing Care payments and has focused on residential care.

The average cost of care is £32,344 a year for a residential placement (PayingForCare, 2019). If this is looked at across the average length of a stay in a care home, it equates to an overall fee of £382,000 (Independent Age, 2017). The two tiers are exacerbated by the shortfall between the true cost of care and the fees paid by the local authority, which may be between £6,000 to £18,000 per placement per year depending on the variables of location and type of care (TSA, 2018). It is not the purpose of this chapter to demonise local authorities by identifying that the fees they pay do not cover the true cost of care; rather, it acknowledges the significant and unsustainable pressures they are working under (LaingBuisson, 2018).

The implications of this shortfall are that several major suppliers of residential care have withdrawn from places funded by public funds (Bottery et al, 2018). For those providers who do accept people at this rate, they will use the income generated by the self-funding individuals to subsidise the local authority rate, and will have a ratio of self-funders to local authority that must be maintained to ensure business continuity (Bottery et al, 2018).

A local authority may pay extra for a person to be near their relative (Age UK, 2019). However, this is not the experience of the author, who has seen people isolated from family in the pursuit of a placement that a local authority can afford and a fee that will be accepted by the provider. One such situation concerned a lady who had been living at home, in rented accommodation, with the support of her family and paid-for carers. She had a fall and did not return to full mobility following a hip replacement, so she was unable to access her bathroom and needed a higher level of care than was deemed safe for her at home. The lady was financially assessed and qualified for the higher level of local authority funding, but none of the care homes in her local area would take her at the fee rate the local authority was willing to offer – despite there being three care homes with vacancies within walking distance of her home. The only placement that could be found for her was 34 miles away. Both her daughters were close to her, and one of them had visited her every day when she was at home, but they were both older people and a round trip of nearly 70 miles each time they wanted to visit was not possible. This was discussed with the social worker, and family members were very vocal about how upset they were. In addition, the manager of the care home the lady was moving to had concerns, but agreed to accept her as she was being supported in an acute general hospital despite being medically fit for discharge, and it was a priority to find her an appropriate placement. The lady was admitted to the care home and found the separation from her daughters distressing. Despite being helped to use Skype and talking to them on the phone, she became anxious and fixated on her relationship with them: she became distressed each time she spoke to them, feeling that they had abandoned her. It was obvious that the lady was very unhappy and her behaviour began to deteriorate, but after a period of five weeks a placement became available in her local area. The lady was moved back and her daughters were able to visit her again. Had she been able to pay for her care, the lady could have moved into one of the three care homes local to her and avoided the disruption of having to move twice in a short period of time. She would have had the choice of three care homes, rather being told she had to go to the only one that would accept her for the fee the local authority was able to pay.

Moving into a care home is stressful for families and the individual alike, and in this instance the lady was not able to receive the reassurance and support that she required from her family. While this is an anecdotal example of the lack of choice afforded to a vulnerable older person and their family, it is not unique; and sadly, while it is the obligation of the local authority to try to provide a placement for people in the place of their choice, this may not be within the financial restraints of the standard local authority rate. To counter this, they will also provide at least one choice of a care home within their funding limit but cannot guarantee the location, owing to the limited number of care homes that offer a placement funded totally by a local authority.

This personal experience demonstrates that limited access to places offered at local authority rate not only limits the choice of care home but can also delay discharge from an acute hospital setting. If access to care is viewed at an earlier stage, prior to crisis, there also appear to be delays and inequality of access to services. There needs to be an understanding that such delays may have contributed to the crisis that led to a hospital admission. An example of this is the story of an 89-year-old gentleman who was living in the community, in rented accommodation with no family support. He had asked the local authority social work team if he could move into a care home as he was very lonely and was becoming increasingly nervous about using the bathroom at night on his own. Support was put in place for him by way of 30 minutes' care to assist him with personal care and a food delivery three days a week. This did not address the issue either of loneliness or insecurity at night. When the gentleman went to go to the bathroom at 1 am one night, he became breathless and fell. He pressed his emergency call button, was attended by paramedics and taken to Accident and Emergency. There was no significant injury, and he was discharged home with no review of his care package. The gentleman fell on two more occasions, and on the last occasion it was deemed appropriate for him to have a higher level of care. It was agreed that a care home placement would be found for him. Although he was medically fit for discharge, a local authority funded emergency respite bed could not be found for him, so he had to stay in hospital for 12 more days until a place in a permanent care home came up.

Home care is seen by some as a panacea to the funding crisis as it is cheaper than residential care (PayingForCare, 2019), and people who are often unwilling to think about how they may age and the support they may require would prefer to live in their own home for as long as possible (The Select Committee on Public Service and Demographic Change, 2013). Home care forms part of The World Health Organization's 2020 Strategy (WHO, 2013), but so does preventing loneliness and isolation, and in this instance the gentleman had outlined that he was lonely. Had he had the money or assets to pay for his care, he would have been able to choose the level of support he had and when he had it; he would have been able to enter a care home when he wanted to, and while this would not have prevented him falling, he would have had the support at hand to deal with it in an appropriate manner – thereby not utilising emergency services for what was essentially a social problem.

These two case studies focus on choice and access to services for people who do not have the means to fund their own care, but one of the other implications is that of the quality of the services provided.

In the discussion about the lady who was placed a long way from her family, she only had one choice of placement and there was no attention to the quality of the care home she was sent to. She needed a place and it was all there was, so she had to slot in with the service. Therefore, the care home's ability to meet all her needs was challenged, and not just the issue of access to her family. Depending on the care home she was sent to, it could be difficult to personalise her care for her; for example, by providing her with the appropriate faith-based interaction or access to a secure garden. These are elements of care that are important to an individual's quality of life and indicate the quality of care provided.

If the shortfall between what the local authority can pay and the true cost of care is not supported by other means such as top up (which will be discussed later on), charitable or self-funding income, it is only common sense to assume that this level of funding will impact on the quality of the service, with the adage that 'you get what you pay for' appearing to be appropriate. Nonetheless, the care home regulator, The Care Quality Commission (CQC), identifies that quality of care across services is being maintained despite financial pressures (CQC, 2018), but this still means that one in six adult care services need to improve (CQC, 2018) and, as already demonstrated, that access to services is inconsistent – with 1.4 million older people not having access to the services they need (CQC, 2018).

There have been several high-profile cases that have meant an increase in scrutiny of the quality of care and the minimum that should be accepted (Department of Health, 2012; Francis, 2013). Moreover, as a society we have increasingly high expectations about the services we receive, and this is no different for care homes (LaingBuisson, 2018). It is certainly desirable to improve quality, but the associated costs in achieving this and keeping pace with the dynamic progression of the care industry fall to the individual care home provider, and it could be argued that this is why there has been a reduction in the number of nursing homes (CQC, 2018). CQC inspect and regulate care homes against the same standards, irrespective of how they achieve their income. Care home providers make a choice about who they admit into their home and how they are funded, and market their product accordingly. Privately funded care homes tend to be luxurious and in affluent areas (LaingBuisson, 2018). While CQC (2018) has outlined a reduction in nursing homes, the self-funding market appears to remain healthy, with new high-end developments in affluent areas demonstrating an optimistic market (LaingBuisson, 2018). There is also a danger that private providers will only be encouraged to take over profitable services (West, 2018), further reducing the local authority funded availability.

The greatest impact on quality is not seen in the care itself but in the incidentals. For example, if a provider takes both local authority and self-funding individuals, they will often keep larger, lighter and more luxuriously furnished rooms for self-funders. Green (2019) supports the idea that there is a flat rate for care that is funded for everybody, but that people who can afford it can pay for additional benefits such as improved food choices, outings and entertainment (Hackett, 2019). It appears that the two-tiered funding system translates into two levels of service; it makes a statement about the value of the people who are accessing care.

Top-up fees and wealth depletion

There is confusion about how social care is funded, with 41 per cent of people believing that the government should be responsible for paying for it (Bottery et al, 2018), making the assumption that social care is either free at the point of entry in the same way the NHS is or that it is heavily subsidised (Bottery et al, 2018). As discussed, the reality is that people who self-fund bear the full cost of their care (Age UK, 2019). For local authority-funded individuals, there is another way in which care homes will try and achieve the actual cost of a placement, and this is through a top-up fee (Age UK, 2019). This affords someone a greater choice of care home, as more will be willing to take the person at the higher fee, but it is a third-party payment that is normally paid by a relative or loved one. The Salvation Army (TSA) found that half of those who rent their property would be agreeable to contribute to the cost of care for a loved one, but 97 per cent said that they did not have the means to enable them to do so (TSA, 2018). A local authority provides someone with a choice of care homes, one of which must be within the local authority fee rate, with the others potentially more expensive options that the local authority are prepared to part-fund with a top-up fee from family. Although it makes sense to offer alternatives, for people without the means to pay it is not a viable option, and therefore only paying lip service to the notion of offering choice. There also needs to be consideration about what happens if the third party paying the top-up fee can no longer afford it. A similar situation arises as people's wealth depletes, and this will be discussed later.

In the author's experience, a provider will ask if loved ones can contribute a top-up fee when they come to view the home before a placement. This causes anxiety at a stressful time, especially if they like the home and feel it would be right for their loved one. They will realise at this point that the only way they can place their relative in the home of their choice is to pay a top-up fee. They may not be able to afford this, and might feel obliged to pay it irrespective of the hardship that this might incur for them. This will become more evident when they have seen several homes, and realise that to pay for the more appropriate home, whether near to them, with a better choice of menu or brighter rooms, that they are going to have to contribute to secure the place. There is no legal obligation for a third party to pay a top-up fee and, as TSA research shows, very few people who rent property are in a position to do so. There is a vicious circle emerging: families who have assets are in a position to help a loved one, but family members are more likely to be self-funders; equally, families who have not managed to get on the housing ladder and rent property are more likely to need the local authority contribution topped up, but they do not have the assets to support this.

While this chapter is about people who don't own their own home, people who do may find themselves in a similar situation once their assets and savings have been utilised to pay for care (CFCS, 2011), and at this point the local authority will step in to assume responsibility for payment. The local authority rate may be considerably lower than the care home had been charging for the person when they were able to pay for themselves, so they may be asked to leave the care home or fund the difference through top-up fees.

While working as a regional manager, the author was involved with a 99-year-old lady who had been supported in a high-quality nursing home in an affluent area on the South Coast for four years. She had sold her flat on admission to the care home and had paid in excess of £300,000 for her care. Over the four years, her assets had diminished to fall below the upper threshold for the local authority to step in and assume responsibility for the fees. The shortfall between the fees set by the local authority and the level that had been paid by the lady as a self-funder was £380 per week. The lady had no close relatives who were willing to fund the shortfall, so discussions were had with the senior management team of the care company to serve notice of termination and ask her to leave. Following lengthy discussions, the lady was allowed to stay in the care home at the local authority rate, because the senior managers were concerned about the negative publicity that would be generated if she moved out and then became unwell or died. In this case, it is sad that the lady's needs were never considered, but the implications of people reaching the threshold to the care home providers cannot be underestimated. The significant loss of income per week from one person has implications on the running of the care home, and it should be considered that if several residents' wealth was depleted at the same time it could threaten the viability of the business. While it is arguably immoral to ask a person to leave somewhere they have made home, it is also understandable that the care home wants to protect their business and the homes of the others who live there. To protect against this, it has become standard practice for care homes to do a financial assessment prior to admission, and ensure that the person has enough assets to pay the fees for a minimum of 24 months.

Conclusion

Older people who do not have the assets to pay for their care should not be subject to marginalisation either in the debates about the long-term plans for social care funding or in the receipt of social care itself, but this appears to be the current reality. Green's report (2019) perpetuates the two-tiered funding model that has the potential to benefit wealthy and fitter people with a higher level of care and disadvantage the poor who, by nature of their social demographic status, may face greater health challenges. While it seems unfair that somebody has to sell their home to fund their care, if they do so they have quicker access, a wider choice of care homes and a more luxurious product. It is also unfair that these people are subsidising those who don't fund their care; but conversely it does not seem acceptable that somebody who rents property has limited choice, limited access to care and limited access to high-quality amenities. As demonstrated, more people are going to find themselves in the position of renting, as victims of increasing house prices, and the message currently being given to them is that it is OK to offer them a second-rate service when it comes to a care home.

Postscript
At the time of writing the author, a registered nurse, has been seconded to the NHS to work with COVID-19 patients as part of her working week as head of Avente Care Homes (Kent). This 60+ hour week prevents her from providing an update on her insight into the crisis in social adult care.

References
Age UK (2019) 'Paying for residential care'. Available from: https://www.aguk.org.uk/infomation-advice/care/paying-for-care/paying-for-a-care-home/ [Accessed 21 February 2019].

Blake, M. (2011) 'Social care reform will rely on good quality care data', National Centre for Social Research (7 July). Available from: http://natcen.ac.uk/blog/social-care-reform-will-rely-on-good-quality-data [Accessed 22 November 2018].

Bottery, S., Varrow, M., Thorlby, R. and Wellings, D. (2018) *A Fork in the Road: Next Steps for Social Care Funding Reform*, London: The Health Foundation.

CQC (Care Quality Commission) (2018) *The State of Healthcare and Adult Social Care in England 2017/2018*, London: The Stationery Office.

CFCS (Commission on Funding of Care and Support) (2011) 'Fairer care funding: the report of the commission on funding of care and support' (The Dilnot Report), London: The Stationery Office.

Department of Health (2012) *Transforming Care: A National Response to Winterbourne View Hospital*, London: Department of Health.

Francis, R. (2013) *Report of Mid-Staffordshire NHS Foundation Trust Public Enquiry Executive Summary*, London: The Stationery Office.

Green, D. (2019) 'Fixing the care crisis', Centre for Policy Studies. Available from: www.cps.org.uk/file/reports/original/190426143506-DamianGreenSocialCareFinal.pdf [Accessed 4 June 2019].

Hackett, K. (2019) 'Conservative MP proposes two-tier social care system', *Nursing Older People*, 31(3): 6.

Independent Age (2017) 'Cost of average length of stay in a residential care home is equivalent to 26 years of family holidays', *Independent Age* (26 October). Available from: www.independentage.org/nes-media/press-releases/cost-of-average-length-of-stay-a-residential-care-home-equivalent-to-26 [Accessed 12 March 2019].

LaingBuisson (2018) 'Care homes for older people UK market report 29th edition flyer'. Available from: www.laingbuisson.com/wp-content/uploads/2018/06/carehomesolderpeople-29-sales-flyer.Pdf [Accessed 4 June 2019].

Marmot, M. (2010) 'Fair society, healthy lives', The Marmot Review, Institute of Health Equity. Available from: http://www.instituteofhealthequity.org/resources-reports/fair-society-healthy-lives-the-marmot-review [Accessed 8 April 2020].

Melican, J. (2018) 'Local authority perspectives on community planning and localism, a case study', in A. Bonner (ed) *Social Determinants of Health: An Interdisciplinary Approach to Social Inequality and Wellbeing*, pp 211–23, Bristol: Policy Press.

MHCLG (Ministry of Housing, Communities and Local Government) (2018) *English Housing Survey – Headline Report 2016–2017*, London: Ministry of Housing, Communities and Local Government.

PayingForCare (2019) 'Paying for care – how much does care cost?'. Available from: www.payingforcare.org/how-much-does-care-cost [Accessed 12 March 2019].

Shelter (2018) 'Grey renting: the rising tide of older private tenants'. Available at: https://blog.shelter.org.uk [Accessed 12 March 2019].

The Select Committee on Public Service and Demographic Change (2013) 'Ready for aging?'. Available from: https://publications. parliament.uk/pa/ld201213/ldselect/ldpublic/140/140.pdf [Accessed 10 April 2020].

TSA (The Salvation Army) (2018) 'The cost of care if you don't own your own home'. Available from: www.salvationaremu.org.uk/old-age-renters [Accessed 22 June 2018].

West, C. (2018) 'Health and social care in an age of austerity', in A. Bonner (ed) *Social Determinants of Health: An Interdisciplinary Approach to Social Inequality and Wellbeing*, pp 325–36, Bristol: Policy Press.

WHO (World Health Organization) (2013) *Health 2020: A European Policy Framework and Strategy for the 21st Century*, Copenhagen: World Health Organization Regional Office for Europe.

13

The Human, Learning, Systems approach to commissioning in complexity

Toby Lowe, Max French and Melissa Hawkins

Introduction

It is now widely accepted that the realm of public service is complex (Haynes, 2003; Bovaird, 2008; Rhodes, 2008; Lowe and Wilson, 2017). This has a number of profound consequences that public servants must address in order to successfully navigate the realm. This chapter will argue that in order to meet these challenges, public servants need new, complexity-informed tools with which to manage the provision of public service.

This chapter will explore what is required of commissioners in order to create positive social outcomes (such as improved wellbeing, increased employment or reduced crime) in complex environments. It will explore this question through the lens of public sector performance measurement and management (PSPMM), and how this has evolved towards increased complexity by moving from an output (activity) to an outcome (results) focus.

It will explore the different aspects of complexity that arise when seeking to commission activity that creates positive outcomes for citizens, and what a complexity-informed response requires. The chapter will then reflect on the way in which these requirements challenge existing public management arrangements, particularly in the field of PSPMM, as it applies to commissioning and performance management.

Finally, the chapter will identify the emergent 'Human, Learning, Systems' (HLS) (Lowe and Plimmer, 2019) approach to the funding, commissioning and management of public service, and provide examples of this approach in action.

The complex nature of creating public service outcomes

It is increasingly common in the broader management literature to understand that managing any 21st-century organisation is a complex task. This can be seen in the prominence of literature concerning management in 'Volatile, Uncertain, Complex, Ambiguous' contexts (Johansen and Euchner, 2013; Bennett and Lemoine, 2014).

This chapter argues that there are four aspects of complexity presented by such problems for commissioners who want to achieve positive outcomes:

- experiential complexity, which results from the variation in how outcomes are experienced by individuals, and the multiplicity of pathways to shared outcomes across the population;
- compositional complexity, which results from the interdependence and interdeterminance of causal factors leading to the creation of outcomes;
- dynamic complexity, which results from the co-evolution of interacting factors and the instability inherent to complex systems;
- governance complexity, which results from the autonomy of public service organisations and other agents, increased by the fragmentation of modern public service landscapes.

These aspects of complexity manifest in particular challenges for commissioners. In this chapter, the detail of how these challenges manifest in respect of the provision of 'human services' – the aspect of public service that involves the provision of services to identifiable people – will be explored. Human services include activity such as social care provision, health care, employment support, criminal justice and education, and these will be used as a lens with which to consider the complexity of public service: it is within this context that the variety of human need and experience is most clearly visible. The authors believe that the sources of complexity identified here also apply to other aspects of public service, such as the provision of public infrastructure (transport, for example) or economic development, but the aspects of complexity in these areas would need to be explored separately in order to develop a contexts-specific understanding.

The purpose of commissioning – to create positive social outcomes

Before the nature of complexity in public service is explored, initial assumptions about the purpose of public service, in the human services context, should be identified. The starting point here is the currently dominant perspective – that the purpose of human services is to create positive social outcomes (Friedman, 2009; Lowe, 2013; Lowe and Wilson, 2017; Borgonovi et al, 2018). For example, in the field of social care, the outcome that people seek could be increased wellbeing; in the area of employment support, the desired outcome could be a greater number of people in work.

This purpose can be observed in the field of PSPMM. Essentially, PSPMM addresses the question of what public servants should be held accountable for. Initially, PSPMM systems were predominantly concerned with output control and process efficiency (Hood, 1991; Heinrich, 2010), and adopted indicators of input, throughput and output as the basis for performance appraisal. Output-based performance measurement and management (PMM) systems became criticised for encouraging a narrow and introspective concern with organisational performance, which jarred with the increasingly fragmented governance landscape under New Public Management (NPM) reforms, and the growing footprint of governance networks and partnerships as contributors of public value (Rhodes, 1997). Outputs also failed to reflect a genuine concern with what mattered to either the lives of service consumers, conflicting with NPM's concern with customer choice and satisfaction (Heinrich, 2010; van Thiel and Leeuw, 2002).

Accordingly, PMM systems in the public and non-profit sectors have increasingly moved towards measures of outcomes, relating to the end value created by services and interventions (Schalock, 2001; Heinrich, 2010; Boyne and Law, 2005; Borgonovi et al, 2018), as the trigger or incentivisation and decision-making in PMM systems. Outcome-based performance management (OBPM) was seen to establish a focus on customer and societal value, and provided the appropriate level of performance indicator for forms of multi-organisational partnerships. Outcomes also supported a move away from a 'command and control' approach to PMM, encouraging managerial entrepreneurialism and helping to establish an outcomes focus across whole organisations (Heinrich, 2010).

Given that the purpose of this form of public service is to create such positive social outcomes, how does complexity manifest? And what is the necessary response of public service to this complexity?

Experiential complexity – variety of demand

In the human services context, experiential complexity is most readily understood in terms of the variety of human needs, strengths and capacities with which public servants are faced when doing this work. In short, each person experiences an outcome in their lives differently – both in terms of the factors that contribute to it, and what those outcomes mean to them.

Let us take the outcome of wellbeing as an example. What wellbeing means will be different to each person. Does socialising with others help create a sense of wellbeing, or do some people like to be by themselves? (And given that the answer to this is likely to be 'both, but at different times', under what circumstances is each appropriate?) Does seeing their family promote their wellbeing, or should they be kept apart? Do they like being outside in nature, or do they prefer the cosy indoors?

Given that the purpose of social care service, for example, can be understood as developing the sense of wellbeing of the person being cared for, then this means that those responsible for this care must know, understand and respond to the particular combination of elements and factors that help to create a sense of wellbeing for each person.

Experiential complexity also results in ambiguity and uncertainty. Human variation creates a variety of perspectives within a social system – different perspectives on what matters to people, different perspectives on how needs should be met, different perspectives arising from access to, and interpretation of, the different information that is available to different people. This creates social systems in which it cannot be assumed that a 'single point of truth' exists – a shared perspective on which everybody agrees.

Required response

The response required of public service to this aspect of complexity is outlined in Ashby's Law of Requisite Variety (Ashby, 1956). This states that if a system is to be stable, the number of states of its control mechanism must be greater than or equal to the number of states in the system being controlled. In the context being discussed, it can be most readily understood through the maxim 'Variety absorbs variety' (Ashby, 1956). In other words, in order to respond to variety in demand, public service must have at least as much variety in the support it offers to people.

This contains the following implications for public service:

- That public servants know and understand the variety with which they are faced. In a human service context, this means that they must know each individual they serve well enough to have a deep understanding of their strengths and needs. This requires a strong relationship between public servant and those they serve. For example, they must know whether seeing their family (which combination of family members, under what circumstances) will help to promote their wellbeing.
- That public servants have the autonomy to respond to variety. The public servant who has the relationship with the person concerned, and who has the in-depth knowledge of the variety of that demand, must have the autonomy to meet that demand in whatever way is appropriate. For example, if not seeing their parents is crucial to a person's wellbeing, the public servant caring for them must have the autonomy to enable that to be the case; they must not be bound by population-level rules that stipulate parental access to their children promotes wellbeing.
- Autonomy requires trust. In order that public servants have the required autonomy to respond to variety, they must be trusted by those who are responsible for managing the work.
- The absence of an assumed single point of truth requires that all voices within a system are heard, so that differences in perspective are made visible and acknowledged. This is necessary so that shared perspectives are constructed, rather than assumed. They must be built through processes of dialogue and negotiation. For example, the desired outcomes for public service should not be assumed in advance; they must be discussed and negotiated both at a political level (what are the legitimate parameters of individual outcome choice? For example, are people allowed to choose their own death?) and within this scope at an individual level.

Compositional complexity

Compositional complexity describes the aspect of complexity that describes the range of factors contributing to the creation of an outcome in the world. This is produced by an enormous range of interdependent factors. Let us consider the challenge of obesity. The work undertaken by Vandenbroeck et al (2007) (Figure 13.1) illustrates that the outcome of obesity – whether people are obese or not – is the product of many interdependent factors. They illustrated this interdependence in the form of a causal-loop diagram:

Figure 13.1: A systems map of the causal relationships between the factors that create the outcome of obesity

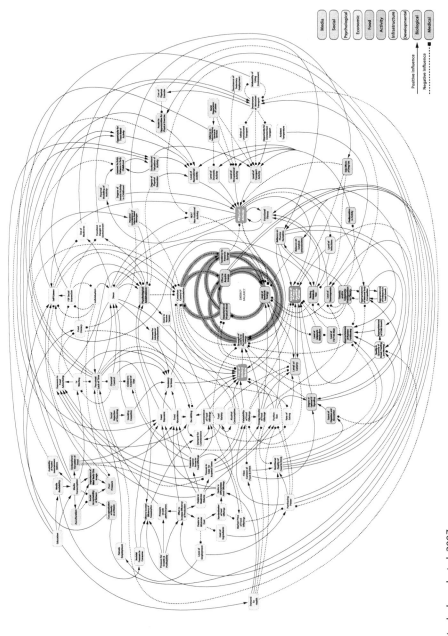

Source: Vandenbroeck et al, 2007

This diagram perfectly illustrates that the social outcomes public service seeks are created by complex systems – of many interdependent elements working in concert. Such systems exhibit emergent properties in which the patterns of behaviour of the whole system (for example, whether it results in obesity or not) are not reliably predictable, even if everything is known about the constituent parts. It is therefore appropriate to say that outcomes are emergent properties of complex systems.

Required response

Finally, emergence and uncertainty requires a different role for 'evidence' in public service, and particularly for evaluation. In complex environments where results are emergent, it is not possible for evaluation evidence to play one of the roles that has classically been demanded of it – to find what works to produce desired social outcomes so that resources can be allocated to programmes that work, rather than those that don't (Schalock, 2001) – because the results produced were contingent on the exact sequence of interactions and relationships between elements in that system at that point in time.

Instead, in complex environments, evaluation and evidence are required to play a different role (Mowles, 2014; Ivaldi et al, 2015). They are tools by which those doing the work reflect, learn and improve. They are learning tools for public servants undertaking the work, rather than information that informs purchasing decisions.

Dynamic complexity

Complex systems are dynamic. They change over time and they change in unpredictable ways. It is not just that the patterns of behaviour of the elements of complex systems are subject to change, but that the patterns of the whole system are also liable to change. A system that was chaotic may flip into a stable state, with seemingly reliable patterns (Boulton et al, 2015). Likewise, a stable system might suddenly become unstable. This is significant when seeking to create positive social outcomes. It means that what works to create an outcome for one person in one place will not necessarily work for a different person in another place. It means that what works for one person at one point in time may not work for that same person at a different time. For example, the combination of housing, welfare payments, mental health support, employment and substance misuse support that enables one homeless person to stabilise their lives and manage a stable tenancy may not work for a different person in a different place; and it may not work for the same person at two different points in their life.

Required response

The required response to dynamicity is to treat public service as an ongoing learning process, a learning process that never arrives at 'the answer'. This means that human services need to shift away from offering standardised and fixed responses that take the form if X is true then we do Y. Public service is required to adapt to changes in context. It turns each encounter between a public servant and the people they serve into a learning situation. And building on the required response to ambiguity, it must be a learning situation in which the public servant and those they serve construct their learning together.

The key shift here for public service is a requirement to shift from a version of management that seeks control over processes that are known to work, and to a version of management that enables experimentation and learning. This can be seen as an extension of the required response to variety. As well as being able to know, understand and have the autonomy to respond to variety of demand, they must have learning mechanisms in place to be able to adapt their response as circumstances change. They must have the learning capacity to recognise change in relevant circumstances, and the ability to reflect on their practice using data and sense-making methods that enable ongoing adaptation.

Governance complexity

The emergent patterns of results produced by complex systems also highlights another aspect of complexity – that results produced by complex systems are beyond the control of any element of that system. The results of complex systems cannot be controlled, they can only be shaped and influenced. For example, a local authority may desire to reduce obesity in the area for which it is responsible. However, obesity (as we see in Figure 13.1) is significantly influenced by a range of factors beyond the control or influence of the local authority; for example, the types of food that are created and distributed, or how food, exercise and body image are represented in the media.

Required response

If the outcomes produced by complex systems are beyond the control of any of the actors in the system, the required response seems to be that actors are able to shape patterns of behaviour in a system (Bellavita, 2006) rather than attempting to control that behaviour. It also suggests that those seeking to create desired outcomes pay attention to the extent to which actors in the system are able to co-ordinate and collaborate effectively. We can refer to the extent of this ability to coordinate and collaborate as the 'health' of the system.

How do the requirements of complexity fit with current public service management practice? We will look at the changes that these requirements place on public service through the lens of performance management practice, as it impacts on the funding, commissioning and delivery of public service interventions.

An end to target-based performance management

The required response from public service to these manifestations of complexity concerns performance management mechanisms. If desired social outcomes – such as reduced obesity, or increased employment, or wellbeing – are emergent properties of complex systems, then it means that outcomes are not 'delivered' by people, organisations or programmes of activity. This means that performance management cannot hold people, teams, organisations or programmes accountable for producing such outcomes, because to do so would be holding them accountable for things they do not control.

Further, this analysis also suggests that it is a mistake to set predefined targets by which to monitor the performance of people who have to make context-sensitive decisions. The desire to set predefined targets comes from a 'control' mentality (Bourne et al, 2017) associated with Principal–Agent Theory (PAT) (Davis et al, 1997). In PSPMM, this has been manifest in the belief that public servants must have their autonomy constrained by targets in order to focus their time and attention on appropriate activities, for fear that if their autonomy is not so constrained, they will act in their own interest (rather than the public interest). This was famously expressed by Le Grand (2010) in terms of the necessity of avoiding 'knave'-like behaviour among public servants.

In complex environments, however, principals cannot effectively constrain the autonomy of agents without undermining their ability to respond to the challenges of variety and dynamism. This requires a shift in the underpinning theory for public service performance management from PAT to Stewardship Theory (Davis et al, 1997; Schillemans, 2013) in which public servants, and those who have authority over them, are viewed as having shared stewardship of the systems that produce social outcomes.

The need to respond to interdependence, variety and dynamism also requires an end to prescriptive commissioning practice. Where public services are commissioned (that is, where they are subject to a purchaser/provider split), commissioners are currently encouraged to specify what is required of a service, either in terms of outputs (the activity that the service should undertake) or outcomes (the results that the activity should achieve). Whether outputs or outcomes (or combinations of these), the service specifications should be expressed in terms of metrics that the commissioner can then use to monitor performance of the provider – are they delivering what they promised to deliver? This is expressed is the 'commissioning cycle' of the United Kingdom (UK) National Health Service (UKNHS, 2019), in Figure 13.2.

However, responding to the interdependence of outcomes requires that particular service providers (or even combinations of service providers) cannot be held accountable for delivering outcomes, because outcomes are not delivered by services, but rather are emergent

Figure 13.2: The National Health Service commissioning cycle

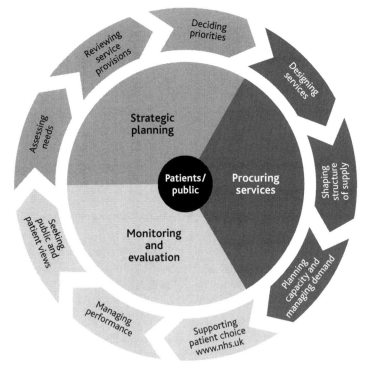

Source: Courtesy of the NHS Information Centre for health and social care. Full diagram available at: www.ic.nhs.uk/commissioning

properties of a broader complex system. Attempting to hold services accountable for outcomes results in gaming of the system (Lowe and Wilson, 2017), in which service providers learn to manipulate data in order to respond to demands to be accountable for outcomes they do not control.

If output (activity) metrics are used to specify contracts, then those services cannot respond effectively to the variety of human strengths and need, and the changing nature of that strength and need. Since neither output nor outcome specification enables an effective response to complexity, an alternative approach is required.

An emerging alternative: Human, Learning, Systems approach

In the UK, a conversation has begun among public servants about how to navigate complexity more effectively (Davidson-Knight et al, 2017; Lowe and Plimmer, 2019; Knowledge Hub Complexities Group, n.d.). This conversation has identified the HLS approach (Lowe and Plimmer, 2019), which creates an alternative paradigm for funding, commissioning and management of human service interventions in complex systems.

Human

Complexity-consistent practice has in all cases encompassed a strong relational dimension with service users. To understand the variety of people's needs and strengths to design appropriate services responses, being human-centred is required of practitioners. Public servants have to be trusted to behave with human compassion in their service delivery efforts rather than with self-interest, while a faith in the goodness of human nature is also required of managers. It has been found that management practice that is implicitly guided by the underpinning assumptions of NPM can crowd out the importance of human relationships, and many public service employees in the empirical work spoke of being deeply uncomfortable with what could be considered common practice, and instead call for the need to 'be more human' (Lowe and Plimmer, 2019).

To explore in further detail what this means, the mnemonic VEST – Variety, Empathy, Strengths and Trust – captures what this means in practice. This is an approach that:

• recognises the Variety of human strengths, needs and experiences;

- builds Empathy between people – so that they recognise, and seek to act on, the emotional and physical needs of others;
- uses Strengths–based approaches – recognising and building on the assets (rather than deficits) of people and places;
- trusts public servants to act on their intrinsic motivation to help others and get better at what they do.

Learning

Learning is a continuous process of adaptation throughout the lifecycle of public service planning, implementation and evaluation. The business literature places learning as a key engine of service improvement in complex environments (Mintzberg and Waters, 1985; Bourne et al, 2017). French and Lowe (2018) also position learning (rather than evidence) as central to responding to complexity, but make the challenge that learning also necessitates moving away from results-based accountability relationships. Lowe and Plimmer (2009) contrast this approach with a process of social innovation in which a public service problem is identified, experiments are undertaken to identify what works in relation to that challenge, and then when what works is known, that solution is taken to scale (Lowe and Plimmer, 2019, p 15; Young Foundation, 2012, p 33).

By contrast, the HLS approach identifies the following ways in which an ongoing learning approach is operationalised (Lowe and Plimmer, 2019):

- an iterative, experimental approach to working with people;
- funding and commissioning for learning, not services – shifting from commissioning specified services to funding organisations' capacity to learn;
- using data to learn – using monitoring data for reflection, rather than target-based performance management;
- creating a learning culture – creating a 'positive error culture' in which people are encouraged to talk with their peers about mistakes and uncertainties in their practice.

Systems

The Systems approach begins with the perspective that outcomes are produced by systems, rather than delivered by organisations (Lowe and Plimmer, 2019). Consequently, systems rather than organisations should be the platform for social interventions. Lowe and Plimmer

(2009) identify the need for a 'system steward' role to ensure that systems can operate effectively to produce desired outcomes.

The report identifies aspects of the role that systems stewards play (Lowe and Plimmer, 2019, pp 37–8). These include:

- building relationships and trust between actors in a system;
- establishing shared purpose;
- developing behaviours, principles and behaviours.

Further, the authors identify the critical role played by commissioners in system stewardship. They assert that how commissioners distribute financial resources (for example, through competitive or collaborative processes) plays a crucial role in whether actors in a system can coordinate their activities effectively (Lowe and Plimmer, 2019, p 24).

Examples of HLS practice that seem to satisfy the requirements of complexity outlined above have been identified.

Responding to experiential complexity: bespoke by default

There has been a significant move towards the provision of human service that is 'bespoke by default' (Lowe and Plimmer, 2019). This refers to a form of relational practice in which the purpose of the support provider is to create an effective human relationship with the person/people who require support, and then to respond appropriately to the strengths and needs that they discover through that relationship.

This bespoke by default approach was highlighted in the Buurtzorg model of nursing care in the Netherlands (Laloux, 2014), in which groups of nurses form self-managing teams to provide appropriate response to the variety of needs they encounter in home-care settings. In the Buurtzorg example, nurses have authority to respond in whatever way they see fit to the people in their care. Each member's actions and judgements are peer-reviewed by other members of the team in order to reflect on and improve performance (Laloux, 2014).

In Gateshead, a local authority in the UK, a similar approach has been developed to create bespoke by default public service. Beginning with experiments to respond differently to those who cannot pay their council tax (the UK's local taxation mechanism), the council has created public service reform (PSR) teams with devolved authority to build relationships with citizens, and to respond to the strengths and needs of those citizens in any way that 'does no harm, and stays legal' (Lowe and Plimmer, 2019).

> Most of the specific things that were done that helped people were small and unspectacular. A coffee, a chat, a food shop whilst benefits were being processed, a bus pass to aid a job search (and just to get people out of the house), some basic clothes... They didn't need supplying for and assessing for, but were decisions made by the workers in the work based upon the specific context of the person and their situation. Public sector change leader. (Lowe and Plimmer, 2019)

A key aspect of this bespoke response is that it is not viewed as a distinct, standardised service. This has two key implications. First, the service has no access or eligibility criteria (anyone who asks for help is entitled to help). Secondly, there is no standardised set of activities which the team undertakes. This means that there is no manual to follow, and the PSR team role requires continuous learning in order to reflect on the appropriateness of the judgements being made by team members.

This bespoke response enabled the PSR team to create better outcomes for 30 of the 42 cases in their prototype. The majority of these people were previously known to public service in the borough, but had been viewed as having complex, intractable needs that could not be effectively met through standard social care or health service responses.

Although it is too early to fully understand the cost implications of a bespoke response, early indications seem to suggest that it creates cost savings across the broader system. Cost savings seem to arise from reducing waste in the system in three ways: (Lowe and Plimmer, 2019)

- Not helping people when they ask for help makes people's problems more entrenched and expensive to help later on.
- Not helping people itself costs money. Providing a standardised service that does not meet the strengths and needs of the people who use it mean that scarce resources are wasted providing the wrong thing. This fits with other evidence that there are significant diseconomies of scale (locality) when providing responses to human need.
- Turning people away from help costs money. Assessment processes that decide whether people's problems are serious enough in order to provide support themselves cost money.

From their initial six-month prototype, the Gateshead team was further able to identify potential cost savings from among the people it had supported (Lowe and Plimmer, 2019):

- The reduction of the likelihood of a child requiring statutory care services. A near crisis has become stable and improving without any intervention from acute services.
- Four people were self-harming and two had considered suicide. Two of these are still struggling but four are improving.
- Seven people had found work or better-paid and/or more sustainable work, thus moving off or needing fewer benefits.
- Three had started to claim benefits when they had no income but were eligible for help, thus reducing the strain on crisis services.
- Five people related to those in the prototype but not within it themselves have also found work or maximised their income to match their entitlement, such that they can better position themselves to find work.
- One person was being financially abused and living in poverty that was materially damaging their health. This trajectory has been dramatically turned around to remove the potential need for sustained acute services.
- Fourteen people are engaging in mental health and/or addiction and recovery support that were previously not engaging with any form of mental health support. Ten of them are responding positively and taking more control of their lives.

Responding to compositional complexity: acknowledging multiple perspectives and negotiating shared purpose

An example of a response to the uncertainty that arises from compositional complexity comes from the city of York in the UK (French and Lowe, 2018). A number of different public services that served the city (housing, emergency services, mental health, social care and homelessness) were all conducting simultaneous system change programmes. Each of these was attempting to get the other services to reorientate around their perspective and priorities.

Through the intervention of a system change associate (French and Lowe, 2018), each of these system change programmes was able to identify that their perspective on the system was only partial, and that they needed to be able to hear and recognise multiple different perspectives in order to enable more effective collaboration. Consequently, public servants in York found themselves in the position of the people in the traditional Indian parable (Figure 13.3) in which each person can only experience a part of the whole, and is unable to recognise the larger picture that multiple perspectives create.

Figure 13.3: The parable of the blind man

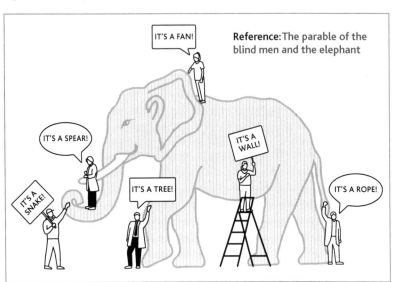

Source: Lowe and Plimmer, 2019

Consequently, public services in York created a Multiple and Complex Needs Network, which brought together all of the respective players into a single conversation; this was able to develop a shared purpose across the actors.

Responding to dynamic complexity: continuous learning and adaptation

In order to respond to dynamic complexity, one of the key changes that those who commission public services must address is that they must move away from purchasing specified services (for example, service X will deliver activity Y to group Z) towards a position in which they 'purchase' the capacity of organisations in order to respond to the changing strengths and needs of the people they serve.

A powerful example of this approach in action is provided by Plymouth City Council and the local Clinical Commissioning Group (CCG), the body responsible for commissioning health care services in the locality). In Plymouth, the contract for provision of support to vulnerable adults does not specify outputs or outcomes to be achieved. Instead, it uses a set of agreed principles as the basis for how the system will function, including ongoing adaptation to support provision based on shared learning.

The key features of this commissioning process were: (Lowe and Plimmer, 2019)

- The council and CCG created an £80 million, ten-year, shared budget to commission a health and care system for vulnerable adults in Plymouth.
- The tender did not specify outputs or outcomes to be delivered. Instead, it focussed on collaboration and learning together.
- This was tendered through an alliance contract model, whereby organisations in the city came together to create a shared response – with organisations jointly liable for the performance of the contract.
- Following the tender process, the council became a signatory to the alliance, formally recognising that they are part of the system.
- The tendering process was conducted as a series of design conversations between the commissioners and providers in the alliance, from which a set of core service principles and activities emerged.
- The signed alliance contract does not specify outputs or outcomes to be achieved. Instead, it uses a set of agreed principles as the basis for how the alliance will function. The details of the service provision are subject to continued adaptation based on shared learning.
- This commissioning process was made possible by four years of system change work, which built relationships of trust between the actors involved.

In this form of commissioning, the contract between commissioner and the alliance of organisations that are providing services does not specify Key Performance Indicators or other targets to be achieved. Instead, the commissioner holds the provider organisations accountable for the quality of their learning and adaptation:

> We want to work with provider(s) to measure and reflect on the outcomes that the system is producing, in order to help the system continuously adapt and improve, and to help organisations understand their particular contributions to these outcomes. Plymouth Council Tender specification document. (Lowe and Plimmer, 2019)

> [The commissioner] didn't specify activities, staffing, where we had to deliver from. Instead they said, 'let's see how we can do this together.'... It's about working together to work out where people are coming from, why things are the way

they are, developing new models. It's about all learning together. Plymouth Provider. (Lowe and Plimmer, 2019)

Responding to governance complexity

The Lankelly Chase Foundation (LCF) provides an interesting example of a response to the lack of control inherent in governing situations that do not have a single, central locus of authority. LCF is a UK-based charitable foundation that distributes approximately £10 million per year in resources to create systemic change for people who experience severe and multiple disadvantage in the UK (LCF).

They have created an 'action inquiry' (French and Lowe, 2018) to explore how to achieve systems change in how places function as systems to support people who have experienced severe and multiple disadvantage. Underpinning the inquiry are nine 'system behaviours' (French and Lowe, 2018) that describe the behaviour of actors in a 'healthy' system. These system behaviours concern perspective, power and participation in a place-as-system (French and Lowe, 2018):

Perspective

- People view themselves as part of an interconnected whole.
- People are viewed as resourceful and bringing strengths.
- People share a vision.

Power

- Power is shared, and equality of voice is actively promoted.
- Decision-making is devolved.
- Accountability is mutual.

Participation

- Open, trusting relationships enable effective dialogue.
- Leadership is collaborative and promoted at every level.
- Feedback and collective learning drive adaptation.

LCF's inquiry begins with the hypothesis that if actors in a system exhibit these behaviours, then the system will better help meet the strengths and needs of people who have experienced severe and multiple disadvantage. The idea is that these behaviours function as principles that enable effective coordination and collaboration in places-as-systems. Hence, they provide a mechanism for coordination and collaboration in the absence of central authority.

To enable this coordination a number of the places that are part of the inquiry are adopting the idea of system stewardship (Hallsworth, 2011; French and Lowe, 2018; Lowe and Plimmer, 2019). This defines the role of system steward as a person (or group of people) who take responsibility for the 'health' of a system (in this case, whether the system behaviours are manifest) and who coordinate actions to understand and promote the health of a system (French and Lowe, 2018). This coordinating role seems to play a crucial role in responding to governance complexity.

Conclusion

Effectively navigating complexity seems to require that public servants adopt a new paradigm for public management – one that leaves behind the conceptual underpinnings of NPM – underpinnings that seek to control public servants and limit their autonomy for fear of unleashing a wave of selfish, 'knave'-like (Le Grand, 2003) behaviours.

On the contrary, navigating complexity requires that public servants are trusted to use their autonomy to act as stewards of common, public goals. It requires that they are able to respond to the enormous variety of human strengths, needs and experiences. It requires that they are able to shape patterns in complex systems that are beyond their control, by finding and promoting behaviours that promote collaboration and coordination of activity. It requires that public servants are able to respond to ambiguity and uncertainty by undertaking activity that enables actors in systems to see the world from one another's perspectives. And it requires that learning is a continuous process of adaptation, in which people are freed from the responsibility to deliver predefined targets, and are instead resourced to learn and adapt to constantly changing contexts. This has been identified as the HLS approach (Lowe and Plimmer, 2019).

This chapter has given examples of what it means to meet each of these requirements in practice. None of these examples provides a complete map to enable complexity to be navigated successfully. However, they function as navigation aids, as points of reference that help to provide familiar landmarks in complex terrain. The commissioners of the 21st century will add to this map with each experiment they make in adopting a HLS approach.

References

Ashby, W.R. (1956) *An Introduction to Cybernetics*, London: Chapman & Hall.

Bellavita, C. (2006) 'Changing homeland security: shape patterns, not programs', *Homeland Security Affairs*, 2(3): 1–22.

Bennett, N. and Lemoine, J. (2014) 'What VUCA really means for you', *Harvard Business Review*, 92(1/2) (Jan/Feb). Available from: https://ssrn.com/abstract=2389563 [Accessed 12 April 2020].

Borgonovi, E., Anessi-Pessina, E. and Bianchi, C. (eds) (2018) *Outcome-Based Performance Management in the Public Sector*, Cham: Springer.

Boulton, J., Allen, P. and Bowman, C. (2015) *Embracing Complexity: Strategic Perspectives for an Age of Turbulence*, Oxford: Oxford University Press.

Bourne, M., Franco-Santos, M., Micheli, P. and Pavlov, A. (2017) 'Performance measurement and management: a system of systems perspective', *International Journal of Production Research*, 56(8): 2788–99. doi:10.1080/00207543.2017.1404159.

Bovaird, T. (2008) 'Emergent strategic management and planning mechanisms in complex adaptive systems', *Public Management Review*, 10(3): 319–40.

Boyne, G.A. and Law, J. (2005) 'Setting public service outcome targets: lessons from local public service agreements', *Public Money & Management*, 25(4): 253–60.

Davidson-Knight, A., Lowe, T., Brossard, M. and Wilson, J. (2017) 'A whole new world: funding and commissioning in complexity', Newcastle University Business School and Collaborate. Available from: http://wordpress.collaboratei.com/wp-content/uploads/A-Whole-New-World-Funding-Commissioning-in-Complexity.pdf [Accessed 12 April 2020].

Davis, J., Schoorman, D. and Donaldson, L. (1997) 'Toward a stewardship theory of management', *The Academy of Management Review*, 22(1): 20–47.

French, M. and Lowe, T. (2018) 'Place Action inquiry: our learning to date'. Lankelly Chase Foundation. Available from: https://lankellychase.org.uk/wp-content/uploads/2019/01/Place-Action-Inquiry-Learning-to-Date-Jan19.pdf [Accessed 12 April 2020].

Friedman, M. (2009) *Trying Hard is Not Good Enough*, n.p.: FPSI.

Hallsworth, M. (2011) 'System stewardship: the future of policy making?', Institute for Government. Available from: https://www.instituteforgovernment.org.uk/sites/default/files/publications/System%20Stewardship.pdf [Accessed 12 April 2020].

Haynes, P. (2003) *Managing Complexity in the Public Services*. Maidenhead: Open University Press.

Heinrich, C. (2010) 'Incentives and their dynamics within public sector performance', *Journal of Policy Analysis and Management*, 29(1): 183–208.

Hood, C. (1991) 'A public management for all seasons?', *Public Administration*, 69(1): 3–19. doi:10.1111/j.1467-9299.1991.tb00779.x.

Ivaldi, S., Scaratti, G. and Nuti, G. (2015) 'The practice of evaluation as an evaluation of practices', *Evaluation*, 21(4): 497–512.

Johansen, B. and Euchner, J. (2013) 'Navigating the VUCA World', *Research-Technology Management*, 56(1): 10–15.

Knowledge Hub Complexities Group (n.d.) Available from: https://khub.net/group/complexity-friendly-system-oriented-commissioning-pilot-project [Accessed 20 March 2019].

Laloux, F. (2014) *Reinventing Organizations: A Guide to Creating Organizations Inspired by the Next Stage in Human Consciousness*. Brussels: Nelson Parker.

Le Grand, J. (2003) *Motivation, Agency, and Public Policy: Of Knights and Knaves, Pawns and Queens*. Oxford: Oxford University Press.

Le Grand, J. (2010) 'Knights and knaves return: public service motivation and the delivery of public services', *International Public Management Journal*, 13(1): 56–71.

Lowe, T. (2013) 'The paradox of outcomes: the more we measure the less we understand', *Public Money and Management*, 33(3): 213–16.

Lowe, T. and Plimmer, D. (2019) 'Exploring the New World: Practical insights for funding, commissioning and managing in complexity'. Newcastle Business School and Collaborate. Available from: http://wordpress.collaboratei.com/wp-content/uploads/Exploring-the-New-World-Report_Digital-report.pdf [Accessed 12 April 2020].

Lowe, T. and Wilson, R. (2017) 'Playing the game of outcomes-based performance management. Is gamesmanship inevitable? Evidence from theory and practice', *Social Policy and Administration*, 51(7) (December): 981–1001.

Mintzberg, H. and Waters, J. (1985) 'Of strategies, deliberate and emergent', *Strategic Management Journal*, 6(3): 257–72.

Mowles, C. (2014) 'Complex, but not quite complex enough: the turn to the complexity sciences in evaluation scholarship', *Evaluation*, 20(2): 160–75.

Rhodes, M.L. (2008) 'Complexity and emergence in public management', *Public Management Review*, 10(3): 361–79.

Rhodes, R.A. (1997) *Understanding Governance: Policy Networks, Governance, Reflexivity and Accountability*, London: Open University Press.

Schalock, R.L. (2001) *Outcome Based Evaluation*, 2nd edn, New York: Kluwer Academic.

Schillemans, T. (2013) 'Moving beyond the clash of Interests: on stewardship theory and the relationships between central government departments and public agencies', *Public Management Review*, 15(4): 541–62.

UKNHS (2019) Commissioning cycle. Available from: https://www.england.nhs.uk/participation/resources/commissioning-engagement-cycle/ [Accessed 20 March 2019].

van Thiel, S. and Leeuw, F.L. (2002) 'The performance paradox in the public sector', *Public Performance & Management Review*, 25(3): 267–81. doi:10.2307/3381236.

Vandenbroeck, P., Goossens, J. and Clemens, M. (2007) 'Foresight tackling obesities: future choices – building the obesity system map', London: Government Office for Science. Available from: www.gov.uk/government/uploads/system/uploads/attachment_data/file/295153/07-1177-obesity-system-atlas.pdf [Accessed 12 April 2020].

Young Foundation (2012) 'Social Innovation Overview: A deliverable of the project: "The theoretical, empirical and policy foundations for building social innovation in Europe" (TEPSIE)', European Commission – 7th Framework Programme, Brussels: European Commission, DG Research.

PART IV

The third sector

Introduction

Alison Navarro

In the earlier parts of this book, the hard structures needed to support healthy communities were reviewed from the perspectives of health and care integration (Part I), the regional specific responses of local government, impacted by austerity budgeting (Part II) and the changing socio-legal dimensions of procurement and commissioning (Part III).

Part IV acknowledges that local authorities are, increasingly, enablers of change, and recognises the role of the third sector in providing the soft structures that are essential for reinvigorated and healthier communities and individuals (see Chapter 16).

The concept of an 'enabling state' was reported by The Carnegie Trust (Wallace, 2013), and describes the shift from a welfare state to an enabling state as being one where the fundamental challenge is creating a new relationship between citizens, communities and the state. The research identified some emerging themes that could contribute to an enabling state:

- Empowered citizens and communities – to use their own capacity to improve community wellbeing and to realise their own aspirations. This could include the community ownership of assets or delivery of services.
- A co-production model for public services – citizens able to share local service provision, with influence over their experience of receiving a service.
- Success where the state has traditionally failed – supporting communities and individuals to address problems where the state has been unable to respond adequately.
- A level playing field – reduce rather than exacerbate inequalities and be effective in recognising and responding to differences in community and individual capacity.

- A holistic approach to public service delivery — a joined-up and preventative approach to service delivery.
- Shared responsibilities — all parts of society have a role in improving our collective and individual wellbeing: welcome effective partnerships between individuals, civil society, businesses and the state.

The third sector plays a fundamental part in supporting this enabler role and the socio-ecological model (see Figure Part IV.1) proposed by Bronfenbrenner. From a practitioner perspective, this model provides an interesting framework and context against which the role of the third sector can be explored.

Part IV begins, in Chapter 14, with an overview of the commissioning of services by local authorities with regard to the role of charities. The third sector delivers these functions as a key feature of civil society (civil society strategy). Chapter 15 provides an example of the role of community-based organisations in supporting young people, and also refers to some ways in which community initiatives can play a role in regenerating the high street while simultaneously building social capital.

Chapter 16 highlights the importance of faith-based organizations in response to Burns's (Chapter 1) promotion of the fundamental need for personal actualisation, self-worth, self-efficacy and hope, the key attributes for unlocking our personal and community's potential,

Figure Part IV.1: A social ecological model

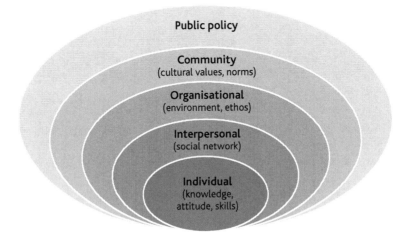

Source: Bronfenbrenner, 1977

which are fundamentally shaped by the depth, duration and nature of our relationships.

Chapter 17 develops our understanding of mutuality, with a particular focus on the importance of voice and effective consultation.

The third sector performs a number of functions to support thriving communities, underpinned by community development:

> where people come together to take action on what's important to them … at its heart, community development is rooted in the belief that people should have access to health, wellbeing, wealth, justice and opportunity. (SCDC, 2019)

The principles that underpin this practice are:

- self-determination – people and communities have the right to make their own choices and decisions;
- empowerment – people should be able to control and use their own assets and means to influence;
- collective action – coming together in groups or organisations strengthens peoples' voices;
- working and learning together – collaboration and sharing experiences.

Working in this way, the third sector:

> is uniquely positioned; an independent and trusted 'bridge' between citizens, communities and statutory agencies. It can act without the constraints public organisations are subject to, enabling it to be more creative in its responses. It creates added value … (Brighton and Hove City Council, 2014)

The term 'third sector' is one of many used to describe a sector that is:

> the eyes, ears and conscience of society. They mobilise, they provide, they inspire, they advocate and they unite. From small local organisations run entirely by volunteers to major global organisations with turnover in the hundreds of millions, their work touches almost every facet of British civic life. (HoLs, 2017)

The National Council for Voluntary Organisations, in the production of its 2019 Almanac (NCVO, 2019), the definitive resource on the state of the voluntary sector, uses the term 'voluntary sector', as it recognises that:

> It's challenging to define what the voluntary sector is or indeed to decide what to call it.

It further states that:

> The term 'voluntary sector' is not widely understood, and neither are alternatives such as 'third sector' or more recently 'social sector'. This is largely because of its huge diversity and the increasing blurred boundaries between the public, private and voluntary sectors.

The 2019 Almanac presents the following data for 2018:

- There were 166,854 voluntary organisations in the UK.
- Smaller organisations made up the vast majority (82 per cent) of the sector. They include micro-organisations, those with an income under £10,000, and small organisations, with an income between £10,000 and £100,000.
- Organisations with an income over £1 million are fewer in number but accounted for more than four-fifths of the sector's income.
- Social services remains the largest subsector in terms of number of organisations and income.
- The distribution of voluntary organisations across the UK is broadly similar to the distribution of the population.
- The majority of voluntary organisations with the biggest assets are based in London.
- Smaller voluntary organisations are more likely to operate solely in their local area.
- The voluntary sector contributed £17.1 billion to the economy in 2016/17, representing around 0.85 per cent of total gross domestic product.
- The sector employs approximately 870,000 people, slightly fewer than in 2017.
- The value of formal volunteering has been relatively stable, and stood at £23.9 billion in 2016.
- 20.1 million people volunteered through a group, club or organisation during 2017/18.
- The voluntary sector workforce has grown by 11 per cent since 2010.

- A majority of voluntary sector employees work in organisations with fewer than 50 paid staff.

The range, breadth and diversity of the third sector and its close relationships to individuals and communities, as well as its capacity and capability to deliver services, provides a vehicle for local authorities to use in driving forward health and wellbeing in its locality. There is evidence that the third sector is a provider of services on behalf of local authorities:

> A considerable proportion of the public income received by charities comes from local government, including through grants and contracts. (HoLs, 2017)

The implementation of the commissioning cycle (see Chapters 9 and 13) should lead to empowering communities – an outcome that is at the heart of community development, a value-based approach that underpins the work of many third sector organisations. From Chapter 4, the role and purpose of charities cannot be seen in isolation:

> Charities should be part of an integrated system that works to improve peoples' [sic] lives. National governments, local government, health commissioners, independent and statutory funders, businesses, politicians and communities themselves each have a role to play. (HoLs, 2017)

References

Brighton and Hove City Council (2014) 'Brighton and Hove City Council Communities and the Third Sector Policy 2014–2020'. Available from: https://www.brighton-hove.gov.uk/sites/brighton-hove.gov.uk/files/BHCCcommunitiesandthirdsectorpolicy%20 2014-20.pdf [Accessed 12 April 2020].

Bronfenbrenner, U. (1977) 'Toward an experimental ecology of human development', *American Psychologist*, 32(7): 513–53.

HoLs (House of Lords) (2017) 'Stronger charities for a stronger society. House of Lords select committee on charities'. Report of session 2016–17 (26 March).

NCVO (National Council for Voluntary Organisations) (2019) 'UK civil society almanac 2019. Data trends insights'. Available from: https://data.ncvo.org.uk [Accessed 12 April 2020].

SCDC (Scottish Community Development Centre) (2019) 'What is community development?'. Available from: https://www.scdc.org.uk/who/what-is-community-development [Accessed 12 April 2020].

Wallace, J. (2013) 'The rise of the enabling state. A review of policy and evidence across the UK and Ireland'. Carnegie Trust, UK. Available from: https://www.carnegieuktrust.org.uk/publications/the-rise-of-the-enabling-state/ [Accessed 12 April 2020].

14

Commissioning and social determinants: evidence and opportunities

Chris O'Leary and Chris Fox

Introduction

Local authorities spend thousands of pounds commissioning services: from professional services, highways maintenance, school meals, housing and social care, as noted in Part II of this book. Local authorities in the United Kingdom (UK) account for a quarter of all public spending (MHCLG, 2018). While much of this expenditure is accounted for by directly employed staff costs, a substantial proportion (around £70 billion in 2016/17 (Booth, 2018)) is used on commissioned services – services delivered by the relevant council, by other parts of the public sector or by external organisations. Local authorities have responsibilities for reducing health inequalities and tackling the social determinants of health, which they can impact at a population level through their key role in early years education, schools, planning, housing, social care, public space, air quality, public transport and community development. Since 2013, they have also had responsibilities for public health (see Chapter 2), following the transfer of responsibilities from the National Health Service (NHS) and creation of health and wellbeing boards (HWBs) under the provisions of the Health and Social Care Act 2012 (see Chapter 4). It has long been recognised that local government plays an important role in shaping social determinants of health (Marks et al, 2015); indeed, the pivotal role of local government has been recognised by the World Health Organization Commission on the Social Determinants of Health (WHO Commission on Social Determinants of Health, 2008). As such, decisions by local authorities about what, how, when and from whom services are commissioned play strategic and significant roles in their local areas.

In this chapter, it is argued that local authorities can and should use their purchasing power strategically to address the social determinants of health that affect their local area. The chapter is structured as follows. First, the authors examine commissioning and procurement as local authority functions, defining these concepts and exploring the conceptual confusion between the two. Secondly, the evidence of current practice of local authorities (with a particular focus on local authorities in the UK) in strategic use of their purchasing power is explored. Core to the argument is the role of local voluntary organisations and small and medium-sized enterprises (SMEs), so there is a particular focus on the commissioning experience of these types of organisations. Thirdly, the case is made for the role that voluntary sector organisations can play in addressing social determinants of health, before drawing some broad conclusions about the way forward.

Conceptualising commissioning and procurement

Commissioning has been central to debates on public sector reform in the UK since the 1980s (Bovaird et al, 2014; Rees et al, 2017). The development of the concept is often associated with the influence of the New Public Management (NPM) (Hood, 1991) reforms of the 1980s and 1990s, which included a splitting of roles between purchaser/provider (in the NHS) and client/contractor (in local government). Because of its early association with NPM, commissioning is seen as a mechanism through which public services are externalised, marketised and privatised, and is therefore often seen as part of 'neoliberalism' – and with the general criticisms made against the public sector reforms in the UK and elsewhere associated with NPM. Through compulsory competitive tendering through to Best Value and onwards to outcome-based commissioning such as Payment by Results, there is a degree of policy continuity across UK governments over the past 30 years, whether Conservative, Labour or Coalition.

Like many such concepts in policy analysis, there is debate about commissioning as a construct. It is 'definitionally fuzzy' (Dickinson, 2015), both about commissioning itself and about its distinctiveness from other related concepts such as partnering and procurement. Perhaps because of this, there is no single agreed definition of commissioning (Bovaird et al, 2014). Many definitions see commissioning as a *strategic* process of understanding the needs of a relevant population and decisions about how and when to address those needs. This is distinct from the process of making decisions about which individual services are needed (sometimes referred to as service commissioning), and organising or contracting for those services.

There is recognition in the literature that this distinction is not made consistently or understood, with commissioning and procurement often used interchangeably (Murray, 2011). This confusion is furthered because UK governments have sometimes combined commissioning and procurement in single definitions (Bovaird et al, 2014) and other times kept them quite separate; and because the term commissioning is inherently confined to the UK context (externalisation, contracting out or privatisation being used outside the UK (Ramia and Carney, 2001)). To add to this conceptual confusion, there is growing academic and real world interest in the use of procurement to further strategic goals (Loader, 2018; Patrucco et al, 2019). Kim Loader, in an article on public sector procurement and SMEs, argues that governments around the world are using their procurement processes and purchasing power to further their economic, social and environmental policy objectives (Loader, 2018).

Commissioning is not just contested conceptually, but also theoretically. Both advocates and critics associate commissioning with marketisation and increasing contestability in public services (Rees et al, 2017), and also with weakening democratic control of public services (Davies, 2008, as cited in Rees et al, 2017). As such, commissioning is often portrayed as a technical/professional process, which is detached from politics (Bovaird et al, 2014). This depoliticisation (Burnham, 2001) is seen as being positive by many, as it is seen to be more objective and evidence-based. There is a plethora of guidance and manuals on the commissioning process (Huxley et al, 2010), much of which sits firmly in the rationalist-scientific tradition. It sees commissioning as a cycle, in which professionals make objective assessments of the needs of local populations, assess and select the most effective interventions to address those needs, undertake open procurement exercises to achieve the highest quality services at the most appropriate cost and undertake ongoing performance monitoring and evaluation, often described as 'analyse–plan–do–review'.

These commissioning cycles are reminiscent of the policy cycles that can be found in numerous government and related guides to public policymaking and in the older public administration literature. There are numerous such policy cycles from which to choose. From Harold Lasswell's seven functions of the policy process (Lasswell, 1956), to Herbert Simon's 'Intelligence, design, choice' (Simon, 1947), through to Brian Hogwood and Lewis Gunn's nine-stage process, which begins with deciding to decide and deciding how to decide, and ends with evaluation and review, and finally termination (Hogwood and Gunn, 1984), there are many examples of attempts to describe and categorise the policy process as a rational-scientific process.

Just like their policy cycle predecessors, these commissioning cycles bear little resemblance to the *actual* process of making strategic policy decisions. For commissioning is inherently a political process (Allen et al, 2011); it is about making choices about where and how to spend limited resources, which needs to prioritise and which interventions are most likely to be workable. It is also inherently context-bound and emotional, because it is about decisions that affect real people's lives. While evidence can and should be part of the commissioning process, it is not the only consideration, and there is not a linear influence of evidence on policy (Black, 2011). There are also different 'cultures of evidence' with which to contend (Milton et al, 2014). It also ignores policy myopia faced by policymakers (Nair and Howlett, 2017); that policy makers are boundedly rational, that they do not concurrently examine the potential policy alternatives to make decisions about which is most likely to address identified policy problems, but rather 'satisfice', assessing options one by one until they find an option that is 'good enough' to meet their needs.

In this chapter, we use the term 'commissioning' to mean population-level decisions about what types and levels of public service provision is needed, how priorities are selected and how this provision should be funded and organised. We see this as being different, though by necessity related, to decisions about what specific services should be contracted for and the process of deciding which service provider should deliver specific services. Commissioning is and should be a political process; it is about 'who gets what, how and when' (Lasswell, 1936). Because of its political and its strategic nature, we argue here that commissioning can and should be used to deliver broad policy and political objectives, such as addressing the social determinants of health.

Local authority commissioning: the evidence

Although there has been much policy and theoretical discussion around commissioning, and particularly around its perceived role in marketisation, the empirical evidence on commissioning is decidedly mixed. In practice, it appears that commissioning has not been the transformative process feared by critics or promoted by advocates (Rees et al, 2017), not least because strategic commissioning decisions have been limited to areas of service that had previously been externalised (Bovaird et al, 2014). There are significant differences in the extent to which local authorities actively and positively engage with commissioning and procurement (Loader, 2018), whether and which policy objectives affect procurement. Commissioning and procurement are organised in many different ways in local authorities across the UK.

There is a dearth of empirical evidence around local authority strategic commissioning, particularly in relation to tackling the social determinants of health. This is surprising. As Dylan Kneale and colleagues identified in a recent systematic review of the use of evidence in public health decision-making in England, local authorities are also responsible for reducing health inequalities, and identified nine non-health areas in which they can achieve this, including early years, education, planning, housing, leisure and communities (Kneale et al, 2017).

Over and above responsibilities in these broad areas of social policy, local government also has specific responsibilities for public health since 2013. These changes include the creation of local HWBs, partnerships between the NHS, public health, adult social care and children's services, tasked with strategic commissioning based on local health needs. A recently published national evaluation of HWBs suggests that they are at risk of becoming 'talking shops', with very little real influence on strategic commissioning decisions (Hunter et al, 2018). There is some evidence around service commissioning undertaken by local authorities around public health. This evidence relates to specific service areas, such as alcohol harm reduction (Martineau et al, 2013), and to the challenges of using evidence in a political decision-making process (McGill et al, 2015; Phillips and Green, 2015; Sanders et al, 2017).

There is also growing evidence of increased joint service level commissioning around adult social care between local authorities and the Clinical Commissioning Groups (King's Fund, 2017), part of the NHS responsible for purchasing urgent and acute hospital services. The King's Fund argues that this joint work, along with developing place-based initiatives and devolution in a number of areas (most notably Greater Manchester), will have a significant effect on commissioning in the future. While promising, much of this is focused on service commissioning, and around specific health and social care services rather than on strategic commissioning on non-health areas that affect health inequalities (such as those identified by Kneale et al, 2017).

Nor is the evidence base more developed in terms of local voluntary sector organisations and SMEs. Despite numerous UK government initiatives to increase procurement of voluntary sector organisations and SMEs to deliver services, there remain a number of significant barriers. Public contracts are growing in size, value and geographical coverage, which disadvantages local charities. Procurement risk aversion favours larger contracts and larger organisations with track records of public sector work (O'Leary, 2018). The recent move to outcome-based commissioning contracts, such as Payment by Results and Social Impact Bonds, can also disadvantage smaller charities. Cundy (2012) and Ward et al (2010) argue that the high up-front costs of bidding and managing such contracts can discourage or prevent smaller and/or local third sector organisations from bidding. There is an increasing evidence base showing that SMEs are similarly at a disadvantage in engaging with public procurement compared to larger suppliers (Flynn and Davis, 2015; Loader, 2016, 2018).

Social determinants, charities and SMEs

There is a considerable body of evidence that links social capital and health (Abbott, 2010), and several studies have suggested that over time, increases in social capital are associated with improved health (Hunter et al, 2011). Social capital is a multifaceted concept, but broadly involves social networks, participation in civil society and community activities, and levels of trust. Over the past twenty years, a significant body of research has examined the role that social capital plays as a social determinant of health. There has been much debate about the concept: how it might be measured; through what mechanisms social capital and health are related; and the value of social capital in addressing the social determinants of health (Moore and Kawachi, 2017). Several authors also suggest that the evidence is less than clear about the role played by social capital. These arguments focus on the type of social capital (particularly individual versus collective social capital), highlighting conflicting findings (Kim et al, 2011) and arguing that more research is needed to understand how social capital affects, and is affected by, social determinants, and what types of interventions might be effective.

Despite this, recent work by the Institute of Health Equity at University College London makes clear that the voluntary sector can directly influence social determinants because of the services they deliver, the communities with which they engage, through informing and engaging with the public, and through their policy and lobbying work (Daly and Allen, 2017). People have better health when they are more comfortable in, and contribute to, their communities (Hunter et al, 2011). In particular, the sector is a significant local source of social capital. Charities provide opportunities for volunteering, which is a means of developing both human and social capital (O'Leary et al, 2018). There is significant evidence that volunteering has positive health outcomes in mental and physical health, wellbeing and life expectancy (Yeung et al, 2017). Third sector has the potential to be more equitable, as it can engage with some groups that government services cannot reach (Paton et al, 2007; Musick and Wilson, 2008).

But there are huge variations in the size, quality and impact of voluntary sector organisations between local areas (Mohan and Bennett, 2019). Areas that are more affluent tend to have larger and more diverse voluntary sector landscapes, while more disadvantaged areas have fewer organisations with smaller resources. Neighbourhoods that lack a vibrant voluntary sector can miss out on a number of benefits, which may be detrimental in addressing health inequalities at the local level. We therefore argue that local authorities using their commissioning and their purchasing power strategically to address social determinants of health should focus on the role of social capital.

Of course, many local authorities already contract with charities to provide a range of services. The sector is involved in the delivery of a large and growing part of public services in the UK (O'Leary and McDonnell, 2019), so that between a third and half of the charities' annual income comes from contracts procured by central and local government. The problem is, this is concentrated in the hands of a small number of very large charities; so that while overall resources in the voluntary sector have increased over the past 20 years, in part thanks to earned income from government contracts, the income for small and medium-sized charities has actually fallen (O'Leary and McDonnell, 2019).

Why is this important? It is important because smaller, more local charities are likely to have a greater impact on neighbourhood social capital than their larger, more national or international counterparts. Smaller charities tend to be more locally focused, and are often directly embedded with the communities they serve. Local charities are the backbone of the social sector; created by local people in response to local issues, and as such are both trusted and have the expertise and knowledge to work effectively (Lloyds Bank Foundation, 2016). They have higher levels of voluntary participation than larger charities (Milligan and Fyfe, 2005; Mohan and Bennett, 2019) and volunteering makes a key contribution locally to social capital. Local charities and SMEs act as 'anchors' that provide local physical, social and economic assets and support local supply chains (Hudson, 2018).

We therefore argue that local authorities should use their strategic commissioning decisions, and their purchasing power, to leverage local voluntary sector organisations and SMEs in action to tackle the social determinants of health. Recognising the complex legal framework around commissioning and procurement, we believe that there are two key mechanisms through which this can be achieved: the Public Services (Social Value) Act 2012 and place-based commissioning.

The Public Services (Social Value) Act requires public bodies to consider securing improvements in economic, social and environmental wellbeing – in social value – when they procure goods and services. Tackling the social determinants of health is a clear social value and should be at the heart of local authorities commissioning strategies. Unfortunately, in its current form, the Act is not delivering on its promise (O'Leary and McDonnell, 2019). In a recent report on the operation of the Act, the Local Government Association found some positive changes in procurement, but little evidence that the provisions were being used to develop local supplier markets or, more importantly, to deliver a more holistic approach to commissioning (LGA, 2017). Other research has found that 40 per cent of NHS commissioners are not using the Act when procuring services (Butler and Redding, 2017) and two-thirds of local authorities are struggling to make use of the Act's provisions, because of insufficient resources, risk aversion and poor procurement practices (Jones and Yeo, 2017). A recent government review of the Act made a number of recommendations for changes (Cabinet Office, 2015). But even under its current provisions, the Act can be used by local authorities to enhance their roles as market makers and as social value enablers, focus strategic commissioning on tackling social determinants and delivering real social value, review procurement processes and procedures, and encourage and support smaller and more local charities and SMEs through the procurement process (O'Leary and McDonnell, 2019).

Secondly, like the Social Value Act, recent moves towards place-based commissioning provide real opportunities to engage with local charities and SMEs to tackle social determinants. Place-based commissioning sees public sector organisations collaborate and integrate within specific area boundaries to jointly commissioning services. Recent work by the King's Fund (Ham and Alderwick, 2015) and the Local Government Association (LGA, 2018) make very positive noises about the potential for place-based commissioning initiatives, and there are several schemes developing across the UK. Again, much of these are focused on service level commissioning, and do not appear to be focused on tackling social determinants of health. But the potential for place-based commissioning to engage with local charities and SMEs in strategic commissioning decisions and in the delivery of local services, and thereby to make a real difference in tackling the social determinants of health, is significant.

Conclusions

Local authorities are key actors in reducing health inequalities and tackling the social determinants of health, which they can impact at a population level through their role in early years education, schools, planning, housing, social care, public space, air quality, public transport and community development. Since 2013, they have also had responsibilities for public health, following the transfer of responsibilities from the NHS and the creation of HWBs under the provisions of the Health and Social Care Act 2012.

Local authorities make strategic decisions about the types of services their local populations need, and spend thousands of pounds commissioning and procuring services. In this chapter, it is argued that local authorities can and should use their purchasing power strategically to tackle social determinants of health. They can do so using the Public Services (Social Value) Act 2012, and through place-based commissioning initiatives.

It is also argued that local charities and businesses can play a key role in tackling the social determinants, through the role they play in social capital. More disadvantaged areas tend to have fewer charities, with smaller resources, compared with more affluent areas. Given the role that local charities and SMEs play in the social capital of communities and the individuals in those communities, and the role that social capital appears to play in reducing health inequalities, it is argued that local charities and SMEs can and should play a key role in tackling the social determinants of health, and that more work is needed to encourage and support them in local commissioning and procurement.

References

Abbott, S. (2010) 'Social capital and health: the role of participation', *Social Theory & Health*, 8: 51–65.

Allen, B., Wade, E. and Dickinson, H. (2011) 'Bridging the divide – commercial procurement and supply chain management: are there lessons for health care commissioning in England?', *Journal of Public Procurement*, 9(1): 505–34.

Black, J. (2011) 'Commissioning policy', House of Commons Health Committee Ev 79, Q 377–81.

Booth, L. (2018) 'Public procurement and contracts, briefing paper no. 6029', London: House of Commons Library.

Bovaird, T., Briggs, I. and Willis, M. (2014) 'Strategic commissioning in the UK: service improvement cycle or just going round in circles?', *Local Government Studies*, 40(4): 533–59.

Burnham, P. (2001) 'New Labour and the politics of depoliticisation', *British Journal of Politics and International Relations*, 3(2): 127–49.

Butler, J. and Redding, D. (2017) 'Healthy commissioning: how the Social Value Act is being used by clinical commissioning groups, Social Enterprise UK and National Voices, UK. Available from: https://www.nationalvoices.org.uk/publications/our-publications/healthy-commissioning-how-social-value-act-being-used-clinical [Accessed 15 August 2019].

Cabinet Office (2015) 'Social Value Act review', London: Cabinet Office. Available from: https://assets.publishing.service.gov.uk/government/uploads/system/uploads/attachment_data/file/403748/Social_Value_Act_review_report_150212.pdf [Accessed 20 August 2019].

Cundy, J. (2012) 'Commissioning for better outcomes: understanding local authority and voluntary sector experiences of family services commissioning in England', London: Barnardo's UK. Available from: https://www.bl.uk/collection-items/commissioning-for-better-outcomes-understanding-local-authority-and-voluntary-sector-experiences-of-family-services-commissioning-in-england [Accessed 15 May 2020].

Daly, S. and Allen, J. (2017) 'Voluntary sector action on the social determinants of health', The Health Foundation, New Philanthropy Capital, Institute for Health Equity, UK. Available from: http://www.instituteofhealthequity.org/resources-reports/voluntary-sector-action-on-the-social-determinants-of-health [Accessed 12 April 2020].

Dickinson, H. (2015) 'Commissioning public services evidence review: lessons for Australian public services', Melbourne School of Government, Australia.

Flynn, A. and Davis, P. (2015) 'The rhetoric and reality of SME-friendly procurement', *Public Money & Management*, 35(2): 111–18.

Ham, C. and Alderwick, H. (2015) 'Place-based systems of care: a way forward for the NHS in England', London: King's Fund.

Hogwood, B. and Gunn, L. (1984) *Policy Analysis for the Real World*, Oxford: Oxford University Press.

Hood, C. (1991) 'A public management for all seasons?', *Public Administration*, 69(1): 3–19.

Hudson, B. (2018) 'Commissioning for change: a new model for commissioning adult social care in England', *Critical Social Policy*, 39(3): 413–33.

Hunter, B., Neiger, B. and West, J. (2011) 'The importance of addressing social determinants of health at the local level: the case for social capital', *Health and Social Care in the Community*, 19(5): 522–30.

Hunter, D., Perkins, N., Visram, S., Adams, L., Finn, R., Forrest, A. and Gosling, J. (2018) 'Evaluating he leadership role of health and wellbeing boards as drivers of health improvement and integrated care across England: final report', London: National Institute for Health Research. Available from: https://research.ncl.ac.uk/media/sites/researchwebsites/davidhunter/Evaluating%20HWBs%20FINAL%20REPORT%20-%20April%202018%20Final.pdf [Accessed 15 August 2019].

Huxley, P., Maegusuku-Hewett, T., Evans, S., Cornes, M., Manthorpe, J. and Stevens, M. (2010) 'Better evidence for better commissioning: a study of the evidence base of generic social care commissioning guides in the UK', *Evidence and Policy*, 6(3): 291–308.

Jones, N. and Yeo, A. (2017) 'Community business and the Social Value Act, Research Institute Report No. 8', London: Power to Change. Available from: https://www.powertochange.org.uk/wp-content/uploads/2017/08/Report-8-Community-Business-Social-Value-Act-1.pdf [Accessed 10 August 2019].

Kim, D., Baum, C., Ganz, M., Subramanian, S. and Kawachi, I. (2011) 'The contextual effects of social capital on health: a crossnational instrumental variable analysis', *Social Science and Medicine*, 73(12): 1689–97.

King's Fund (2017) 'What is commissioning and how is it changing?', London: King's Fund. Available from: https://www.kingsfund.org.uk/publications/what-commissioning-and-how-it-changing#summary [Accessed 15 August 2019].

Kneale, D., Rojas-García, A, Raine, R. and Thomas, J. (2017) 'The use of evidence in English local public health decision-making: a systematic scoping review', *Implementation Science*, 12(53). Available from: https://implementationscience.biomedcentral.com/articles/10.1186/s13012-017-0577-9 [Accessed 12 April 2020].

Lasswell, H. (1936) *Politics: Who Gets What, When, How*. New York: McGraw-Hill.

Lasswell, H. (1956) *The Decision Process: Seven Categories of Functional Analysis*, College Park, MD: University of Maryland Press.

LGA (Local Government Association) (2017) 'Encouraging innovation in local government procurement', Local Government Association, London.

LGA (Local Government Association) (2018) 'Shifting the centre of gravity: making place-based, person-centred health and care a reality', Local Government Association, London.

Lloyds Bank Foundation (2016) 'Commissioning in crisis: how contracting and procurement processes threaten small charities', London: Lloyds Bank Foundation.

Loader, K. (2016) 'Is local authority procurement supporting SMEs? An analysis of practice in English local authorities', *Local Government Studies*, 42(3): 464–84.

Loader, K. (2018) 'Small and medium-sized enterprises and public procurement: a review of the UK coalition government's policies and their impact', *Environment and Planning C: Politics and Space*, 36(1): 47–66.

Marks, L., Hunter, D., Scalabrini, S., Gray, J., McCafferty, S., Payne, N., Peckham, S. and Thokala, P. (2015) 'The return of public health to local government in England: changing the parameters of the public health prioritization debate?', *Public Health*, 129(9): 1194–1203.

Martineau, F., Graff, H., Mitchell, C. and Lock, K. (2013) 'Responsibility without legal authority? Tackling alcohol-related health harms through licensing and planning policy in local government', *Journal of Public Health*, 36(3): 435–42.

McGill, E., Egan, M., Petticrew, M., Mountford, L., Milton, S., Whitehead, M. and Lock, L. (2015) 'Trading quality for relevance: nonhealth decision-makers' use of evidence on the social determinants of health', *BMJ Open*, 2015;5:e007053. Available from: https://doi.org/10.1136/bmjopen-2014-007053 [Accessed 18 May 2020].

MHCLG (Ministry and Housing, Communities and Local Government) (2018) 'Local authority revenue expenditure and financing: 2017/18 final outturn, England, statistical release', London: Ministry and Housing, Communities and Local Government.

Milligan, C. and Fyfe, N. (2005) 'Making space for volunteers: exploring the links between voluntary organizations, volunteering and citizenship', *Urban Studies*, 42(3): 417–34.

Milton, S., Petticrew, M. and Green, J. (2014) 'Why do local authorities undertake controlled evaluations of health impact? A qualitative case study of interventions in housing', *Public Health*, 128: 1112–17.

Mohan, J. and Bennett, M. (2019) 'Community-level impacts of the third sector: does the local distribution of voluntary organizations influence the likelihood of volunteering?', *EPA: Economy and Space*, 51(4): 950–79.

Moore, S. and Kawachi, I. (2017) 'Twenty years of social capital and health research: a glossary', *Journal of Epidemiology and Community Health*, 71(5): 513–17.

Murray, J. (2011) 'Third sector commissioning and English local government procurement', *Public Money and Management*, 31(4): 279–86.

Musick, M., and Wilson, J. (2008) *Volunteers: A Social Profile*. Bloomington: Indiana University Press.

Nair, S. and Howlett, M. (2017) 'Policy myopia as a source of policy failure: adaptation and policy learning under deep uncertainty', *Policy & Politics*, 45(1): 103–18.

O'Leary, C. (2018) 'The lesson to be learnt from Carillion is that we need more private sector and charities involved in delivering public services, not fewer', MetroPolis blog, Manchester Metropolitan University. Available from: https://mcrmetropolis.uk/blog/the-lesson-to-be-learnt-from-carillion-is-that-we-need-more-private-sector-and-charities-involved-in-delivering-public-services-not-fewer/ [Accessed 15 August 2019].

O'Leary, C. and McDonnell, D. (2019) 'Procurement and commissioning in the non-profit sector', in D. McDonnell (ed) *Innovation and Change in Non-Profit Organisations: Case Studies in Survival, Sustainability and Success*, pp 49–60, Shoreham on Sea: Pavilion Publishers.

O'Leary, C., Baines, S., Bailey, G., McNeill, T., Csoba, J. and Sipis, F. (2018) 'Innovation and social investment programmes in Europe', *European Policy Analysis*, 4(2): 294–312.

Paton, R., Mordaunt, J. and Cornforth, C. (2007) 'Beyond nonprofit management education: leadership development in a time of blurred boundaries and distributed learning', *Nonprofit and Voluntary Sector Quarterly*, 36(suppl. 4): 148S–162S.

Patrucco, A., Walker, H., Luzzini, D. and Ronchi, S. (2019) 'Which shape fits best? Designing the organizational form of local government procurement', *Journal of Purchasing and Supply Management*, 25(3).

Phillips, G. and Green, J. (2015) 'Working for the public health: politics, localism and epistemologies of practice', *Sociology of Health and Illness*, 37(4): 491–505.

Ramia, G. and Carney, T. (2001) 'Contractualism, managerialism and welfare: the Australian experiment with a marketised employment services network', *Policy & Politics*, 29(1): 59–80.

Rees, J., Miller, R. and Buckingham, H. (2017) 'Commission incomplete: exploring the new model for purchasing public services from the third sector', *Journal of Social Policy*, 46(1): 175–94.

Sanders, T., Grove, A., Salway, S., Hampshaw, S. and Goyder, E. (2017) 'Incorporation of a health economic modelling tool into public health commissioning: evidence use in a politicised context', *Social Science and Medicine*, 186: 122–9.

Simon, H. (1947) *Administrative Behavior: A Study of Decision-Making Processes in Administrative Organization*, New York: Macmillan.

Ward, E., Sample, E. and Roberts, M. (2010) 'Testing the waters', *Druglink*, 25(6): 11–15.

WHO (World Health Organization) Commission on Social Determinants of Health (2008) 'Closing the Gap in a Generation: Health Equity through Action on the Social Determinants of Health'. Final Report of the Commission on Social Determinants of Health. Geneva: WHO.

Yeung, J., Zhang, Z. and Kim, T. (2017) 'Volunteering and health benefits in general adults: cumulative effects and forms', *BMC Public Health*, 18(1): 8.

15

Future generations: the role of community-based organisations in supporting young people

Adam Bonner

Introduction

In 2020, there is a reported high level of employment in the United Kingdom (UK). However, there are major concerns regarding high levels of youth unemployment in many parts of the UK. The recent COVID-19 global pandemic is only likely to exacerbate this challenge as 'experts predict the coronavirus pandemic will trigger the worst economic slump since the Great Depression of the 1920s' (Stubley, 2020).

Regional differences, across Wales, Scotland and England (see Chapters 5, 6, 7, 9 and 21) in youth unemployment and other demographic factors, including race and disability, are issues that need to be considered by local and national governments. This chapter presents two non-statutory approaches aimed at engaging young people in the community.

The Youth United Foundation (YUF) supports the development of well-established community-based organisations including the Scouts, Guides and Boys' Brigade joined, recently, by the creation of new uniformed youth organisations, including Fire and Police Cadets, to help significantly increase opportunities for young people from the most disadvantaged communities.

For many young people, the local high street provides a safe meeting place for young people, who can no longer 'hang out' in the youth clubs of past years. However, with the demise of the traditional high street major challenges are presented to local authorities, which increasingly rely on generating business rates from hard-pressed shops under threat from the tidal wave of online retailing.

Building on the place-based policies of the London Borough of Sutton (see Chapter 6), Sutton Community Dance (SCD) is an example of reimagining the high street and prioritising shared places as an important context for building intergenerational bridges. Such a model of reimagination and creative agility will be critical in helping already challenged town centres to develop new possibilities for reform post the COVID-19 pandemic. This all-age inclusive development makes a significant contribution to the social determinants of health in this South London borough, through improvements in health and wellbeing (see Bonner, 2018, part 2) and the promotion of self-actualisation (see Chapter 1 in this volume).

Reductions in youth services

An important consequence of central government austerity budgeting and restrictions in funding available to local authorities is the 18 per cent drop in council spending on young people's services. A reduction of £90 million between 2014/15 and 2019 has been reported by the Chartered Institute of Public Finance and Accountancy (CIPFA) (Brady, 2019). Cuts in services for early intervention for vulnerable young people increase risks for substance misuse, teenage pregnancy and youth crime. Local authority services such as community centres, parks and after school programmes have been removed from communities, resources that had been developed by councils over many years. In cycle after cycle of council cuts, their discretionary services have been sacrificed in order to protect statutory services. Rob Whiteman, chief executive of CIPFA, has commented that 'much like libraries, the statutory role of local authorities to provide youth services is unclear, labelled simply as a "duty to secure access to positive activities"'. There is a general trend to prioritise acute needs over preventative services, with the unintended consequences of increasing the demand for statutory social care including child protection (Atkins, 2019).

In the report 'Youth Services at Breaking Point', the public service union UNISON draws attention to the loss of 900 youth worker jobs and a reduction of £13.3 million from youth services between 2016 and 2019, resulting in a loss between 2012 and 2018, of 4,500 youth worker jobs and over 760 youth centres (UNISON, 2018). These services help with employment, training and education, increase resilience for mental health and contribute to reductions in alcohol and other drug misuse, thus saving future public sector money in many areas of local authority activities.

Differences in the reduction of youth services across England and Wales have been reported by the YMCA, which concluded that local authorities are so focused on complying with statutory requirements for young people that during a time of shrinking council budgets these long-term benefits accrued from youth services are often overlooked in the process-making decisions about council budget planning.

Opportunities outside school and positive activities that support learning and personal development were taken for granted by previous generations (YMCA, 2019). There has been a 46 per cent funding reduction in London's youth services since 2011/12. This has resulted in the closure of 104 youth centres and a reduction of 562 youth worker jobs (Berry, 2019). Unemployment and lack of youth engagement is thought to motivate young disadvantaged people, in Northern Ireland, to become influenced by paramilitary groups (Black, 2015).

Currently a 'social emergency' has been declared by MPs working within the All Party Parliamentary Group on Knife Crime (APPG), who report that the government has failed young people in the most 'devastating way' (APPG, 2018). Growing numbers of school exclusions and children taken into care are just some of the factors to be taken into account when considering the contributory factors leading to the number of under-18s admitted to hospital with knife crime injuries, which increased by a third between 2013/14 and 2017/18 (Figure 15.1).

The APPG report shows a 68 per cent increase in annual recorded knife crime offences from March 2014 to September 2018. A response of 70 per cent from 154 councils to a Freedom of Information enquiry by the All-Party Parliamentary Group on Knife Crime has revealed a

Figure 15.1: Knife crime injuries, 2011–19

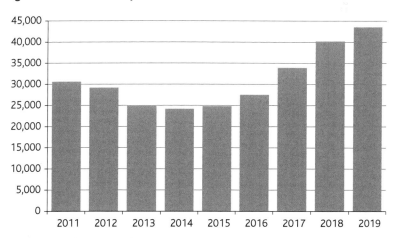

Source: Home Office, year ending March. Figures exclude Greater Manchester. Quoted in https://www.bbc.co.uk/news/uk-42749089

40–91 per cent real terms cut in spending on youth services by local councils over the same time period. Areas that had the highest cuts had some of the highest increases in knife crime. Youth services in City of Wolverhampton cut youth services by 91 per cent, Cambridge County Council by 88 per cent and Wokingham Borough Council by 81 per cent. Increased demands in statutory child protection and other children's services have meant that councils have had to divert their limited funds away from preventative work (APPG, 2018).

Cuts in local services and adverse childhood experiences

The costs of not addressing these issues will continue to unlock antisocial behaviour, including drug-taking, gang-related violence, youth suicide and increased vulnerability to human trafficking and modern slavery. Adverse early childhood experiences and the lack of affordable housing for young people mitigate against some young people reaching their potential.

The fundamental importance of early childhood experiences and the development of social networks, which have a major impact on later life health and wellbeing, have been reviewed (see Bonner, 2018, chapter 1). This critical issue impacting on the wellbeing of young people is addressed in the Well-Being of Future Generations Act (WFG Act) 2015 (see Chapter 20).

What works for young people?

There is a statutory duty for councils to 'secure, so far as is reasonably practicable, sufficient provision of education and recreational leisure-time activities for young people', as noted in Section 507B of the Education Act 1996 (HMG, 1996). There has been a range of responses by local authorities to the huge cuts imposed on them by integrating youth services with other support for young people and their families and by targeting vulnerable groups. In the report 'Bright Futures: Our Vision for Youth Services, the Local Government Association has presented a long-term vision for youth services. The six key principles of this vision include:

- *Youth-led* listening to the needs of local young people by offering both universal, open-access provision, and targeted support for those considered to be at risk, disadvantaged or with higher needs.
- *Inclusivity, equity and diversity* no young person should feel marginalized or isolated as a result of disability, sexuality, nationality,

socioeconomic status, special educational needs, mental health issues, religion or any other characteristics.

- *Respect* young people are valued and respected as part of the community. They are actively encouraged to participate in their communities, enjoy opportunities without fear of judgement or negative stereotyping.
- *Quality, safety and well-being* [services provided by staff with appropriate safeguarding training, linked to a wider network of support…. Helping to keep young people safe and supporting their mental, emotional and physical health, improves their social and economic wellbeing, with access to education, non-formal learning and recreation].
- *Empowerment* service to empower young people to progress and engage in employment, education and training, and take an active role in their local communities. Young people are listened to and can make positive demonstrative changes to their communities and understand how to engage with the democratic process
- *Positivity* services should be strength-based and focus on developing the skills and attributes of young people, rather than attempting to fix a problem. (LGA, 2019)

Mentoring of disaffected young people has been developing over recent years. A report based on findings from research undertaken by Shiner and others (Shiner et al, 2004) from the London School of Economics, published by the Joseph Rowntree Foundation, has reviewed ten Mentoring Plus programmes run by Crime Concern and Breaking Barriers. These one-to-one services, using volunteer mentors from the local community, provide education and training and social activities. Four hundred young people aged 12–19 were recruited and 57 per cent of those recruited went on to engage with the programme on a monthly basis. Many of those recruited had substantial disruption in their schooling and family lives, were at significant risk of social exclusion and were not engaging in the community. Many had left school without any qualifications and their lifestyles often included illicit drug use and contact with the criminal justice system. The programme was particularly effective in engaging with Black African/Caribbean young people at risk of social exclusion and involved sensitive relationship-building around low-key social interactions with little reference to their challenging issues or behaviours. The greatest impact of the programme was in relation to engagement in education, training and work. Although many of the relationships between the volunteer mentors and the mentees did not develop beyond 'mundane' social interactions, many of the young people felt positive about the mentoring and the Plus, social activities element of the programme. Impact on offending, family relationships, substance use and self-esteem was not clear from this research.

Non-statutory approaches that support and empower young people

In 2012 the Coalition government undertook a review of councils' spending on youth services, but since that time there has been a reduction of more than £400 million in funding for youth services and youth centres have been closed as noted previously. In this review, 'Positive for Youth', section 507B of the Education Act was reiterated. A review of the guidance to councils (DDCMS et al, 2018), freshly articulated the statutory duty placed on local authorities to provide appropriate local youth services. In this new strategy, 'the government recognizes the transformational impact that youth services and trained youth workers can have, especially for young people facing multiple barriers and disadvantage'. This is good news as local councils had been forced to deprioritise youth services in their attempts to balance diminishing budgets. The strategy includes ways to 'fully embed' the National Citizen Service within the youth sector, to consider the expansion of uniformed youth groups in disadvantaged areas and to support positive citizenship by cross-government measures. To assist young people facing barriers to work, the strategy aims to create a new organisation independent of government to oversee the distribution of a £90 million Big Lottery Fund, extracted from dormant bank accounts. The aim of this is to 'harness the experience of grassroots youth workers, business and other local services to build a strong partnership of support around each young person' (Big Lottery Community Fund, 2018).

Young people as assets, not problems

Over recent years, a critical factor in the development of healthy communities has been the increasing adoption of the assets-based approach to youth work and to broader community work. While differing language has been used to describe the values base, the assets-based approach seeks to always begin any consideration of interventions by first identifying the strengths of an individual or community and then mutually agreeing what further strengths or 'assets' can and should be developed (see Chapters 6, 7 and 8). Such an approach has also become increasingly important and transformative in the arena of wider health development, as shown in Scotland (NHS Scotland, 2011).

When focusing on the development of transformative community work with young people and when seeking to understand how collective work can improve the social, mental and physical health of young people, the assets-based approach offers a rich lens and set of tools through which to truly develop a holistic approach. As a pioneering London borough using this approach, Sutton published a detailed breakdown of 40 individual assets from family support to positive peer influence and 32 community assets ranging from public participation in decision-making to high-quality streets (LBS, 2013).

The range of assets identified as critical by the London Borough of Sutton is used throughout both the delivery of youth and community work (and work with older people) as well as the actual commissioning of such work in the first place and the work's evaluation as appropriate.

Building assets and developing trust takes time

As with the most successful interventions for young people and communities, the assets-based approach works best when the work can be properly planned and evaluated. Other key prerequisites include the need for building long-term relationships and a consistent offer, so young people, their parents and carers are able to know those with whom they are working to establish meaningful levels of trust. Such long-term approaches are essential in both the statutory provided services from local authorities as well as the support offered by voluntary organisations, such as faith-based groups and uniformed youth groups.

The long-term approach isn't only about ensuring consistency of relationship between individuals involved within the youth or community work on the micro-level but also to provide the context through which organisations, funders and regulators can develop feedback loops and an established knowledge base of the most impactful work. Conversely, the tendency for funders is often to focus on brand new projects, programmes and providers who present, often excellent, innovative ideas and new solutions to the ongoing challenges for disaffected youth and broken communities, referred to throughout the other chapters in this book.

Uniformed youth foundation

One positive example of long-term support for young people and families is the role played by the uniformed youth organisations across the UK. Well-known organisations including the Scouts, Guides and Boys' Brigade have been joined by the more recent groups, including Fire and Police Cadets. Such organisations have an incredible strength by being both embedded long term in many UK communities as well as being largely run by a vast array of volunteers, generating the essential social capital referred to by authors and academics including Robert Putnam (Putnam, 2000).

A new £5 million Uniformed Youth Fund was announced by the Department for Community Culture Media and Sport in August 2019 to be distributed by YUF.

YUF is a network of 11 youth organisations that deliver work across the UK. The network seeks to provide opportunities for young people through local uniformed youth groups. The network, which includes some of the biggest youth organisations in the country, delivers direct opportunities to 1.5 million young people on a regular basis.

Long-term youth organisations reducing isolation and loneliness

Experiences of loneliness can be a normal part of human development. It is very likely that the feelings and responses we have to feeling lonely will change over time and as we mature. That said, for some young people loneliness can be an ever-intensifying state, where they increasingly feel isolated, distant and outside relationships with their peers, families and communities they live in.

Loneliness is different from social isolation, and young people can feel incredibly lonely even when we might otherwise regard them as being socially connected or very sociable (Sharabi et al, 2012). As such, it is possible for a young person to feel lonely even when they are surrounded by people they call 'friends'. This form of 'in-group loneliness' arises when someone's own life experiences, values, beliefs, thoughts and feelings are not recognised, or do not resonate, with their peers or adults around them.

What is the role of uniformed youth organisations?

Evidence shows that uniformed group activities can give young people the resources and skills they need to feel connected and valued. For example, uniformed group programmes in schools have been shown to have positive wellbeing outcomes, including a rise in levels of children's and young people's empathy, resilience, collaboration and career aspirations (Gorard and Siddiqui, 2017). More widely, youth participation enhances character formation, and increases self-esteem.

As well as benefits during childhood and adolescence, participation in uniformed youth organisations may have a protective effect on participants. Analysis from an ongoing cohort study of people born in the UK in a single week in 1958 found that, even when controlling for early life factors, those who were members of the Scouts/Guides had better mental health in later life than their non-attending peers. These positive effects appeared particularly strong for children growing up in low social position households, ameliorating inequalities in later life probability of mental health based on childhood socio-economic position (Dibben et al, 2017).

There are wider benefits for the mental health and wellbeing of adult volunteers, with studies showing volunteering can provide important social connectivity and social capital benefits (Linning and Jackson, 2018). Other evidence suggests that volunteering may be more strongly associated with enhanced mental wellbeing, and that this grows with age (Tabassum et al, 2016).

Every blade of grass has its angel that bends over it and whispers, 'Grow, grow'. This beautiful line from the Talmud is the epigraph to social activist Hilary Cottam's 2018 book, which argues for a reinvention of the welfare state (p 3) so that all feel supported and can 'live to our true and shared potential'. The post-war welfare state ('an original and brilliant experiment', p 20) is unable to deal with the reality of modern life: it has become a 'management state' (p 12)in which 80 per cent of the resource is spent on gate-keeping. A fundamental change is needed in which 'the emphasis is not on managing need but on creating capability' (Cottam, 2018).

The chapter has thus far explored the critical theme of isolation, violence, loneliness and the marginalisation of young people. The response of YUF is highlighted as a model that successfully aims to increase the level of meaningful and relevant support through the network of well-established uniformed youth groups. These highly credible groups provide a specific and well-travelled road for intervening within the lives of young people, seeking to provide 'angels' present in the lives of young people to help them grow as per the quote from the Talmud.

Such groups, as discussed, provide a long-term community benefit through being deeply embedded in many communities across the UK.

Yet, as commented upon throughout this publication, the challenges and opportunities that the UK now faces in terms of health and wellbeing require a response focused on far wider social cohorts than just those of young people.

Reimagining the high street and prioritising shared places as an important context for building intergenerational bridges

Increasingly, an urgent phenomenon requiring attention is the decline of UK high streets and the longer-term effect this decline is likely to contribute to the state of health and wellbeing.

The Office for National Statistics (ONS) informs us that 'there are nearly 7,000 high streets in Great Britain, defined by a cluster of 15 or more retail addresses within 150 metres.'

The nature of UK high streets is significantly shifting and doing so now with pace. Between 2012 and 2017, the number of high street retail jobs fell in every country and region except London. New research also indicates the top 150 UK retailers have 20 per cent more store space than they need and can afford (Simson, 2019). Critically, it is noted in ONS analysis that 'in 2017, the retail sector provided between 25 per cent and 31 per cent of high street employment in all regions and countries of Great Britain except London'. From March 2016 to 2019, UK retail lost 106,000 jobs according to the British Retail Consortium. Researchers at A&M and Retail Economics suggest that during the past five years, companies have had to spend 10.8 per cent more on overheads such as business rates, increasing wages and rents.

However, the high street's decline as a centre for retail opportunity and employment isn't simply a change for those seeking work or looking for local shops. The growing shift from town centres (generally) and high streets (specifically) away from retail and towards residential property signifies the changing nature of these places as hubs for community. Coupling this with the ONS's latest research, indicating that 'around 2 per cent to 3 per cent' of high street properties are currently leisure or community facilities (ONS, 2019), it is clear that the broader observable shift is away from public shared spaces to private individual spaces being focused at the geographical heart of UK communities. Coupling the well-documented closure of youth services and youth centres with the decline of high street activity, a conclusion can be drawn about a spiral of growing abandonment, or an opportunity for creative community responses.

Sutton Community Dance (SCD)

This section includes early observations from an innovative, all-inclusive community regeneration project. SCD was launched in August 2019 with the intention of creating a hub for social change through the vehicle of dance. The broadly reported physical and mental health benefits for individuals taking part in dance are widely reported and somewhat obvious. Any safe physical exercise should be easily evidenced as adding to the individual's health, and increasingly dance is observed to add particular value (above simply attending gyms) in contributing positively to individuals' mental health.

Swedish researchers studied more than 100 teenage girls who were struggling depression and anxiety-related issues. Half of the girls attended weekly dance classes, while the other half didn't. The results showed the girls who took the dance classes improved their mental health and reported a boost in their mood. These positive effects lasted up to eight months after the dance classes ended. The researchers concluded that dance could result in a very positive experience for participants and could potentially contribute to sustained new healthy habits (Duberg et al, 2013).

Whereas many excellent dance schools focus upon helping to develop the individual, typically girls aged 5–12, SCD deliberately set out (based on the Director of Dance's experience and skills) to be a dance hub for all ages, from 18 months to senior citizens of all ages. Furthermore, the organisation was established with a strong focus on including children, young people and adults with additional needs both physical and intellectual.

Informed and inspired by the work of Putnam (2000), SCD was launched in 2019 with the aim of making a difference within its community through the focus on developing bridging social capital. Putnam (2000, p 65) defined social capital as 'features of social organization such as networks, norms, and social trust that facilitate coordination and cooperation for mutual benefit'. Bourdieu (1986, p 248) defined it as 'the aggregate of the actual or potential resources which are linked to possession of a durable network of more or less institutionalized relationships of mutual acquaintance or recognition'.

Putnam identifies two key components of social capital development – bonding and bridging. Many well-established community activities contribute to the growth of bonding social capital by providing shared interest groups in which people with similar backgrounds or interests can join together. However, the work of researchers such as Zhang et al (2011) have evidenced the far more significant social, economic and political outcomes created through activities targeting the development of bridging capital – increasing connections with those who, to put it simply, are very different from each other.

Within the first five months of operating, SCD created a programme that already had over 600 people enrolled in weekly classes across every age group, from a range of local postcodes (across a diversity in income levels) and with over 30 per cent of those enrolled reporting an additional need.

This presents an encouraging picture of diversity, but deeper level early observations also show a reported increasing of social connections. The figure is currently anecdotal, but at least three-quarters of members have noted new friendships that have developed since they began to attend classes.

Arguably, of even greater longer term interest to the borough is SCD's deliberate choice of location, within the town centre's large shopping centre in a derelict and spacious two-level former Mothercare retail unit (floor area 550 m²) within Sutton's St Nicholas Shopping Centre (see Figures 15.2 and 15.3). SCD states that its intentions are to grow personal wellbeing through dance and to enrich the local community's health and sustainability by encouraging a renewed focus on shared experiential activity within the heart of the town. Noting the growth in empty units (the St Nicholas Centre's retail units are 40 per cent empty at the time of writing), it is easy to simply point to the proven convenience and lower prices offered by shopping online without considering the negative consequences of a reduction in public spaces to meet in, and the importance of beginning to create bridging bonds of social capital.

Figures 15.2 and 15.3: St Nicholas Centre, London Borough of Sutton. Former Mothercare store (two floors 550 m²) converted into three dance studios and a 'Wait and Create' space, all developed by SCD and paid for with its own crowdfunded campaign involving 138 supporters, together raising £19,000

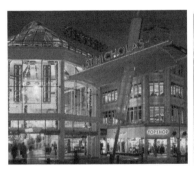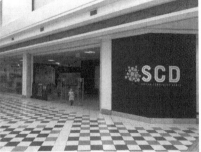

Source: Author

Business rates, energy costs, rents and well-reported drops in footfall can easily dissuade organisations from investing in town centre hubs. Indeed, these factors can add further detriment to already challenged business models, and yet these times offer both an opportunity and present a need for individuals, agencies and organisations to look again at the new market for experiential activities that all have the opportunity to engage with.

With SCD, for example, the 660 people taking part in weekly classes also represent an additional 800 people attending as parents, friends, partners and carers (see Figures 15.4 and 15.5). If this cohort visits out of town, smaller and residential street-based venues for activities such as dance, far fewer opportunities are presented for such individuals and families to bump into each other and find other secondary activities in which to partake within the same geographical context. This isn't just about boosting the local economy through direct financial investment into local outlets, but includes boosting local jobs and nurturing further shared spaces, particularly on an intergenerational level.

To quote a recently joined member of SCD, 'we've never been a dance family, we didn't think it was our thing or affordable to us but walking past SCD on the way to Primark we couldn't resist having a look and we've now joined. My dad had felt isolated since my mum died last year but is so much happier now he attends the weekly Club 60 Class and my daughter attends Ballet every Wednesday.'

SCD will develop more established methods of assessing its impact, especially to inform its reflection, development and future focus, as well as making the business model sustainable. However, a recent survey demonstrated that more than 70 per cent of members were not visiting the shopping centre prior to joining SCD classes.

Figures 15.4 and 15.5: All ages, all abilities inclusive dance programmes, 60 programmes operating each week, engaging 1,460 members of the community, 660 of whom participate in dancing every single week

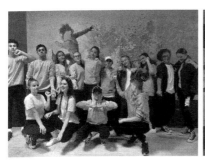 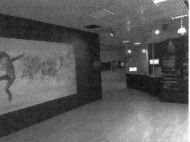

Source: A.M. Bonner

Through increasing bonding social capital through a shared interest in dance, SCD wants to help people 'get by' by encouraging reciprocity and collaboration: isolation is reduced and friendships are grown. The organisation continues to aspire to add greater value by focusing on the development of bridging social capital, allowing people to flourish more deeply both on the individual and social level – by providing access to resources, networks and opportunities that are simply otherwise unavailable if people aren't able to find contexts in which they can transcend their social and demographic boundaries.

Conclusion

The impact of the loss of public spaces and facilities for young people, previously provided by local authorities, has a significant adverse effect on the community health of young people. Reductions in social mobility and stratification will have a significant socio-economic influence on health and wellbeing in the UK's post-Brexit landscape (see Bonner, 2018).

Clearly, there is a role for community organisations in addressing youth disaffection, highlighting the need for mutuality. (For the fair distribution of burdens, as an organising principle to strengthen relationships in communities and support sustainability, see Chapter 17.)

Although various schemes, such as apprenticeships and other approaches, are available, there is a need for a greater understanding of what works to engage young people and how new innovative employment opportunities may be developed. Community-based approaches such as the Prince of Wales Trust and linked organisations such as Youth United Foundation seek to engage with young people across diverse communities and regions in order to provide meaningful skills and experiences in order to give hope, and help in building healthy socially integrated communities now and in the future.

The community regeneration project examined here, SCD, provides a good example of a small-scale local entity that is responsive to local needs (see Chapter 14) and is supporting health and wellbeing across all age ranges and abilities. This innovative project delivers the added value of bringing people into a shopping centre, thus becoming a critical factor in the regeneration of the high street and thereby promoting social capital and building intergenerational bridges.

These community projects are locally grounded and provide *soft structures* that impact more directly on people than the *hard structures* provided by statutory authorities. This idea is developed further in Chapter 16.

Postscript

The COVID-19 pandemic and subsequent lockdown has inevitably led to the closure of the St Nicholas Shopping Centre, including SCD. Anticipating the lockdown, SCD launched during the last week of March 2020 to offer live-streaming of classes 6 days a week.[1] During the last two weeks of March, just before and after the Government-mandated lockdown took effect, SCD lost 10 per cent of its membership. However, the online classes proved to be a lifeline for many and, with an overhaul of the membership structure, the following two weeks saw a surge in membership enrolments as siblings, parents, grandparents and friends were encouraged to log on and join in. In these days of isolation and anxiety the medium of dance has once more proved to be effective in promoting wellbeing and improving mental health, as reported by many of the participants – across all age and income demographics. SCDTV has been able to continue promoting inclusion, which has been particularly important for those families who have family members having to be shielded and experience social isolation due to their increased vulnerability. The high levels of participation in a wide range of classes throughout this crisis have demonstrated the strong sense of community which had already been engendered by SCD, and this community has transferred successfully to a virtual platform due to the strength of the social capital already created. SCDTV has also developed a partnership with the Local Authority's Public Health Team (at the LA's invitation) to create video content for the School's Nursing Service to offer within their programme of support.

Note
[1] For SCDTV see https://scd.org.uk.

References

APPG (All Party Parliament Group) (2018) 'Cross-party campaign to prevent knife crime', All Party Parliament Group on knife crime. Available from: http://www.preventknifecrime.co.uk [Accessed 31 August 2019].

Atkins, G. (2019) 'Children's social care: 10 key facts', Institute for Government. Available from: https://www.instituteforgovernment.org.uk/explainers/childrens-social-care-10-key-facts [Accessed 15 May 2020].

Berry, S. (2019) 'London's youth service funding black hole is getting worse', Mayor of London, London Assembly (22 March). Available from: https://www.london.gov.uk/press-releases/assembly/sian-berry/youth-service-funding-black-hole-is-getting-worse [Accessed 12 April 2020].

Black, R. (2015) 'Disaffected youth turning to paramilitaries', *Belfast Telegraph* (4 March). Available from: https://www.belfasttelegraph.co.uk/news/northern-ireland/disaffected-youth-being-driven-to-paramilitaries-31041155.html [Accessed 12 April 2020].

Big Lottery Community Fund (2018) '£1.2 million fund open to help grass roots community groups offering support for young people facing barriers to employment', Big Lottery Fund (11 October). Available from: https://www.tnlcommunityfund.org.uk/news/press-releases/2018-10-11/1-2-million-fund-opens-to-help-grassroots-community-groups-offering-support-to-young-people-facing-barriers-to-employment [Accessed 12 April 2020].

Bonner, A. (2018). 'The individual growing up in society', in A. Bonner (ed) *Social Determinants of Health: An Interdisciplinary Approach to Social Inequality and Wellbeing*, Bristol: Policy Press.

Bourdieu, P. (1986) 'The forms of capital', in J. Richardson (ed) *Handbook of Theory and Research for the Sociology of Education*, pp 241–58, Westport, CT: Greenwood.

Brady, D. (2019) 'Council spending on young people's services drops 18%', *Public Finance* (March). Available from: https://www.publicfinance.co.uk/news/2019/03/council-spending-young-peoples-services-drops-18 [Accessed 12 April 2020].

Cottam, H. (2018) 'Radical help. How can we remake the relationship between us and revolutionise the welfare state'. Available from: https://www.theguardian.com/books/2019/jun/07/radical-help-hilary-cottam-review-revolutionise-welfare-state [Accessed 12 April 2020].

Dibben, C., Playford, C. and Mitchell, R.J. (2017) 'Be(ing) prepared: Guide and Scout participation, childhood social position and mental health at age 50—a prospective birth cohort study', *Journal of Epidemiology and Community Health*, 71: 275–81.

Duberg, A., Hagberg, L. and Sunvisson, H. (2013) 'Influencing self-rated health among adolescent girls with dance intervention: a randomized controlled trial', *Archives of Pediatrics and Adolescent Medicine*, 167(1): 27–31. Available from: https://jamanetwork.com/journals/jamapediatrics/fullarticle/1390784 [Accessed 12 April 2020].

Gorard, B.S. and Siddiqui, N. (2017) 'Does participation in uniformed group activities in school improve young people's non-cognitive outcomes?', *International Journal of Educational Research*, 85: 109–20.

HMG (UK Government) (1996) Section 507B of the Education Act 1996.

DDCMS (Department for Digital, Culture, Media and Sport), OCS (Office for Civil Society), Crouch, T. and Wright, J. (2018) 'Civil society strategy: building a future that works for everyone', policy paper, 9 August, London: Cabinet Office. Available from: https://assets.publishing.service.gov.uk/government/uploads/system/uploads/attachment_data/file/732765/Civil_Society_Strategy_-_building_a_future_that_works_for_everyone.pdf [Accessed 15 May 2020].

LBS (London Borough of Sutton) (2013). 'Sutton's Developmental Assets book', London Borough of Sutton. Available from: https://www.sutton.gov.uk/downloads/file/1325/suttons_developmental_assets_booklet [Accessed 12 April 2020].

Linning, M. and Jackson, G. (2018) 'Volunteering, health and wellbeing: what does the evidence tell us?', Volunteer Scotland. Available from: https://www.volunteerscotland.net/media/1436178/volunteering__health___wellbeing_-_full_report.pdf [Accessed 12 April 2020].

LGA (Local Government Association) (2019). Must for youth services LGA Ref 15.64. Available from: https://www.local.gov.uk/must-know-youth-services [Accessed 12 April 2020].

NHS Scotland (2011) 'Asset based approach to health improvement' (October). Available from: http://www.healthscotland.com/documents/5535.aspx [Accessed 12 April 2020].

ONS (Office for National Statistics) (2019) 'High streets in Great Britain: mapping the location and characteristics of high streets'. Available from: https://www.ons.gov.uk/peoplepopulationandcommunity/populationandmigration/populationestimates/articles/highstreetsingreatbritain/2019-06-06 [Accessed 12 April 2020].

Putnam, R. (2000) *Bowling Alone: The Collapse and Revival of American Community*, New York: Simon & Schuster.

Sharabi, A., Levi, U. and Margalit, M. (2012) 'Children's loneliness, sense of coherence, family climate, and hope: developmental risk and protective factors', *The Journal of Psychology*, 146(1–2): 61–83.

Shiner, M., Young T., Newburn, T. and Groben, S. (2004) 'Mentoring disaffected young people', Joseph Rowntree Foundation. Available from: https://www.jrf.org.uk/sites/default/files/jrf/migrated/files/1859351646.pdf [Accessed 12 April 2020].

Simson, E. (2019) 'High street. How many shops have closed?' BBC News (23 October). Available from: https://www.bbc.co.uk/news/business-49349703 [Accessed 12 April 2020].

Stubley, P. (2020) 'When will the coronavirus recession begin and what will the likely economic impact be?', *Independent*, 4 May. Available from: https://www.independent.co.uk/news/business/coronavirus-recession-economy-what-is-when-uk-us-a9498306.html [Accessed 15 May 2020].

Tabassum, F., Mohan, J. and Smith, P. (2016) 'Association of volunteering with mental well-being: a lifecourse analysis of a national population-based longitudinal study in the UK', *BMJ Open*, 2016: 6:e011327. Available from: https://bmjopen.bmj.com/content/bmjopen/6/8/e011327.full.pdf [Accessed 15 May 2020].

UNISON (2018) 'Axing millions from your work puts futures at risk' (December). Available from: https://www.unison.org.uk/news/press-release/2018/12/axing-millions-youth-work-puts-futures-risk-says-unison/ [Accessed 12 April 2020].

YMCA (2019) 'Youth consequences'. Available from: https://www.ymca.org.uk/research/youth-and-consequences [Accessed 31 August 2019].

Zhang, S., Anderson, S. and Zhan, M. (2011) 'Differential impact of bridging and bonding social capital of economic wellbeing: an individual level perspective', *Journal of Sociology and Social Welfare*, 38(1): 119–42.

The role of the third sector working with the hard and soft structures of public–private partnerships to promote individual health and reinvigorated, healthier communities

Tony Chasteauneuf, Tony Thornton and Dean Pallant

Introduction

In this chapter, the authors consider how a recommitment to the 'local authority' of citizens and beneficiaries offers the possibility of revitalised and healthier individuals and reinvigorated and healthier communities, which are unachievable through the hard and soft structures of the commissioner/provider statutory approach. The pivotal dynamic of one-to-one relationships in these processes and their association with health outcomes (emotional, physical, spiritual) is identified alongside the opportunities and challenges in agencies engaging/re-engaging with the agency of citizens and beneficiaries. The chapter explores the tension between the 'agency' of citizens and beneficiaries that constitutes bottom–up power and 'agencies' with top-down power. The authors look at the benefits of embracing the expertise and investment of individuals and their communities in their personal and shared lives, how this can be supported and how it can be undermined.

People, relationships and communities

The origins of the quote that 'Love is spelled T I M E' may be disputed, but the truth of which it speaks is seldom in doubt (Ziglar, 1984). Time spent with others and others' time spent with us can have a significant influence on wellbeing. The depth, duration and nature of our relationships is fundamental to a healthy society. Our sense of self-worth, self-efficacy and hope, the key attributes for unlocking our personal and community's potential, are fundamentally shaped by the depth, duration and nature of our relationships. Evidence from research in areas ranging from attachment theory (Bowlby, 1969) and adverse childhood experiences (Public Health Wales, 2016) through to the importance of keyworker/client relationships (for example in effecting positive outcomes in homelessness services, see Macdonald and Jackson, 1998) or the impact that just a few extra minutes with our general practitioner (GP) has on added value to health and wellbeing (Siddique, 2016) all support this idea.

The challenge for the empiricist is that one can measure time but not love. The empiricist's challenge is the commissioner, trustee, benefactor and fundraiser's frustration. Why? Because 'love' provides, supports, improves, inspires, motivates, energises, develops, heals and sustains. It is the means and the ends. It doesn't define the method, but we all know it changes our lives; body, mind and soul. We can evaluate and possibly measure at least some of those 'love outcomes'. This might be better understood if we substitute the word 'love' with the word 'relationship'.

Relationships are essential in daily living, in order to meet our physical needs. We instinctively know that healthy relationships make us happy and are good for us (Parnham, 2018). We cannot be healthy on our own. Lacking social connections is as damaging to our health as smoking 15 cigarettes a day (Holt-Lunstad, 2015); and social networks and friendships help us to recover when we get ill (Hari, 2018). Making relationships is a significant aspect of human development, the outcomes of which have a fundamental influence on later life mental health and wellbeing (Bonner, 2018).

When considering the social determinants of health, 'relationships' and, more precisely, the interdependence, depth, duration and nature of the relationships of those individuals are important. Institutions can provide the means of channelling, organising and directing vital resources and, of course, institutions are managed and governed by people. However, it is the contact between people that is the most critical element in our wellbeing. This isn't just about contact with health or support professionals, something that has been recognised at least in part in the relatively new approach to 'social prescribing' (NHS England, 2019). It is much more than employing 'link workers' to support GP patients to navigate and access community facilities.

In Chapter 2, Harry Burns reviewed the importance of salutogenesis, a focus on supporting an individual's capacity to use physical and social resources to facilitate problem-solving in order to achieve a sense of coherence (Antonovsky, 1993). This well-established concept in health and health promotion is supported by a relational world view based on Maslow's Hierarchy of Needs, which has been reinterpreted by Cross (2007), a Native American child welfare expert, from a cultural perspective, expressed as breath of life theory (Blackstock, 2011); see Figure 16.1. Cross (1997) proposes that 'spirituality is the unique force differentiating human life from other forms of life, defining our individual and collective experience. Spirituality should not be misinterpreted to mean organized religion; rather a personally defined force that centres one's sense for the purpose of the *breath of life theory*'.

A healthy appreciation of the nature of a person is essential for a healthy appreciation of relationships. A person is not simply an autonomous rational individual. From the perspective of theological anthropology, humans bear the divine image so that in and through their relationships they reveal something of the Creator, as bearers of the divine image, and are called to act in *loco Dei* (McArdle, 2006). 'Healthy persons' are therefore not defined as 'individuals' but rather as 'persons-in-relation' (Pallant, 2012).

Empowered individuals are good for individual and community health. Strengths-based practice in one-to-one support work and the assets focus of community development, exist because of the application of the 'empowerment' approach (GCPH, 2011). How empowered are we really ready or willing for our target individuals and cohorts to be?

One may or may not accept the theory of linguistic relativity, that language influences thought (Whorf, 1940), but how many of us have still at some point considered how the term 'local authority' has increasingly come to represent less the concept of a dynamic democratic bridge to help transport community life to a more satisfactory state

Figure 16.1: Holistic model representing Cross's world view principles (2007)

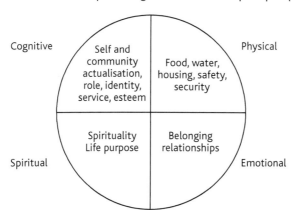

Source: Author/Chastenuef, T., adapted from Cross (2007)

303

and more of a bureaucratic dead end in our quest for reinvigorated community life? Is this why we find ourselves gravitating increasingly to the term 'community'? Against the backdrop of stubbornly low local election turnout (Dempsey, 2017), is this why we are increasingly drawn to concepts of engagement, empowerment and citizenship? Is our experience telling us that it is through the exercise of power through communities rather than the statutory power of local authorities that the health of individuals truly benefit because of the community benefits of 'community' – people living in healthy relationships.

But what authority are our institutions ready or willing to relinquish, or at least share, for individuals and communities to take more control of their capacity for wellbeing, their individual and community resources, as expressed through their relationships with each other and the institutions that seek to affect their lives? What or who should be the 'local', with whom should be the 'authority' and how should it be expressed?

TSA provides a unique and rich context for exploring the nature, impact and potential of relationships across a range of power and authority dynamics. A Church and welfare agency – part of a global movement – it is increasingly reconfiguring its understanding of 'community' within the context of enduring and ever-deepening theological understanding and its practical approaches to 21st-century engagement by integrating belief and faith into all attitudes and actions. The following three examples of Salvation Army activities in the North of England show the evolving approach of this organisation in response to changing individual and community needs, and the cultural changes in local authority planning, budgeting and commissioning (see Box 16.1).

Box 16.1: Salvation Army activities in the UK

The international Salvation Army operates in 135 countries providing practical support and services to address:
- homelessness
- modern slavery
- poverty
- addiction
- older people
- community, debt advice, unemployment isolation

Also promotes social justice by influencing social policy.

In the UK, The Salvation Army:

- provides over 3,000 places every night for homeless people in residential Lifehouses
- 2018–19 helped 1,208 people through the Salvation Army Employment Plus Service
- supported 2,267 victims referred to Salvation Army-managed slavery services
- brought together 5,690 people at Salvation Army lunch clubs

Swan Lodge – Sunderland

Swan Lodge, in Sunderland, is one of the 82 residential centres (Lifehouses) operated by The Salvation Army, and it provides accommodation-based support for single people (males and females) at risk of homelessness. Most homelessness services have historically been reliant on local authorities for funding, and still are. The advent of the Supporting People programme in 2003 provided new funding for homeless services. The political will and opportunity to address the fundamental causes of homelessness recognised the expertise and passion of staff to properly invest in the futures of each individual beneficiary through an unapologetically holistic and long-term support approach, delivered by increasingly skilled support workers, employed by ever more joined-up and quality assured charities. As charity profiles, standards and community understanding were raised, language changed from the language of purpose, charity and beneficiary to the language of strategy, agency and client; funding moved from grant to contract, and funding partnerships and programmes became commissioned and sub-contracted services.

In Sunderland, this saw TSA's Swan Lodge Lifehouse deliver a step-change in its range of preventative services, such as floating support and accommodation-based services, including a 65-bed unit accommodation project for single people at risk of homelessness. Sunderland City Council commissioned The Salvation Army to develop a whole systems approach to their homelessness services, encompassing Swan Lodge Lifehouse as well as a number of other services for single people and families: immediate access service including assertive outreach, further accommodation-based support and floating support. The opportunity for TSA to gain the position of Prime Contractor for 'Housing Related Support for People with Multiple Needs and Exclusions, including Families, enabled the retention of Swan Lodge and the management of a supply chain of subcontractors to deliver other service strands within the contract.

Service pathways and treatment for those at high risk were developed through partnership working across the city; multiple forms of multi-agency meetings and working groups taking place across voluntary and statutory agencies on a regular basis. The challenges faced in providing suitable supported accommodation to the client group cannot be met by commissioned housing-related support organisations alone. Strong links with external agencies such as drug and treatment services and adult services are essential. In partnership, the service offered isolated, vulnerable and homeless people and families pathways out of exclusion, and the opportunity to fulfil their potential and move towards an independent future.

Driven by innovation and a passion for vocation, Swan Lodge has provided integrated, holistic support delivered by exceptional teams, who are recognised by clients and commissioners as delivering the finest quality services and achieving the most successful outcomes; identifying gaps in existing provision and sourcing funding to create innovative new activities that enable socially excluded people and families to achieve their optimum level of independence and realise their potential (see https://www.salvationarmy.org.uk/safc-garden-of-light).

However, the hidden value and untapped potential of the sector and, by implication, the individuals with whom the sector had been engaging for so many years, which had formed such a key part of the justification for the new Supporting People programme, had been radically underestimated by Whitehall. The initial estimated cost of £800 million ended up being exceeded by over 100 per cent. The political will to tackle homelessness requires a rare degree of insight, empathy and political capital. Almost overnight, the Supporting People focus turned from effectiveness to efficiency. In 2009, the ring fence around the Supporting People funding stream was removed. In 2011/12, Supporting People funding was rolled into the Formula Grant – a single grant given by central government to local authorities. At the same time, the Department for Communities and Local Government ended the requirement that local authorities collect or submit client data. Research in 2012 (Homeless Link, 2013) showed that the local authority is the primary funding source for over 70 per cent of homelessness services, previously via Supporting People Funding that is no longer ring fenced, managed by local authority community commissioners.

In Sunderland, at the end of TSA's three-year contract, the city council withdrew all housing related support contracts within the city. Today, the funding received by Swan Lodge Lifehouse comes entirely through housing benefit, reducing the support provided to some of the most vulnerable people in the community and leaving provision 'on the brink'. Yet the Salvation Army's commitment is covenantal in nature, not transactional – kin not contract; it will remain. However, the capacity to provide the required response is not guaranteed. What is the hidden opportunity cost, direct cost, human and community capital cost of a commissioner/provider contract relationship, not least given the bipolar policy environment that gives rise to them with all the thrills of the highs and institutional and individual demoralisation of the lows? The local community is the source of the volunteers, funding, opportunities, encouragement, advocacy, action, the relationships that endure and upon which the most excluded depend, not for the duration of a one-to-one, a treatment episode or funding contract – but for life.

Victory Programme – Crook, County Durham

TSA has had a presence in Crook going back many years. Yet, while the church congregation of recent years is diminished and ageing, the local community's engagement with and through The Salvation Army is growing, as is the impact on individuals' wellbeing. Nowhere is this more visible than in the achievements of The Salvation Army's Victory Programme.

The Victory Programme was launched in Crook in 2014. Initially, it was a response to the cooking and budgeting challenges faced by those accessing food parcel support. However, the design of the programme reflected an understanding, sensitivity and knowledge of the local community informed by the insights of several volunteers who had spent their lives in Crook, plus the teaching and marketing experience of The Salvation Army's leaders in Crook at that time. Therefore, the Victory Programme was designed to be a fun, free, shared learning experience as opposed to anything looking or sounding like a classroom, and/or a church for that matter! The objectives were to build confidence and competence through affirming relationships and learning, resulting in healthier and happier lives. Along the way, not only have these outcomes been achieved but also has an almost tangible increase in community capacity.

The Victory Programme is based on the Second World War campaign 'Dig for Victory'. In practice, it has three main components:

- Dig for Victory: participants are provided with the tools, seeds and information to learn how to grow fresh vegetables at home in their own gardens or on a community allotment.
- Eat for Victory: participants learn together in hands-on sessions how to make nutritious, cost-effective meals based on wartime recipes with their produce or carefully budgeted produce from local shops. Participants are provided with everything they need to cook and enjoy recipes that they can make at home. They also get to take home free of charge what they make in the sessions.
- Budget for Victory: participants learn how to budget with their income, however much that might be; this also includes learning valuable tips from older generations about making sure that every penny counts. Sessions include viewing and discussing old newsreel footage on wartime austerity.

The programmes run one day a week for six weeks with the optimum group size being six to eight people.

The impact of the programme on individuals is evaluated through participant feedback and monitoring. This includes participants scoring themselves on a scale of 1–10 regarding how they felt before starting the programme and then how they feel having completed the programme, across a range of prompts.

However, the value of the programme is probably most vividly seen in the story of the woman who is now responsible for the delivery and ongoing development of the programme. This local mother of two was a graduate of the very first Victory Programme in Crook. She very nearly turned around at the front door owing to her high levels of anxiety and lack of confidence, but was accompanied by a friend who encouraged her to give it a try as 'just a bit of fun'. Having not been employed for years, within months of completing the programme, she was given the job of coordinating it. With her local knowledge, insights into the stresses and strains for many but also the many positives within the local community, combined with her own capability and the skills she has developed as a mother, and the credibility this has brought to her engagement with participants and local organisations, the programme has gone from strength to strength. This can be seen not least in the relationship that she has built with local organisations and, more precisely, the individuals working within those local organisations.

Over the last few years, one of the features of this relationship with the local council has been a steady trickle of funding. Yet this has not significantly affected how the Victory Programme otherwise would have organically developed. The funding has offered welcome encouragement, publicity and opportunity to innovate, but the relationships, the sharing of learning and collaboration with colleagues within the council and the wider community have not been impeded by the dynamics of the commissioner/contractor framework; hence, for example, the development of a holiday hunger version of the Victory Programme for families in collaboration with local schools and other local charities. During this time, The Salvation Army's 'ownership' and commitment to underwriting the Victory Programme has only increased. Similarly, the local community's 'ownership' has grown and continues to grow, as evidenced by the number of volunteers being generated through the Victory Programme and the development of a Victory Graduate Programme in response to demand from those completing the Victory Programme.

The positive impact of this small local programme on the health of hundreds of individuals and the community as a whole seems set to continue well into the future through the local commitment, mutual dependence and autonomy of the key stakeholders.

Copper Beech – Bramley, Leeds

The slow disintegration in recent decades of local physical and social structures, or at least participation in those structures that had previously provided 'community', from churches to sporting and social clubs, has led to the growing realisation that facilitating 'community' now requires a different and more intentional approach.

At a macro-level, this disintegration might be viewed as more of a disaggregation, whereby the relationships between structures/institutions have weakened or broken down or have simply died. The nature and importance of those relationships is key to the associated discussion of 'social capital' (Putnam, 1995) that has developed in recent years; a discussion that inevitably leads back to a focus on the commitment and continuity of local relationships as well as how representative those local relationships are of the communities whose interests they seek to promote at a time when participation seems to be declining. The Salvation Army is not alone as a faith-based organisation (FBO) in being faced with the realisation that if it is to continue to facilitate 'community' it must adapt to cultural and attitudinal changes in how people engage, develop a sense of belonging and identify as a community. This creates the usual internal change management challenges one would expect but also the opportunity to rediscover and renew values, beliefs and mission.

This was the challenge and opportunity with which The Salvation Army's Yorkshire Division was presented as it considered plans for the development of its Copper Beech site in Bramley, Leeds, in the early 2010s. The site included The Salvation Army's early years Copper Beech nursery with approximately 100 places, a vacant hostel that had previously been used by the Salvation Army to accommodate and support young single mothers and their children and a large area of disused land. Discussion with The Salvation Army Housing Association (SAHA) quickly highlighted the opportunities to develop the site for affordable housing. SAHA manages the properties used by The Salvation Army's Homelessness Services Unit and has an awareness of the support needs of vulnerable tenants and associated funding challenges that extended beyond the usual housing officer/tenancy management approaches. At the same time, The Salvation Army's Yorkshire Division was keen to ensure that any housing development would offer residents the opportunity to be a 'community' and not just a group of residents; to be a new 'community' expression of The Salvation Army that was looking more towards the asset-based approaches of community development than the more traditional ready-made programme approach. While it was acknowledged that this would be much more of a 'slow burn' engagement approach, it was anticipated that it would result in greater levels of ownership, sense of belonging, wellbeing and enduring community capacity. To fulfil The Salvation Army's vision, therefore, it was agreed that the organisation would work with nursery families, residents, neighbours and partner agencies to help develop 'a community continually growing together in joy. The sharing and hope centred on the Mission of The Salvation Army and the talents, interests and ideas of our community', with the name Copper Beech extended to the whole community. Working closely with Leeds City Council, SAHA delivered 83 new low-cost/affordable housing units. However, crucially, the development also included a newly refurbished community centre and the appointment by The Salvation Army of a full-time leader and a live-in part-time community worker to promote community connectedness and support the development of pop-up community activities among residents, nursery families and neighbours. While it is still very early days for this initiative, the levels of engagement and initiative already being taken by residents and nursery families in day-to-day activities (from tea and toast get-togethers to planting and harvesting fruit and vegetables from the community's raised beds) and the planning and delivery of community events are very encouraging for the future development of this as a self-sufficient, connected and healthy community. Interestingly, this has in turn led to the development of relationships with other organisations – particularly those with similarly empowerment-focused and low-threshold orientations to engagement, including a new formal church partnership under the name of Connect@CopperBeech between TSA and a local Baptist missional community with historic connections to the site – not an insignificant feat for church communities from different denominations.

In prioritising the nurturing of 'relationships with and between community members, a sense of ownership, confidence and ultimately a contagious sense of belonging', TSA has developed and invested heavily in an expression of its mission in Bramley. This recalibration of approach that refocuses on the development of relationships, asset-based community development and sustainability can be seen as part of broader ongoing discussions within and between various FBOs; discussions that are in turn leading to interest and involvement in the related area of community organising and the development of what might be termed 'grass roots community capital' as distinct from the more institutionally oriented/dependent social capital. This is not without its challenges for organisations such as The Salvation Army, not least in reimagining how governance of purpose and objectives are operationalised in a contemporary beneficiary-led charity as opposed to the hierarchical institution of the 19th century.

Lessons in togetherness

There is 'time' that we might spend alongside each other and then there is 'quality time' that we can share together. We can be alongside each other without really connecting. However, it is in our connecting that our individual and community wellbeing can be transformed beyond a simple aggregation of our individual wellbeing into 'togetherness'. If 'love is spelled T I M E' (Ziglar, 1984), then that time can be understood as consisting of some essential characteristics that connect us and form the basis of 'relationship', including:

- shared vulnerability, shared values, common interests, shared experiences, shared resources, empathy (DEPTH);
- time to develop and last as long as parties choose, ongoing commitment (DURATION);
- shared power, ongoing empowerment of parties, justice, dynamism – open to change (NATURE).

If one had to choose just one underpinning competency, characteristic, value then it would surely be 'listening'. The consultative approach is being adopted by a number of local councils (see Chapters 6, 7 and 8). To what extent does 'consulting the electorate' extend to listening to their needs?

Organisations wishing to promote, support and improve the wellbeing of communities and the individuals who make up those communities need to mould their approaches so that the manner of their engagement reflects, promotes, supports and improves the depth, duration and nature of community and individual relationships fundamental to the realisation of their aims and purposes. The challenge of designing and delivering strategies and operations based on 'relationship' and the 'agency' of local communities and the individuals of those communities applies to local charities and not just 'local authorities'. Community anchor organisations can be effective in increasing volunteering and socio-economic benefits (for example, stimulating active citizenship and civic participation, bringing together diverse groups and engaging marginalised people). Aligning a 'community-led' approach with the predetermined aims, ambitions and aspirations of the local organisation/charity/church requires honest, open, flexible and sensitive discussion, reflection and navigation – intra- and inter-organisation and community. This is what partly characterises any healthy relationship. Diverse and at times competing interests are not inconsistent with a healthy relationship. Indeed, if the relationship is dynamic and the parties are open to change, this can be a driver for personal, community and organisational growth; indeed, mutual transformation. The challenge comes in the practical application. A major UK charity, such as TSA, offers an extensive and resilient infrastructure that small charities often lack, while at the same time provides for enduring, heavily localised presence, commitment and relationships across the UK and Ireland, offering so many opportunities for individual and community wellbeing.

At the same time, TSA recognises the increasing need to actively navigate, evaluate, discuss and adapt the vertical and horizontal compatibility of its hard and soft governance and operational structures in light of its developing understanding of contemporary community work (from asset-based community development to community organising), an evolving and challenging policy context (from austerity to individualised budgets) and the need to remain true to its foundational, versus its habitualised traditions and strategic competencies.

The strategic and operational challenges for a local authority are larger and more complex in moving to a relationship-focused approach to the wellbeing of its communities (see Chapter 15).

However, the benefits would no doubt justify the investment, given a local authority's capacity to not only engage directly with individuals and neighbourhoods but also other local organisations, groups and charities. Partnership working, within a Social Determinants of Health framework provides clarity and intentionality in joint working. 'Professional' relationships in the social service and community sectors, intentionally and unintentionally, will shape the way we engage our target groups and beneficial outcomes (Chasteauneuf, 2011). Charities such as TSA must also play their part in delivering such shifts in approach through the demands they make of local authorities regarding commissioning practices, and the degree to which they collude or stand firm in the face of commissioning practices and contracts that fail to meet the standard of a relationship-focused approach.

Love, faith and hope for the future

Third-sector organisations work closely with people and communities, understand the needs of service users and communities, and play an important role in working with public services in addressing 'wicked issues'. A key attribute of charities, particularly so for FBO, is that they are driven by compassion, a fundamental aspect of the loving relationships referred to in this chapter. Compassion literally means 'to suffer together' and is regarded by psychologists as the feeling that arises when someone is confronted with another person's suffering and motivated to relieve that suffering (Keltner, 2019).

From a national strategic social policy perspective, FBOs and the individuals who subscribe to their associated belief frameworks represent a vital strategic core competence to be supported, nurtured and carefully developed. FBOs and the faith sector have provided and continue to provide a rich and sustainable source of activity, innovation and insight regarding the challenges facing communities and effective responses to immediate and long-term need, including the 'wicked issues' of today and tomorrow. A belief system, such as Christianity, that promotes the solidarity and togetherness of individuals within our communities, offers real life hope amid such contemporary Western concerns as the mental health impacts of the increasing isolation of individuals and inequalities in the distribution of wealth and income.

The holistic and timeless concept and pursuit of social justice within the Christian context even extends to the pressing global environmental crisis of climate change. As summarised by Archbishop Denis Hart (Roman Catholic Archdiocese of Melbourne) in 2014, 'The love of Jesus … extends not only to human beings, but to the whole of creation ... a true "healing for the whole of the world". For this reason, we cannot divorce care for the integrity of the earth and care for the integral development of human beings here and now from our hope in the age to come' (Hart, 2014). Catherine Booth, one of the founders of TSA, grasped this larger vision of God's work in the world when she preached about holiness in the 19th century: 'It is not a scheme of salvation merely – it is a scheme of restoration ... [God] proposes to restore me – brain, heart, soul, spirit, body, every fibre of my nature to restore me perfectly, to conform me wholly to the image of his Son' (Booth, 1881). This truth is captured in official Salvation Army teaching, which encourages people 'to treat every relationship as a holy covenant' (Salvation Army, 2010).

How fitting, therefore, that the three case studies discussed here include Swan Lodge, which includes its 'Garden of Light' opened in 2018, Crook's Dig for Victory scheme and the raised beds at the Copper Beech community hub, providing the focus for community interaction and development founded on the restoration of relationships – including our relationship with the Earth.

Conclusion

A recommitment to the 'local authority' of citizens and beneficiaries offers the possibility of revitalised and healthier individuals and reinvigorated and healthier communities, unachievable through the hard and soft structures of the commissioner/provider statutory approach. The pivotal focus should be the dynamic of one-to-one relationships and their association with health outcomes (emotional, physical and spiritual). Public, private and third-sector institutions should consider the relationships of their target cohorts and not try to force those individuals to fit their relationships into hard and soft structures of those institutions (including contrived service user/customer committees/consultations). Furthermore, institutions should be adapting how they work with 'partners' so as to develop similarly healthy inter-organisational relationships. Powerful organisations can co-opt partners, resulting in relationships becoming commodified and/or instrumentalised (Pallant, 2012). Faith-based organisations need resilient habits and practices as well as systems and strategies to ensure they faithfully sustain healthy and enduring relationships with all their partners.

Major charities such as The Salvation Army, with significant infrastructure alongside strong local presence, should be a significant part of the framework that helps inform, support and improve the micro-relationships of the community 'front line'. These micro-expressions benefit from being free of long-term and/or high levels of externally contracted funding and associated government/business type administrative requirements/justifications. While there should be an evidence base and accountability for how resources are invested, impact assessments of types of initiatives delivered to certain standards/criteria should form the basis of 'investment' rather than outcome measures and associated targets.

In turn, charities such as The Salvation Army need to be wary of adopting an internal quasi-commissioning approach and failing to tread carefully in where and how they choose to adopt quasi-therapeutic frameworks that lead them away from the mutual one-to-one and group relationships at local community level. This is not to say that there are no benefits to either of these approaches, but their haphazard or unrestrained implementation/adoption presents the risk of adopting outdated subjective and temporary outcome measures for health-oriented interventions and related policies that prioritise a professional engagement over a human connection/relationship; that provide a 'be-friend' rather than a 'friend'. Problems soon arise when the focus is not on the goal of 'healthy persons' thriving in a healthy environment but is subverted by powerful forces seeking lesser outcomes. Such subversion leads to injustice, and the price is paid by individuals as well as the wider society.

A fundamental challenge for local authorities and many charities is to embrace the bottom-up 'agency' of citizens and beneficiaries within the context of 'agencies' accustomed to the exercise of top-down power, so those agencies can use their capacity (such as their structures and funds) to:

- honour (acknowledge, encourage, magnify) the commitment of citizens and beneficiaries rather than seek to create it;
- encourage community-based groups – including those from faith communities – who appreciate and encourage a holistic vision of healthy persons in all aspects of life;
- invest in individual and community capacity rather than seek to buy sustainability through short-term contracts;
- look to the dynamic of one-to-one relationships to navigate opportunities and challenges in ways that 'honour' and 'invest' rather than 'exploit' and 'deplete', underpinned by a passion for listening, learning and our shared story; for each other.

References

Antonovsky, A. (1993) 'The structure and properties of the sense of coherence scale', *Social Science and Medicine*, 6: 725–33.

Blackstock, C. (2011) 'The emergence of breath of life', *Journal of Social Work Values and Ethics*, 8(1). Available from: https://jswve. org/download/2011-1/spr11-blackstock-Emergence-breath-of-life-theory.pdf [Accessed 15 May 2020].

Bonner, A.B. (2018) 'The individual, growing into society', in A.B. Bonner (ed) *Social Determinants of Health: An Interdisciplinary Approach to Social Inequalities and Wellbeing*, pp 3–15, Bristol: Policy Press.

Booth, C. (1881) *Godliness: An Address on Holiness, Exeter Hall*, London: The Salvation Army.

Bowlby, J. (1969) *Attachment and Loss*, vol. 1, New York: Basic Books.

Chasteauneuf, T. (2011) 'The outcome business', *Parity*, 24(7): 18–19. Available from: https://search.informit.com.au/documentSummary; dn=394604360730046;res=IELHSS [Accessed 19 August 2019].

Cross, T. (1997) 'Understanding the relational worldview in Indian families', *Pathways Practice Digest*, 12(4).

Cross, T. (2007) 'Through indigenous eyes: rethinking theory and practice', paper presented at the 2007 Conference of the Secretariat of Aboriginal and Island Child Care in Adelaide, Australia (20 September).

Dempsey, N. (2017) 'Local Elections 2017', House of Commons Library Briefing Paper Number CBP 7975, 8 May. Available from: https://commonslibrary.parliament.uk/research-briefings/cbp-7975 [Accessed 15 May 2020].

GCPH (Glasgow Centre for Population Health) (2011) 'Asset based approaches for health improvement: redressing the balance'. Briefing paper 9. Concepts series, Glasgow Centre for Population Health.

Hart, D. (2014) 'Social justice and the Gospel', *Kairos*, 25(18): 4–5. Available from: https://melbournecatholic.org.au/Portals/0/kairos/ kairos_v25i18/files/assets/basic-html/page4.html [Accessed 28 July 2020].

Hari, J. (2018) *Lost Connections*, New York: Bloomsbury.

Holt-Lunstad, J. (2015) 'Loneliness and social isolation as risk factor for mortality: a meta-analytic review', *Perspectives in Psychological Science*, 10(2): 227–37.

Homeless Link (2013) 'Who is supporting people now? Experiences of local authority commissioning after supporting people', Homeless Watch. Available from: www.homeless.org.uk/take-a-step [Accessed 13 April 2020].

Keltner, D. (2019) 'What is compassion?' Available from: https://greatergood.berkeley.edu/topic/compassion/definition [Accessed 13 April 2020].

Macdonald, D. and Jackson, A. (1998) *Skills for Life: A Good Practice Guide to Training Homeless People for Resettlement*, London: Crisis.

McArdle, P. (2006) 'The relational person within a practical theology of health care', PhD diss., Australian Catholic University, 2006.

NHS England (2019) 'Social prescribing and community-based support. Summary guide'. Available from: https://www.england.nhs.uk/wp-content/uploads/2019/01/social-prescribing-community-based-support-summary-guide.pdf [Accessed 13 April 2020].

Pallant, D. (2012) *Keeping Faith in Faith-Based Organizations – A Practical Theology of Salvation Army Health Ministry*, Eugene, OR: Wipf and Stock.

Parnham, A. (2018) 'Wholistic well-being and happiness: psychosocial–spiritual perspectives', in A.B. Bonner (ed) *Social Determinants of Health: An interdisciplinary approach to Social Inequalities and Wellbeing*, pp 29–40, Bristol: Policy Press.

Public Health Wales (2016) 'Well Wales adverse childhood experiences'. Available from: http://www.wales.nhs.uk/sitesplus/888/page/87836 [Accessed 13 April 2020].

Putnam, R.D. (1995) 'Bowling alone: America's declining social capital', *Journal of Democracy*, 6(1): 675–8.

Salvation Army (2010) *Handbook of Doctrine*, London: Salvation Army.

Siddique, H. (2016) 'GP appointments should be five minutes longer, says BMA', *Guardian* (28 August). Available from: https://www.theguardian.com/society/2016/aug/28/doctor-appointments-15-minutes-bma-overweight-population [Accessed 13 April 2020].

Whorf, B.L. (1940) 'Science and linguistics', *The Technology Review*, 42(6): 229–31, 247–8.

Ziglar, Z. (1984) *Raising Positive Kids in a Negative World*, Nashville, TN: Nelson.

Mutuality in the public, private and third sectors

Richard Simmons

Introduction

This chapter explores the concept of mutuality and the ways in which it may be applied to the social determinants of health in local government. The chapter attempts two things: first, to set out the scope of the concept and its potential applications; secondly, to examine these applications (relative to alternative options) through a novel heuristic framework and brief analysis of how mutuality in this context has evolved over time.

Mutuality is defined broadly in the *Oxford English Dictionary* as the sharing of a feeling, action or relationship between two or more parties, upon which cooperation is based. In turn, cooperation may be defined as 'acting together, in a co-ordinated way, in social relationships, in the pursuit of shared goals, the enjoyment of the joint activity, or simply furthering the relationship' (Argyle, 1991, p 15). Meanwhile, coordination is considered here through the lens of governance, or 'the *process of steering for collective action* with respect to an issue in private and public affairs' (Briassoulis, 2019, p 419; author's emphasis). In this formulation, mutuality provides a basis for cooperation, and cooperation works reciprocally to renew mutuality. This is particularly important when cooperation provides a clear basis for coordinated activity (relative to alternative bases of, say, coercion or competition; see Figure 17.1).

With regard to governance, different expressions of mutuality and cooperation arise, but are often conflated, in the literature. These include orthodox notions of governance as a *coordinative structure* (for example, adversarial, managerial, collaborative); modes of governance as different *logics of coordination* (for example, hierarchy, market, network); or governance arrangements as specific forms of *organisational structure* (for example, public–private partnerships, cooperatives, community organisations) (Lelièvre-Finch, 2010). Such notions of

Figure 17.1: Mutuality, cooperation and coordination

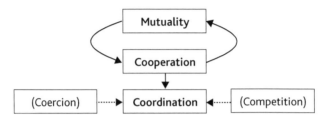

governance may also be applied in different contexts, whether *spatial* (for example, global, national, local or urban, rural, coastal); *sectoral* (for example, health, social care, housing, education); or *issue-based* (for example, poverty, lifestyle, lifecourse). In each case, the literature also often assesses the quality of governance (for example, as 'good governance' or otherwise) (Briassoulis, 2019).

This chapter examines mutuality from these different perspectives for the social determinants of health in local government. There is no presumption here that the invocation of mutuality per se results in an inherently superior quality of governance. Instead, the chapter takes a more modest position; that is, that mutuality is properly considered in conditions where its contribution may be productive, and that where mutuality meets this condition, it should be employed as productively as possible. The chapter looks at some of the empirical evidence, which suggests that this is not always the case.

Accordingly, this chapter addresses such questions as:

- When is mutuality more or less appropriate?
- How strong is the evidence base for mutuality?
- Where mutuality is considered to be appropriate, what can be done to develop its role and potential?
- How 'radical' might local government be in developing notions of mutuality to address the social determinants of health?

The chapter starts from broad perspectives of *governance*, narrowing through the place and role of mutuality in *modes of governance*, to how it is expressed in specific *governance arrangements*. While space constraints prevent more detailed and varied accounts of mutuality within particular spatial, sectoral or issue-based contexts, the intention throughout is to provide useful insights for actors at the local level interested in mobilising mutuality to address the social determinants of health.

Mutuality and 'governance': relational and collaborative perspectives

Mutuality connects with some important currents in modern governance. Broadly, as the sharing of a feeling, action or relationship between two or more parties, upon which cooperation is based, mutuality connects with what Bartels and Turnbull (2019, p 1) describe as 'an ever-growing interest in the 'relational' properties of exchanges between administrative actors'. This more relational set of conditions is commonly associated with what Osborne (2010) has termed the 'New Public Governance' – in which

> public administration is a more dynamic and fluid activity than ever before, marked by networks and multi-actor dependencies between public sector organizations, private companies, third sector organizations, and citizens ... The relational quality of public administration is central to studies of network governance, partnerships, co-production, contracting, social welfare, citizen participation, and so on. (Bartels and Turnbull, 2019, p 1)

In this way, mutuality also connects with notions of 'collaborative governance', a form of governance that has:

> emerged to replace adversarial and managerial modes of policy making and implementation, [which] brings public and private stakeholders together in collective forums with public agencies to engage in consensus-oriented decision making. (Ansell and Gash, 2008, p 543)

It is important to locate expressions of mutuality in this broader context, as it is in these 'networks and multi-actor dependencies' that its strongest impact in relation to the social determinants of health might be anticipated. Here, mutuality may be seen as an adaptive response to encounters with the uncertainty and complexity that can arise.

Uncertainty and complexity are widespread in the contemporary governance systems (for example, Geyer and Cairney, 2015). Phenomena such as bounded rationality (Simon, 1955) and 'wicked' policy problems (Rittel and Webber, 1973) mean that:

> Policymakers must often act in the face of irreducible uncertainty – uncertainty that will not go away before

> a judgment has to be made about what to do, what can
> be done, what will be done, what ought to be done.
> (Hammond, 1996, p 11)

Such complexity and 'wicked problems' impact frequently on the social determinants of health – for example, in the complex interactions between levels of inequality and disadvantage, service provision and intervention that can lead to unpredictable and uncertain outcomes for individuals and communities (Bonner, 2018).

Importantly, one leading commentator – Keith Grint (2005, p 1477) – directly and explicitly associates 'increasing uncertainty about the solution to the problem' with an 'increasing need for collaboration in resolving the problem'. This reflects what Huxham and Vangen (2005, p 7) describe as a 'moral imperative' underpinning the pursuit of greater collaboration and cooperation, which rests on the belief that many really important public service issues simply cannot be tackled by acting alone. For Cleaver (2004, p 272), this is not just about morality, but explicitly 'the mutuality and interdependence of people with multiple identities'. Such conditions create conducive incentive structures for mutuality and cooperation as the basis for coordination.

Mutuality and 'modes of governance'

Nevertheless, within governance, mutuality must find its place alongside other potential coordinating mechanisms for the 'steering for collective action'. While mutuality is particularly associated with highly networked and relational conditions, this does not capture the full range of possibilities. Concisely, according to one popular perspective, such mechanisms (or modes of governance) include hierarchies and markets as well as network ideal-types (see, for example, Thompson et al, 1991; Tenbensel, 2005). Each gives rise to different broad patterns of social relations that may be preferred by particular actors. Hence, ideal-types of hierarchy and bureau-professionalism may be promoted as efficient and effective owing to their emphasis on specialisation, expertise, standardisation, formal procedures and clearly defined, centralised chain of command (du Gay, 2000, 2005). Alternatively, market-based ideal-types may be claimed to respond to a plurality of individual preferences more efficiently and effectively than other modes of governance (for example, Hayek, 1976). Correspondingly, the tendency within hierarchies is toward command-and-control and more *coercive* forms of relations; within market-based conditions it is toward *competitive* forms of relations, in which actors are cast as self-interested, utility-maximising individuals. Such patterns of relations stand in contrast with those network-types in which mutuality is prevalent (Simmons and Birchall, 2007b), where individual potential is viewed as dependent on connection to a community, cohering around values such as solidarity, fellowship and association, and processes such as *cooperation* and participation (Birchall, 2001).

When is mutuality appropriate?

What guides the prevalence of, and preference for, particular patterns of relations? Ideological commitments? Pragmatic concerns? Patterns of interest and identity? There is no straightforward answer to this question. However, various contributions within the literature provide useful insights. For example, while Grint (2005) identifies an association between 'wicked problems' and more collaborative and cooperative patterns of relations, he acknowledges that command-and-control solutions may be more appropriate in the face of urgent and time-bound 'critical' problems, and comparatively straightforward managerial solutions (based on incentivising self-interested – skilled or unskilled – individuals) more appropriate in the face of 'tame' problems (Rittel and Webber, 1973). Given that each of these problem-types are still widely encountered in relation to the social determinants of health – in local government, and beyond – it may therefore be imprecise to claim that 'collaborative governance' has 'emerged to *replace* adversarial and managerial modes of policy making and implementation' (Ansell and Gash, 2008, p 543; author's emphasis). In short, there is no 'silver bullet'. Mutuality and cooperation may be advocated for dealing with the complexity and uncertainty associated with 'wicked problems', but less so under other conditions.

In a further useful contribution, Quinn and Hall (1983) also identify uncertainty as one of the key conditions (along with competition) that make movements toward one or other of the above ideal-types more likely than another (see Table 17.1).

Here, mutuality and cooperation are most strongly advised in contextual conditions of *low competition* and *high uncertainty*. Such

Table 17.1: Contextual conditions and associated 'prescriptions'

	Low competition	High competition
Low uncertainty	*Hierarchy* ('Controlling')	*Market-based* ('Competing')
High uncertainty	*Mutuality* ('Collaborative')	*Adhocracy* ('Creative')

Source: Quinn and Hall, 1983

conditions are not uncommon in the current public service context. The high uncertainty associated with 'wicked problems', such as those impacting on the social determinants of health, has already been identified. However, various factors also work to preclude extensive competition in many areas of local government activity – for example, legal or capital barriers, constraints on the provision of choice or market failure in public procurement (Dunleavy and Hood, 1994; Greener, 2003; OGC, 2008). As a result, there is sustained empirical evidence of reduced competition and greater collaborative working in a number of public service contexts (for example, Lowndes and Skelcher, 1998; Entwistle and Martin, 2005; Osborne et al, 2015). Again, there is no silver bullet; when the conditions of competition and uncertainty combine in other ways, other solutions (that is, hierarchy, market-based and adhocracy) are foregrounded. Yet in the right conditions, mutuality remains a clear option for effective governance and coordination.

Various similar frameworks identify the value of mutuality. One further, final example that will be explored here is Christopher Hood's (1995, 1998) examination of bureaucratic control, in which he uses Mary Douglas's 'Cultural Theory' (1970, 1982; Thompson et al, 1990) to identify four approaches that correspond broadly with those in Table 17.1 (see Table 17.2).

Again, Hood (1995) presents various prescriptions when particular sets of conditions prevail. Mutuality is indicated as a basis for coordination in conditions where there is a strong sense of groupness (high social integration), but as yet few authoritative rules or standards by which progress might be definitively judged (low social regulation) – so that the group must decide these as it goes along. Interestingly, Hood (1995, 1998) associates mutuality with particular forms of public service organisation, which are characterised by their commitments to collegiality, co-production and organisational democracy. Notably, for the first time this associates notions of governance as a *coordinative structure* with those of governance arrangements as specific forms of *organisational structure* – a point to which this chapter will return.

Table 17.2: Mutuality and bureaucratic control

		Social integration	
		High	Low
Social regulation	High	*Hierarchical oversight*	*Contrived randomness*
	Low	**Mutuality**	*Competition*

Source: Hood, 1995, 1998

Mutuality and Shared Learning

The cultural theory upon which Hood's (1995) analysis is based offers further useful insights; in its 'requisite variety condition', which states that all four approaches should be expected to be present at any time (however attenuated any of them might be in any particular given context), and compatibility condition, which states that each of the cultural biases has something to offer each of the others, as well as representing a potential threat.

The requisite variety condition is generally reflected in everyday experience – it is rare to find pure empirical examples of any of the above ideal-types (including mutuality). Moreover, there is also considerable evidence that if one approach is sufficiently dominant in a particular context to shut out other contributions, this may result in sub-optimality or dysfunctional momentum (Perri 6 et al, 2002). Hence, while each dominant perspective in the above frameworks may lead to a preferred position or 'default strategy', contingencies often demand a more balanced 'repertoire of problem-framing and problem-definition strategies' (Hoppe, 2011, p 115). In this way, Quinn (1988, p xv) distinguishes between one approach to decision-making that is 'purposive, static and entropic' (expected to 'give the right answers'), and another that is 'holistic, dynamic and generative' (expected to 'ask the right questions'). Policy actors' purposive frame is the equivalent of their default strategy; in their holistic frame, they draw more widely on a range of competing perspectives. This places a premium on not only sound, purposive judgement, but also the holistic ability to *question, learn and adapt*, so that:

(i) recognition is given to what each approach offers and claims;
(ii) conflicts, contradictions and incongruencies between them are appropriately managed.

The first of these requires openness to *mutual sharing and learning* between different perspectives. In turn, this requires acceptance that (a) each perspective produces valid information for decision-making (Argyris, 1976, p 365), and that (b) none holds more than a portion of such information (Perri 6 et al, 2002, p 83).

The second requires *mutual adjustment and support* for emergent strategies and practices. In turn, this requires (a) receptivity to the corrective feedback provided by each perspective (Argyris, 1976, p 365), without (b) conceding wholly to any such perspective (Perri 6 et al, 2002).

In sum, even in contexts where hierarchy is dominant (for example, low competition, low uncertainty or high social integration, high social regulation) or where market-based perspectives are dominant (for example, low uncertainty, high competition or low social integration, low social regulation), mutuality may bring new ways of thinking and doing that strengthen these other approaches. For example, there may be something considerable to be gained from drawing more creatively on the more relational and collaborative approaches associated with mutuality – such as adding notions of partnership, co-production and citizen participation – where these are currently excluded or underdeveloped. In relation to the social determinants of health, this may be the case in addressing patterns of inequality, or issues of multiple exclusion and community wellbeing (Bonner, 2018), where greater mutuality may have a positive effect at the level of values, systems and practices (although whether this is sufficient to achieve tangibly better outcomes remains an empirical question).

Moreover, there is evidence that in practice, different perspectives may be seen as representing a potential threat to dominant, purposive frames (whether for particular patterns of social relations, cognitive frames or operational practices). For example, various arguments have been presented against citizen and user participation (Burton et al, 2004; Andrews et al, 2008), and the collaboration and co-production literature often has as much to say about collaborative inertia or process loss as it does about collaborative advantage (Huxham and Vangen, 2005). Work is therefore required to achieve acceptance from each different perspective that each of the others produces valid information and also make policy actors receptive to such corrective feedback. For example, work is often necessary to bridge between different institutional spheres, with divergent viewpoints, interests and values, to enable collaboration (cf. Lawrence and Suddaby, 2006; Cloutier et al, 2016). Accordingly, Huxham and Vangen (2005) identify various success factors for collaborative advantage, including access to resources, coordination and seamlessness, shared risk and mutual learning. In this sense, mutual sharing, learning, adjustment and support are always achievements.

Overall, there are a number of contributions in the literature from which mutuality and cooperation emerge as a useful basis for coordination. Broadly, the above frameworks provide indications of its potential value in addressing some of the 'wicked problems' associated with the social determinants of health, especially when there is a combination of either high uncertainty and low competition or high social integration and low social regulation. Under such conditions –

for which there is considerable empirical evidence in relation to the social determinants of health in local government – mutuality holds a legitimate and continuing interest.

In this way, this chapter has considered the role and potential of mutuality and cooperation in relation to governance (as a *coordinative structure*) and modes of governance (as different *logics of coordination*). At these levels of abstraction, mutuality is indicated as having a legitimate place at the table, however expansive or attenuated its actual role might be in particular contexts.

Yet a key question that follows might be whether we need a little mutuality or a lot. If it is a little, then its insights still might be added to approaches that are dominated by other perspectives. As we have seen, at the level of values, systems and practices this can have important effects – although usually as policy or managerial, rather than structural, adjustments (Toonen and Raadschelders, 1997). So what about structures? The next section considers mutuality in relation to governance arrangements (that is, as specific forms of *organisational structure*). Hence, if a lot of mutuality is required, it may be employed as a preferred position or default strategy and explicitly designed into governance arrangements.

Mutuality and governance arrangements: re-examining organisational structure

While mutuality and cooperation are often associated with the organisational forms of mutuals and cooperatives, principles of mutuality and cooperation can feature strongly in a range of organisational, institutional and systemic settings. Thus, it should be noted that while mutuals and cooperatives are generally built on principles of mutuality and cooperation, it is not the case that principles of mutuality and cooperation only find their expression in mutuals and cooperatives. Nevertheless, the decision to build governance arrangements around arrangements where mutuality is explicitly 'designed in' is an active choice, and this must be justified accordingly.

Aligning incentive structures: an heuristic framework

This chapter offers a novel framework for thinking about these issues, based on the incentive structures created by three different sets of interests: *collective interest* (CI: where provision is judged to have benefit for society as a whole, and there is willingness from the state to pay for welfare), *self-interest* (SI: where provision is judged to have benefit for particular individuals, who are willing to pay for their own welfare), and *collective self-interest* (CSI: where benefits for individuals are dependent on collective action, and there is a willingness to make collective contributions and participate in collective processes). In combination, these three sets of interests generate eight broad possibilities (see Figure 17.2). Each of these ideal-type governance arrangements are in common use in many localities, and each may have an effect on the social determinants of health.

Mutuality might be expected to have least effect here when collective self-interest is low (Boxes C, D, G and H); in general, this seems to be the case. Briefly, Box D represents classic market provision, based predominantly in organising for the welfare of self-interested individuals in the absence of any sufficient form of collective interest. Box G represents classic public goods, based on a clear public interest but insufficient levels of self-interest or collective self-interest for welfare to be organised beyond the public sector, funded by taxation. Box C represents the need to provide for individuals who, despite their willingness to do so, cannot themselves easily organise their own welfare. They must therefore rely on the public sector to coordinate or otherwise resource provision, including differing levels of subsidy according to the level of public interest. Box H represents redundant provision, in which there is apparently insufficient interest from any party to avoid decommissioning (although pockets of interest may emerge to revive such provision in the face of such withdrawal).

Conversely, mutuality might be expected to have most effect when collective self-interest is high (Boxes A, B, E and F); again, in general, this seems to be the case. Box B represents perhaps the 'purest' type of mutual or cooperative organisation. Here self-interest combines with collective self-interest to ensure provision for individuals who cannot themselves easily organise their own welfare, and where there is insufficient collective interest for the public sector to coordinate or otherwise resource this provision on their behalf. Often called self-help and mutual aid, this has been a significant form of welfare provision for more than a century through mutual organisations such as friendly societies and building societies and various forms of cooperative as member-owned or people-centred businesses (Birchall, 2011, 2012). As businesses, they must often compete in the market with investor-owned businesses, where, to remain viable, members must be persuaded that the mutual or cooperative generates greater overall welfare than the alternatives (relative to their contributions). Meanwhile, Box F also represents a situation where there is insufficient collective interest for the public sector to coordinate or otherwise resource provision on

Figure 17.2: Incentive structures and ideal-type governance arrangements

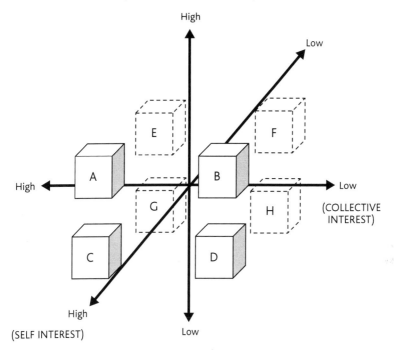

(COLLECTIVE SELF INTEREST)

	CI	SI	CSI	'Ideal-type' governance arrangements
A	High	High	High	**Multi-Stakeholder Mutual**
B	Low	High	High	**Single Stakeholder, Fully Mutual, perhaps competing with the market**
C	High	High	Low	'Best Value' provision, perhaps with (subsidised) user fees
D	Low	High	Low	Market provision
E	High	Low	High	**Community Co-production**
F	Low	Low	High	Local Organisation/Interest Group
G	High	Low	Low	Public goods
H	Low	Low	Low	Decommissioning

people's behalf, but also where there is insufficient self-interest for a viable people-centred business to be established. Collective self-interest is sufficient, however, to sustain the provision of welfare through, for example, membership of voluntary organisations and interest groups, in which principles of mutuality and cooperation may play an important part. In Box E, collective self-interest combines with collective interest to bring representatives from different aggregations of collective self-interest together with representatives from the public sector. This allows the combination of a range of complementary resources (for example, finance, authority, knowledge and solidarity) in support of 'community co-production' of welfare through a range of potential organisational structures. Finally, Box A represents the combination of collective self-interest, collective interest and self-interest. This adds an additional layer of complexity in ensuring that an effective balance is maintained between these sets of interests, in order to defeat any attempt to capture private contributions for public benefit or vice versa. Collective self-interest can play an important role here as 'honest broker'. As Birchall (2001, p 3) explains:

> Kellner (1998, p 9) suggests that mutuality mediates between the three basic principles of liberty, equality and fraternity: they can be achieved only if we develop a culture of mutual responsibility. More exactly, it might be used as a (gender neutral) synonym for fraternity ... It is a kind of honest broker between the claims of liberty and equality, supplying the goodwill needed to secure people's assent to political decisions that are not in their individual short term interest.

Under these conditions, a 'multi-stakeholder mutual' might be proposed, in which each set of interests may be represented in membership, conferring each with rights of ownership, benefits and control – but in which coercion and competition are not viable bases for coordination, so that each must learn to cooperate. Examples include certain of the new leisure trusts developed in many local authority areas since the mid-1990s (Simmons, 2008).

Mutuality and partnerships

Various forms of local partnership, formal and informal, are notably missing from the above analysis. Nonetheless, these are also common where the public interest and at least one other set of interests are aligned – that is, public–private partnerships (Box C), community partnerships (Box E) and/or multi-stakeholder partnerships (Box A). Throughout this book, there are important arguments for more relational partnering, particularly with regards to public–private partnerships, and an important new research initiative is currently in development. This chapter acknowledges these perspectives, suggesting how 'mutuality' might help inform such an approach. In short, there are some important messages here about where and how different interests might be aligned, how cooperation and collaboration (rather than coercion or competition) might be established as the dominant basis for coordination, and how this might be sustained through the ongoing renewal of mutuality in the partnering relationship.

Seeing new possibilities?

The framework in Figure 17.2 results in some readily identifiable organisational structures. It is provided as a brief heuristic for identifying where mutuality might be more or less likely to have a notable effect. However, there are various hybrid structures, both 'organic' and 'enacted' (Billis, 2010a) which would add nuance to the diversity of approaches listed (e.g. Simmons et al, 2007; Billis, 2010b; Vickers et al, 2017; Edmiston and Nicholls, 2018). Sometimes these hybrids are not intuitive, but can make good sense in creatively aligning the above incentive structures and bringing different sets of interests together in governance arrangements. For example, in an ongoing EU research project (Strength2Food), the interests of private organic farmers are being connected in a supply cooperative for public food procurement in primary schools in Serbia. There is a clear public interest here for the local authority in improving the quality of school meals for young children and in supporting the strategically important local agriculture sector. There is also self-interest from consumers (parents and children) in getting healthy, high-quality food at little or no additional cost. And there is collective self-interest from the organic farmers in forming the supply cooperative, given that none of them individually is able to guarantee supply across the public procurement contract. Creative partnerships are now being formed to make this happen, in what might be seen as an example of harnessing mutuality to address a key social determinant of health (Simmons, 2019). Yet while all parties were aware of each other (to at least some extent), prior to the research project there was no attempt to bring them together for this purpose. The underlying message here is that the creative alignment of incentive structures can generate interesting alternatives, and that sometimes local government may be limited only by its inability to see them.

Mutuality (and the social determinants of health in local government): where has it come from, where is it now and where is it going?

Mutuality has a long history in relation to the social determinants of health. Formally, prior to the development of the modern welfare state, for example, friendly societies provided access to health care and other welfare benefits for those who could not afford the high entry costs to the market. As the role of central government increased, so these earlier forms became marginalised. Mutuality rose again in the 1960s and 1970s in response to this 'big government' – for example, in community resistance to slum clearances through the formation of mutual forms of organisation to rehabilitate their homes, but also the establishment of community health councils and the appointment of parent governors in education to participate directly in school governance. By the 1990s, among a range of 'new' forms of participation, such as user groups, forums and committees (Stewart, 1996), the large-scale voluntary transfer (LSVT) of housing stock to new agencies gave opportunities for tenants to become board members, and some social care providers began to seek partnership with service users as co-producers (Birchall and Simmons, 2004). The 1997–2010 Labour government brought further impetus. As Reddel (2002, p 50) observes:

> In recent times, terms such as 'social capital', 'community engagement', 'community regeneration and renewal', 'community capacity building', 'social partnerships', and 'social entrepreneurship' reflect a growing re-emergence in discourse of the ideas and values of community and citizen participation.

Moreover, the new millennium saw new expressions mutuality being designed into the fabric of service delivery agencies – such as leisure trusts, tenant management organisations, foundation hospital trusts and co-operative schools (Simmons and Birchall, 2009). This wave of enthusiasm in the early 2000s, which was dubbed the 'new mutualism' (Birchall, 2001), has been joined in the last decade by further waves, initially in response to the 'big society' agenda (Birchall, 2011), and more recently as a potential response to austerity (Davies and Pill, 2012; Bailey and Pill, 2015). This has seen a range of important developments in the enabling environment, including the right to manage (whereby public service staff can apply to set up a new mutual), centralised support (initially from the cabinet office and now from the Department for Digital, Culture, Media and Sport, plus the establishment of an arm's-length Mutuals Taskforce) and the encouragement of community and social enterprises in public procurement.

Nevertheless, since the 'creeping nationalisation' of the friendly societies began more than a century ago (Mabbett, 2001), mutuality has perhaps more often been used as a strategic defence against larger, more powerful forces, rather than as a strategic offence, as an equal and legitimate force in addressing the social determinants of health. Despite some sympathetic experts who began to put the word 'community' in front of their specialism (community planners, architects and workers), early attempts to respond to 'big government' were often countered by a deeply entrenched resistance to change amongst public service professionals (Birchall and Simmons, 2004). Subsequent participatory forums, from community health councils, to school governing bodies, to LSVT housing associations, to other user groups, forums and committees, have often found themselves similarly marginalised or manipulated by bureaucrat-professionals who have found ways to continue to control the agenda (Barnes et al, 2003). Strategic defence here has taken the form of somehow fighting back against this bureaucratic/professional power, often against the odds.

The more recent use of mutual structural organisational forms, such as leisure trusts and other public service 'spin outs' (Simmons, 2008; Sepulveda et al, 2018), has often had its origins in a different form of strategic defence – *dynamic conservatism* (or changing to stay the same) – as a way for local authorities and service professionals to avoid the privatisation or decommissioning of services in the face of financial constraints (Simmons, 2008). However, evidence that changes in structural form have led to more mutual values, systems and practices often remains partial and/or unconvincing, particularly with regard to organizational democracy (Simmons, 2008). This has also been the experience in foundation trusts (as public benefit corporations deliberately based on cooperative principles) (Allen et al, 2012). In each case, communities may have benefited substantially; for example, services have been saved from closure, or increased collegiality has developed among staff whose collective self-interest has been served in the process of spinning out. However, in real terms the basic underlying nature of services has often remained unchanged, so that service users and communities are unable to see any meaningful acknowledgement of themselves in any supposed transformation. Hence, where people have been mobilised to participate in various structures by the relational promise offered by supposedly more mutual relationships, in practice a number of them have been left feeling unenthused, unenthralled and unengaged (Newman and Clarke, 2009, p 182). By comparison, when structures align better with people, this can be generative, rewarding, effective and even constitutive (Tunstall, 2001; INVOLVE, 2005). For example, one set of governance arrangements that consistently comes out well in evaluations relative to non-mutual forms of provision is that of tenant management organisations (TMOs); a wide diversity of cooperative and mutual housing types that have evolved over time in different ways to meet particular needs, assisted by different enablers and invested firmly bottom-up in communities – which they generally serve to renew through quite intensive member participation and involvement that is able to direct services towards the things members care most about (Cairncross et al, 2002; Simmons and Birchall, 2007a). Despite their relative success, however, TMOs account for only a small proportion of the overall sector. Bliss (2009) attributes this, at least in part, to 'housing establishment perceptions that ordinary people and communities can't be trusted to make decisions'. There is, then, a sense in some quarters that such options are somehow dangerously radical. Nevertheless, in her book entitled *Radical Help*, prize-winning author Hilary Cottam (2018) turns this assertion around the other way:

> The challenges we face today cannot be cured by an expert or a process that is done to us. What is common to these problems is that the solutions require our participation. Solutions require us – communities, the state, business and citizens – to work together, drawing on new ideas and above all on each other to create change. But our post-war institutions were not designed to help us collaborate or to come together to sustain changed ways of living. In fact, they were more often designed to keep us out, at arms' length, where we could be managed.

Perhaps this is a place to start if mutuality is to move from strategic defence to strategic offence? However, from networks and multi-actor dependencies, to procurement and relational partnering; from individual and community co-production, to new mutuals and even cooperative councils/cooperative places (Kippin and Randle, 2017); in practice, how radical can these solutions be?

In principle, the above narrative suggests there are certain contexts where limits may be perceived on the value of mutuality. Yet the contexts in which mutuality might be more highly valued remain many and varied – arguably increasingly so, especially in relation to 'wicked problems' associated with the social determinants of health. Provided appropriate safeguards are put in place, for example around relative autonomy (rather than unconditional trust) and appropriate regulation (based predominantly on horizontal, peer review rather than adversarial or managerial forms of accountability) (Hood, 1995), more radical expressions of mutuality and cooperation – including various hybrids of and partnerships between public, private and third-sector actors – provide a valuable approach.

However, the enabling environment is important, and there is evidence that entrenched attitudes and a lack of familiarity with such ways of working can mean that any successes are often gained despite, not because of, the support that is offered. The use of mutuality to address the social determinants of health may therefore fall foul of '3 Cs': incompatible values and attitudes (culture); a lack of ability (competence); or a lack of willingness (commitment) (Simmons and Brennan, 2017). In this sense, if mutuality is to be employed as productively as possible, there is a need to develop a more open, skilled and committed approach.

This applies equally to the relations that exist between actors within different parts of an overall service system, as it does to those within specific organisational settings. For example, with regard to intergovernmental relations, Landy and Teles (2001, p 414) invoke a 'principle of mutuality' in which 'It should be the obligation of each level of government as it participates in joint decision-making to *foster the legitimacy and capacity of the other*' (emphasis added). This principle (itself quite radical given the dominance of a performance-managed orthodoxy with ring-fenced accountabilities?) might be usefully applied across the boundaries between any of the 'two or more parties … sharing a feeling, action, or relationship … upon which co-operation is based'. For example, in relation to the recent promotion of 'new mutuals', the government-endorsed Mutuals Taskforce, chaired by Professor Julian Le Grand (2012), states that:

> The balance of focus on central Government Departments, the parent bodies of employees exploring mutualisation, the employees themselves and commissioners is crucial. For without the drive and support of any one of these groups, mutualisation is likely to prove more, and unnecessarily, challenging. Establishing mutuals requires collective effort.

This 'joined-upness' may sound like hard work. However, this need not be the case. Indeed, it may actually prove to be the opposite if it involves a lot of people doing a relatively small amount to build governance arrangements based on mutuality and cooperation; as compared with alternatives where a relatively small number of people (experts, entrepreneurs) do a lot. A key point here is that while mutuality can help address 'wicked problems', the establishment of mutuality as a coordination mechanism is itself often a tame one. The distinguished local government scholar John Stewart (1999, p 3) once pointed out that: 'the impossible suddenly becomes possible when you can see it from another point of view'. Similarly, what currently seems radical often becomes less so when people realise it is possible – and, indeed, sometimes preferable.

Conclusions

Mutuality is examined in this chapter as the basis for relational contact between two or more parties, whereby *cooperation* is sustained as the basis for coordination – rather than, for example, forces of *coercion* or *competition*. Aligning with prevailing notions of relational and collaborative logics of coordination and sets of governance arrangements, mutuality has recently become something of a hot topic. However, the concept is nothing new in governance at the local level. Going back over a century, friendly societies were present at the very origins of the welfare state, providing affordable alternatives to the market. Interest in mutuality has waxed and waned in the intervening period, as central government has first assumed greater post-war responsibility for welfare and then sought to roll back on this commitment. However, while these waves of interest have recently intensified and become more frequent, scope is perhaps emerging for them to move from more strategically defensive to more strategically offensive positions.

This chapter draws on conceptual frameworks that suggest mutuality is particularly important in the face of 'wicked problems', and in contexts where, for example, there are combinations of high uncertainty and low competition, or high social integration and low social regulation. This places mutuality in an excellent position to contribute to addressing the social determinants of health, given such conditions are now widely encountered in local government (and beyond). Such contributions may be more or less radical in their departure from prevailing structural and cultural norms, and such departures may be more or less well supported by the enabling environment. However, in situations where the incentive structure is conducive and effective practical arrangements are put in place, relationships based on mutuality and cooperation can survive and thrive in ways that are generative, rewarding, effective and constitutive. This is far from guaranteed, and there are plenty of examples of, for example, collaborative inertia, process loss and failed participatory initiatives. However, the moral imperative identified by Huxham and Vangen (2005, p 7) – that many really important public service issues simply cannot be tackled by acting alone – means that calls for greater mutuality are highly unlikely to go away. As these calls arrive, there may be a further legitimate imperative: to establish and deepen the relational culture, competence and commitment for mutuality to succeed.

References

Allen, P., Keen, J., Wright, J., Dempster, P., Townsend, J., Hutchings, A., Street, A. and Verzulli, R. (2012) 'Investigating the governance of autonomous public hospitals in England: multi-site case study of NHS foundation trusts', *Journal of Health Services Research and Policy*, 17(2): 94–100.

Andrews, R., Cowell, R., Downe, J., Martin, S. and Turner, D. (2008) 'Supporting effective citizenship in local government: engaging, educating and empowering local citizens', *Local Government Studies*, 34(4): 489–507.

Ansell, C. and Gash, A. (2008) 'Collaborative governance in theory and practice', *Journal of Public Administration Research and Theory*, 18(4): 543–71.

Argyle, M. (1991), *Cooperation: The Basis of Sociability*, London: Routledge.

Argyris, C. (1976) 'Single-loop and double-loop models in research on decision-making', *Administrative Science Quarterly*, 21: 363–75.

Bailey, N. and Pill, M. (2015) 'Can the state empower communities through localism? An evaluation of recent approaches to neighbourhood governance in England', *Environment and Planning C: Government and Policy*, 33(2): 289–304.

Barnes, M., Newman, J., Knops, A. and Sullivan, H. (2003) 'Constituting "the public" in public participation', *Public Administration*, 81(2): 379–99.

Bartels, K. and Turnbull, N. (2019) 'Relational public administration: a synthesis and heuristic classification of relational approaches', *Public Management Review*. Available from: https://doi.org/10.1080/14190 37.2019.1632921 [Accessed 13 April 2020].

Billis, D. (2010a) 'Revisiting the key challenges: hybridity, ownership and change', in D. Billis (ed) *Hybrid Organizations and the Third Sector*, pp 240–62, Basingstoke: Palgrave Macmillan.

Billis, D. (2010b) (ed) *Hybrid Organizations and the Third Sector*, Basingstoke: Palgrave Macmillan.

Birchall, J. and Simmons, R. (2004) *User Power*, London: National Consumer Council.

Birchall, J. (2001) (ed) *The New Mutualism in Public Policy*, London, Routledge.

Birchall, J. (2011) *People-Centred Businesses*, Basingstoke: Palgrave Macmillan.

Birchall, J. (2012) 'The comparative advantages of member-owned businesses', *Review of Social Economy*, 70(3): 263–94.

Bliss, N. (2009) *Bringing Democracy Home*, West Bromwich: Commission on Co-operative and Mutual Housing.

Bonner, A. (2018) *Social Determinants of Health: An Interdisciplinary Approach to Social Inequality and Wellbeing*, Bristol: Policy Press.

Briassoulis, H. (2019) 'Governance as multiplicity: the assemblage thinking perspective', *Policy Sciences*, 52(3): 419–50.

Burton, P., Goodlad, R., Croft, J., Abbott, J., Hastings, A. and MacDonald, G. (2004) *What Works in Community Involvement in Area-Based Initiatives?* London: Home Office.

Cairncross, L., Morrell, C., Darke, J. and Brownhill, S. (2002) *Tenants managing: an evaluation of tenant management organisations in England*, London: ODPM.

Cleaver, F. (2004) 'The social embeddedness of agency and decision making', in S. Hickey and G. Mohan (eds) *Participation – From Tyranny to Transformation?*, pp 271–7, London: Zed Books.

Cloutier, C., Denis, J., Langley, A. and Lamothe, L. (2016) 'Agency at the managerial interface: public sector reform as institutional work', *Journal of Public Administration Research and Theory*, 26(2): 259–76.

Cottam, H. (2018) *Radical Help: How We Can Remake the Relationships between Us and Revolutionise the Welfare State*, London: Virago.

Davies, J. and Pill, M. (2012) 'Empowerment or abandonment? Prospects for neighbourhood revitalization under the big society', *Public Money and Management*, 32(3): 193–200.

Douglas, M. (1970) *Natural Symbols: Explorations in Cosmology*, London: Barrie and Rockliff,

Douglas, M. (1982) *In the Active Voice*, London: Routledge,

du Gay, P. (2000) *In Praise of Bureaucracy*, London: Sage,

du Gay, P. (ed) (2005) *The Values of Bureaucracy*, Oxford: Oxford University Press.

Dunleavy, P. and Hood, C. (1994) 'From old public administration to new public management', *Public Money and Management*, 14(3): 9–16.

Edmiston, D. and Nicholls, A. (2018) 'Social impact bonds: the role of private capital in outcome-based commissioning', *Journal of Social Policy*, 47(1): 57–76.

Entwistle, T. and Martin, S. (2005) 'From competition to collaboration in public service delivery: a new agenda for research', *Public Administration*, 83(1): 233–42.

Geyer, R. and Cairney, P. (2015) *Handbook on Complexity and Public Policy*, Cheltenham: Edward Elgar.

Greener I. (2003) 'Who choosing what? The evolution of the word "choice" in the NHS and its implications for new labour', *Social Policy Review*, 15: 49–67.

Grint, K. (2005) Problems, problems, problems: the social construction of "leadership"', *Human Relations*, 58(11): 1467–94.

Hammond, K. (1996) *Human Judgment and Social Policy: Irreducible Uncertainty, Inevitable Error, Unavoidable Injustice*, Oxford: Oxford University Press.

Hayek, F. (1976) *The Mirage of Social Justice*, London: Routledge.

Hood, C. (1995) 'Contemporary public management: a new global paradigm?', *Public Policy and Administration*, 10(2): 104–17.

Hood, C. (1998) *The Art of the State*, Oxford: Oxford University Press.

Hoppe, R. (2011) *The Governance of Problems: Puzzling, Powering and Participation*, Bristol: Policy Press.

Huxham, C. and Vangen, S. (2005) *Managing to Collaborate: The Theory and Practice of Collaborative Advantage*, London: Routledge.

INVOLVE (2005) *The True Costs of Participation*, London: Involve.

Kellner, P. (1998) *New Mutualism: The Third Way*, London: Co-operative Party.

Kippin, H. and Randle, A. (2017) *From Co-operative Councils to Co-operative Places*, London: Collaborate.

Landy, M. and Teles, S. (2001) 'Beyond devolution: from subsidiarity to mutuality', in K. Nicolaïdis, and R. Howse (eds) *The Federal Vision: Legitimacy and Levels of Governance in the United States and the European Union*, pp 413–26, Oxford: Oxford University Press.

Lawrence, T. and Suddaby, R. (2006) 'Institutions and institutional work', in S. Clegg, C. Hardy, T. Lawrence and W. Nord (eds.) *Handbook of Organizational Studies*, pp 215–54, London: Sage.

Le Grand, J. and the Mutuals Taskforce (2012) 'Public service mutual: the next steps', discussion paper. London: Cabinet Office. Available from: http://eprints.lse.ac.uk/44579 [Accessed 28 July 2020].

Lelièvre-Finch, D. (2010) 'The challenge for public leadership arising from mixed modes of governance' in S. Brookes and K. Grint (eds) *The New Public Leadership Challenge*, pp 283–9, Basingstoke: Palgrave Macmillan.

Lowndes, V. and Skelcher, C. (1998) 'The dynamics of multi-organizational partnerships: an analysis of changing modes of governance', *Public Administration*, 76(3): 313–33.

Mabbett, D. (2001) 'Mutuality in Insurance and social security: retrospect and prospect', in J. Birchall (ed) *The New Mutualism in Public Policy*, London: Routledge, 118–31.

Mutuals Taskforce (2012) *Public Service Mutuals: The Next Steps*, London: Mutuals Taskforce.

Newman, J. and Clarke, J. (2009) *Publics, Politics and Power: Remaking the Public in Public Services*, London: Sage.

OGC (Office for Government Commerce) (2008) *Competitive Dialogue in 2008*, London: Office for Government Commerce.

Osborne, S. (2010) The New Public Governance: Emerging Perspectives on the Theory and Practice of Public Governance, London: Taylor and Francis.

Osborne, S., Radnor, Z., Kinder, T. and Vidal, I. (2015) 'The SERVICE framework: a public-service-dominant approach to sustainable public services', *British Journal of Management*, 26(3): 424–38.

Perri 6, Leat, D., Seltzer, K. and Stoker, G. (2002) *Towards Holistic Governance: The New Reform Agenda*, Basingstoke: Palgrave Macmillan.

Quinn, R. (1988), *Beyond Rational Management*, San Francisco, CA: Jossey-Bass.

Quinn, R. and Hall, R. (1983) 'Environments, organizations, and policy makers: toward an integrative framework', in R. Hall and R. Quinn (eds) *Organization Theory and Public Policy: Contributions and Limitations*, Beverly Hills, CA: Sage Publications, pp 281–98.

Reddel, T. (2002) 'Beyond participation, hierarchies, management and markets: "new" governance and place policies', *Australian Journal of Public Administration*, 61(1): 50–63.

Rittel, H. and Webber, M. (1973) 'Dilemmas in a general theory of planning', *Policy Sciences*, 4: 155–69.

Sepulveda, L., Lyon, F. and Vickers, I. (2018) '"Social enterprise spin-outs": an institutional analysis of their emergence and potential', *Technology Analysis & Strategic Management*, 30(8): 967–79.

Simmons, R., Powell, M., Birchall, J. and Doheny, S. (2007) '"Citizen governance": opportunities for inclusivity in policy and policy-making?', *Policy and Politics*, 35(3): 455–75.

Simmons, R. and Birchall, J. (2007a) 'Tenant participation and social housing in the UK: applying a theoretical model', *Housing Studies*, 22(4): 573–95.

Simmons, R. and Birchall, J. (2007b) 'The role of co-operatives in poverty reduction: network perspectives', *Journal of Socio-Economics*, 37(6): 2131–40.

Simmons, R. and Birchall, J. (2009) 'The public service consumer as member', in R. Simmons, M. Powell and I. Greener (eds) *The Differentiated Consumer in Public Services*, Bristol: Policy Press, 57–76.

Simmons, R. and Brennan, C. (2017) 'User voice and complaints as drivers of innovation in public services', *Public Management Review*, 19(8): 1085–1104.

Simmons, R. (2008) 'Harnessing social enterprise for local public services: new leisure trusts in the UK', *Public Policy and Administration*, 23(3): 278–301.

Simmons, R. (2019) 'Short-food-supply-chains and public procurement: primary school meals in Serbia', paper presented at the International Conference on Public Policy, Montreal, June.

Simon, H. (1955) 'A behavioral model of rational choice', *Quarterly Journal of Economics*, 69(1): 99–118.

Stewart, J. (1996) 'Innovation in democratic practice in local government', *Policy and Politics*, 24(1): 29–41.

Stewart, J. (1999) 'Oral evidence to parliamentary select committee on public administration report', *Innovations in Citizen Participation in Government*, London: Stationery Office.

Tenbensel, T. (2005) 'Multiple modes of governance – disentangling the alternatives to hierarchies and markets', *Public Management Review*, 7(2): 267–88.

Thompson, G., Frances, J., Levacic, R. and Mitchell, J. (eds) (1991) *Markets, Hierarchies and Networks: The Co-ordination of Social Life*, London: Sage.

Thompson, M., Ellis, R. and Wildavsky, A. (1990) *Cultural Theory*, Boulder, CO: Westview Press.

Toonen, T. and Raadschelders, J. (1997) 'Public sector reform in western Europe', *Conference on Comparative Civil Service Systems*. Available from: http://www.indiana.edu/~csrc/toonen1.htm [Accessed 20 December 1997].

Tunstall, R. (2001) 'Devolution and user participation in public services: how they work and what they do', *Urban Studies*, 38(13): 2495–2514.

Vickers, I., Lyon, L., Sepulveda, L. and McMullin, C. (2017) 'Public service innovation and multiple institutional logics: the case of hybrid social enterprise providers of health and wellbeing', *Research Policy*, 46: 1755–68.

PART V

Socio-economic political perspectives

Introduction

Lord Peter Hain

Devolution and local empowerment

If the objective is to empower everyone, regardless of who they are or what their income is, then it is essential to bring decision-making closer to citizens through devolution and decentralisation. But that has been undermined by a decade of austerity since 2010, severely cutting local government budgets. The fad for 'neoliberal' economics – that is to say, favouring market forces wherever possible and tolerating state regulation and public investment only where absolutely necessary – has meant getting government as small as possible and out of the way to leave space for a free market free-for-all.

In schools, for example, instead of empowering parents, teachers and school governors within a framework of strong resource support for and enforcement of minimum standards by local and national government, to ensure equal opportunities for all, the aim has been to 'free' schools to compete in a contrived marketplace – while teachers are required to work to more centrally determined frameworks than ever before.

In parallel came former Prime Minister David Cameron's concept of 'the Big Society'. But that became little more than a soon-forgotten ruse to dump responsibility for providing community services onto a voluntary sector itself experiencing a huge capacity collapse driven by government.

Surely, power can only be spread downwards in an equitable manner if there is a national framework where opportunities, resources, wealth and income are distributed as equally as possible, and where democratic rights are constitutionally entrenched?

Surely empowering local communities means establishing high minimum levels of public provision – affordable housing, public transport, social services, nursery schools, care services for the elderly, childcare and so on – and enabling these to be 'topped up' by local decisions?

Until now, at least, the incontrovertible advantage of modern Britain has been its 20th-century innovation: the pooling and sharing of risks and resources across the whole of the United Kingdom (UK) to ensure common welfare and decent standards of life for all citizens, regardless of nationality or where you live – common welfare standards first introduced by Liberal governments and subsequently consolidated by Labour governments up until 2010 – ensuring common economic and social standards: common UK-wide old age pensions, common UK social insurance (sick pay, health insurance, unemployment insurance and labour exchanges), common UK child and family benefits, a common UK minimum wage and a UK system of equalising resources, so that everyone irrespective of where they live has the same political, social and economic rights, and not simply equal civil and political rights.

Pooling and sharing the UK's resources also enables redistribution from richer to poorer parts of the UK, such as the coalfield communities of the South Wales Valleys or North-East England. That is especially important since around 40 per cent of UK gross domestic product is concentrated in London and the South-East of England. Insights into devolution of powers to the Scottish Parliament and the Welsh Assembly are presented in Chapters 19 and 20, with respect to housing and wellbeing. Despite devolution to Scotland, Wales and Northern Ireland, the UK remains one of the most centralised states in Europe – especially in England outside London, which has its own elected mayor and assembly. Devolution for England through the English regions, cities and city regions, according to their own boundary preferences, ought to be prioritised.

But it is important to be clear about attempts to present devolving budgets to cities after 2010. These have not been so much acts of empowerment as mechanisms to shrink the Whitehall state, offloading as much responsibility as possible onto individual citizens to fend for themselves, outsourcing to private providers and subcontracting tax and spending to devolved cities and legislatures; as it were, economic devolution in neoliberal terms.

The theme has been to preach localism but practise centralism. Spending in England has been financed from Whitehall, for many years, and it has constantly interfered with and controlled local government, while substantially cutting local council budgets, forcing cuts in services. That was preceded by decades of steady erosion of local government powers and standing.

In Chapter 18, Bennett reviews the emergence of local government, which originated in part to address the needs of people in poverty and the control of infectious diseases, and the contemporary 'ironic localism, deregulation'. Tackling the social roots of ill health requires *collective* action and societal responsibility, not simply the preaching of *individual* responsibility. If the National Health Service ambition of reducing health inequalities and improving population health is to be realised, the focus must shift to addressing the causes of poor health and wellbeing rather than simply managing the consequences (see Chapter 1). As this book shows, that will require a new relationship with local government and also a change to the way in which public spending is accounted for. Traditional public accounting rules reinforce the tendency to act late; to spend on consequences rather than to invest upstream in tackling causes.

Instead of Whitehall setting local authorities' annual budgets, there should be long-term funding settlements so councils can plan ahead, improve their services and reinvest the savings. For instance, local government should be given new powers and access to additional central funding to keep elderly and vulnerable people out of hospital with locally managed integration of health and social care programmes.

Here, the ideological contrast between an 'empowering' and a 'neoliberal' government is starkly revealed. The great majority of individuals need the state on their side, but not on their backs. They need active government that intervenes to curb market excess and market power. They need the assistance of strong communities.

They need the solidarity that comes from acting collectively to exercise influence over the decisions that shape their lives, and to experience the fulfilment of active citizenship. Above all, they need power to be decentralised.

In the final chapter, Chapter 21, Nigel Ball reflects on the cycles of reform and cultural change and the changing relationship between local and central government.

18

From front-line defence to back-foot retreat: the diminishment of local government's role in social health outcomes

Michael Bennett

When I first came to consider local government, I began to see how it was in essence the first-line defence thrown up by the community against our common enemies – poverty, sickness, ignorance, isolation, mental derangement and social maladjustment. The battle is not faultlessly conducted, nor are the motives of those who take part in it all righteous or disinterested. But the war, I believe, is worth fighting. (Winifred Holtby, in a letter to her mother, Alderman Alice Holtby, 1935)

Introduction

Modern local government in the United Kingdom (UK) was born out of a growing concern about the links between social conditions and the state of public health. Yet while 'social determinants of health' has become a global discipline, local government has ceded its role over the last decade as its capacity has withered during the time of austerity. The COVID-19 crisis of 2020 has shown the capacity of local government to mobilise anew around public health issues, but its fundamental fiscal and constitutional weaknesses show that a new settlement is needed more than ever.

The story of local government and public health

One way of interpreting the last 150 years of English local government is through the lens of inequality and wellbeing – or what we are now calling the social determinants of health. As the Industrial Revolution developed and England grew wealthier, the health and welfare of its workers deteriorated. Between 1801 and 1841, the population of London doubled and that of Leeds nearly tripled. But such growth in urbanisation was deadly. Between 1831 and 1844, the death rate per 1,000 increased in Birmingham from 14.6 to 27.2, in Bristol from 16.9 to 31 and in Liverpool from 21 to 34.8 (Bryant and Rhodes, 2019). This crisis was the result of a terrible mismatch between the increase in the urban population and available housing. Overcrowding and poor living conditions led to widespread disease and poor health.

The shock of these negative effects on public health led to significant sanitary reforms in the 19th century and subsequently to the establishment of public health institutions.

During the 19th century, the new and growing cities and towns gained powers from Parliament to create municipal corporations (city-based all-purpose councils) with significant powers of taxation. By 1900, 'most public provision was in the hands of these councils or special-purpose authorities. Local government and school boards were responsible for the provision of almost all early public services such as hospitals and schooling and set the property taxes which funded them' (Travers, 2018).

Local government developed across this period to address poor health, poverty, water supply, sanitation, housing, street cleansing and access to gas and electricity. Local government in the late Victorian and Edwardian period evolved out of fragmented structures towards modern, county governance with a larger, more strategic footprint.

English local government, in other words, existed to meet social problems – and what today we call the social determinants of health. By the 1930s, the social and health responsibilities of local government had expanded to include a wider range of actions than is covered by current National Health Service (NHS) public health practice (Gorsky et al, 2014). To characterise the 1930s as a Golden Age for public health would be mistaken – serious health inequalities and high maternal mortality rates persisted. However, the impact of an active public health policy, informed by emerging science and supported by respected democratic institutions, led to life expectancy increasing from 40 years in the 1850s to 60.8 years in 1930 (Gorsky et al, 2014).

Common enemies and social evils

This is the story we see taken up in Winifred Holtby's letter to her mother. Struck down by disease, Holtby was at that time hurrying to finish her groundbreaking novel, *South Riding*. She would lose her own battle and die later that year, aged only 37. Published posthumously in 1936, *South Riding* draws partly on her mother's experiences as the first woman alderman in local government in East Riding, and explores the social nature of poor health and the role of elected councillors in leading the fight for improved conditions in their communities. The novel has one of the best descriptions of public health services (or lack of them), 'where the impact of tuberculosis, maternal mortality, lack of access to cancer services, and the impact of infectious disease are all vividly presented' (Neville, 2012).

Prior to the language of social determinants of health, we see in Holtby's account a deep and fundamental connection between the activities and purpose of local government and the war against poor health and social conditions.

These conditions focused attention on a range of social challenges not just as matters of voluntary action 'but as active dangers to the overall 'health' of the wider body politic. The central theme of this wave of concern was not just mass poverty, but – much more speculatively and sensationally – the possible link between such poverty and the spectre of social breakdown, economic failure and national decline' (Harris, 2009).

Modern government and radical improvements in population health

The 20th century led to radical improvements in public health across England and the UK. In common with other advanced industrial countries, public health measures such as pure food and clean water, the development of immunisations against many serious diseases such as polio and smallpox, and enhanced economic conditions, are together credited with substantial reductions in the burden of infectious diseases (Fielding, 1999).

Particular advances were made in infant mortality. Indeed, much of the improvement in mortality rates since the 18th century occurred in the 20th century. The drop in the number of deaths of children aged four and under is a prime illustration of the dramatic change in childhood mortality over the century (Fielding, 1999).

In 1915, there were 89,380 deaths of children aged under one, compared with just 2,721 in 2015. The number of deaths of children between one and four years of age was 55,607 in 1915, while it was 460 in 2015. By 2000, 83 per cent of all deaths in England and Wales occurred at ages 65 and over compared with less than 25 per cent a century earlier. Infant mortality accounted for 25 per cent of all deaths in 1901, but less than 1 per cent at the end of the century (ONS, 2003): see Figure 18.1.

Clearly, these advances in public health cannot be solely attributed to local government. Effective public health action requires a range of interventions, including political commitment to population level change, research to produce knowledge, institutions to galvanise and resources to enable intervention (Gray et al, 2006). This range of interventions is captured in the theoretical framework based on the interconnected and interdependent domains of the rainbow model of social determinants of health (Dahlgren and Whitehead, 1991). The fullest treatment of this is provided in Adrian Bonner's comprehensive collection (Bonner, 2018).

The interdisciplinary approach to understanding the social determinants of health includes the 'interconnectedness and interdependence of socio-economic, cultural, environmental, living and working conditions, social and community networks, and lifestyle choices that contribute to a person's health and well-being' (Bonner, 2018, p xxi). There is no claim that they are exclusively attributable to local government. However, the history of modern Britain and the development story of local government show that councils, working collaboratively with their partners in public, private and third sectors,

Figure 18.1: Childhood death numbers, England and Wales, 1915–2015

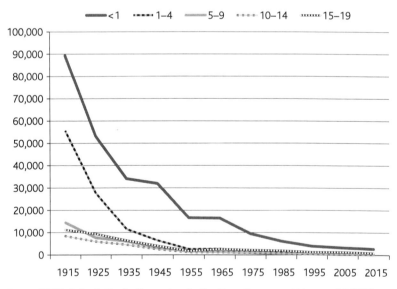

Source: UK Statistics Authority licensed under the Open Government Licence v3.0 (ONS, 2017, https://www.ons.gov.uk/peoplepopulationandcommunity/birthsdeathsandmarriages/deaths/articles/causesofdeathover100years/2017-09-18

can clearly impact significantly across this interconnected issue of social determinants of health and wellbeing.

Indeed, as Sir Michael Marmot, author of the government's review of health inequalities in England (2010a) has argued, 'the key policy areas – the social determinants of health – where action is likely to be most effective in reducing health inequalities' are very much in areas where local government has a key influencing role. Marmot focuses on:

- early child development and education;
- employment arrangements and working conditions;
- social protection;
- the built environment;
- sustainable development;
- economic analysis;
- delivery systems and mechanisms;
- priority public health conditions;
- social inclusion and social mobility.

As he says, 'In every single one of these areas, local government has a significant role to play in working with the NHS and other partners in improving health' (Marmot, 2010b).

Still front-line defence?

Following the global financial crisis of 2008, the UK's economy was plunged into the deepest recession of recent times with the sharpest fall in gross domestic product (–5 per cent) in a calendar year since records began (Allen, 2010). In turn, the government pursued a policy of strict fiscal 'austerity'. Even while government spending as a whole was restrained, it has been local government in England that has borne the biggest burden.

The Institute for Fiscal Studies (IFS) shows that local government spending was cut by 21 per cent in real terms between 2009/10 and 2017/18. This followed a cumulative increase of 57 per cent in real terms between 2000/1 and 2009/10.

However, the IFS shows (see Figure 18.2) that these cuts in funding were not spread evenly across councils but were significantly 'larger for councils serving more deprived communities than for those serving less deprived communities' (Amin-Smith and Phillips, 2019). Cuts averaged 31 per cent for the most deprived fifth of council areas, compared with 17 per cent for the least deprived fifth of council areas. Spending per

Figure 18.2: Service spending by English local authorities, 2000/1–2017/18

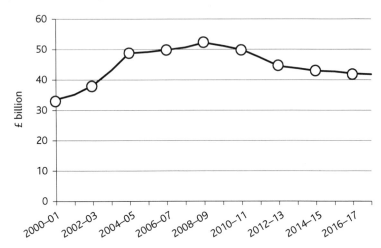

Source: Chart author's own, based on Amin-Smith and Phillips, 2019

person in the most deprived areas has fallen from 1.52 times that in the least deprived areas on average in 2009/10 to 1.25 times in 2017/18 (Amin-Smith and Phillips, 2019). The withdrawal and targeting of this investment on the grounds of austerity has impacted on some councils' ability to provide the social determinants of good health.

A result of this severe cutback in funding has been for councils to target their reductions in discretionary services in order to provide relative protection for statutory and more acute services. Figure 18.3 shows that councils' net expenditure on planning and development and housing services is down more than 50 per cent, and that on highways and transport and on cultural and leisure services is down more than 40 per cent. However, spending on adult social care services has been cut by just 5 per cent and spending on acute children's social care services (such as social work, safeguarding and fostering) is actually up around 10 per cent (Amin-Smith and Phillips, 2019). While the periods of improvement in public health resulted from heavy investment in social conditions for children, the last ten years have seen a rapid withdrawal from this area by local authorities.

Digging deeper, the IFS shows another level of prioritisation: a narrower group of population with highest need. Therefore, while spending on acute children's social care services has risen, spending on more general children's services, such as Sure Start, has fallen by more than 60 per cent. Looking at housing services, while budgets for homelessness have increased, budgets for housing advice, for the

Figure 18.3: Real-terms changes in local government service spending by service area, 2009/10–2017/18

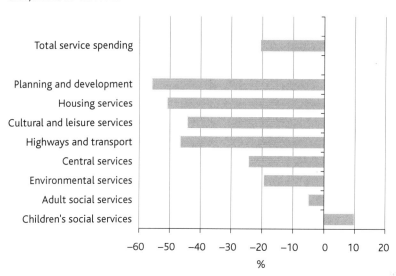

Source: Amin-Smith and Phillips, 2019. Reproduced with permission from Institute for Fiscal Studies

Supporting People programme and for improving and renewing private-sector housing have fallen by around two-thirds. And the numbers of people receiving adult social care services have fallen much more than spending, as support has been focused on those with the highest care needs (Amin-Smith and Phillips, 2019). Local authorities, in other words, have radically reduced their social health services to the childhood population, concentrating solely on those with the acutest need; or to put it another way, on those to whom they have a legal obligation to support.

One example of this can be seen in the ever greater resources that local authorities are spending on children with child protection plans, which means those children who are in crisis (DfE, 2019), and the dramatic cutbacks that saw two-thirds of spending on the Sure Start programme cut between 2009-2019. Evaluation of Sure Start's impact on child health found reduced hospitalisations, including a reduction in infection-related hospitalisations, and that its significant preventative impact benefited children living in disadvantaged areas most (Cattan et al, 2019). As the Children's Commissioner for England has argued, 'Mainstream and acute services such as age 4–16 education and provision for children in care have been protected at the expense of targeted preventative services, removing vital safety nets for some very vulnerable children' (Kelly et al, 2018).

The number of children looked after declined dramatically between 1981 and 1994 as children's policy changed and local authorities sought other ways of supporting young people, which did not involve removing them from their home environments (Rowlands and Statham, 2009).

The recent rise sees England returning to levels of children in care not seen since 1984. Even more remarkably, the figures show that the number of children requiring protection has increased by 85 per cent in ten years, from 29,000 in 2008 (Laming, 2009) to 52,260 in 2019 (DfE, 2019).

Indeed, England now spends nearly half of its entire children's services budget on 73,000 children in the care system (Kelly et al, 2018). As the Children's Commissioner argues, 'Children do not arrive in extreme need overnight and many could be prevented from getting to that point if we helped them sooner in a more effective way. We are, in effect, attempting to manage and contain crisis in children's lives after allowing it to escalate' (Longfield, 2018). This shows a dramatic move away from local government's tradition of focusing on the creation of good social conditions for health and development towards dealing with the problems of poor conditions.

In February 2019, the House of Commons Public Accounts Committee published an official lamentation of the UK government's 'unacceptable lack of ambition for the sector, with no aspiration for improving local finances beyond merely "coping"'. Indeed this seemed to be mirrored in the words of Melanie Dawes, Permanent Secretary, Ministry of Housing, Communities & Local Government, who in evidence to the committee stated that 'We believe the sector as a whole is sustainable if the amount of resources that are available to it can deliver the statutory services which it is required to do' (Ford, 2018). Sustainability is therefore cast as fulfilling legal obligations, not creating outcomes acceptable or desirable to society.

What we see is an ever-tightening rationing, with scarce resources being focused on a narrower group of people with highest care needs at the expense of prevention and wider social benefits. While entirely understandable and logical from local authorities' point of view, it runs contrary to the social model of health where there is an 'interconnectedness and interdependence of socio-economic, cultural, environmental, living and working conditions, social and community networks, and lifestyle choices that contribute to a person's health and well-being' (Bonner, 2018, p xxi).

One way of interpreting the current positioning of local government is that its new and limited *raison d'être* is to focus simply on fulfilling minimum standards required by statutory duties, whereas its role as transformer of the social conditions of local populations has been given up in all substantive ways. Local government has in effect ceded its role in creating the determinants of good health. How did this happen?

Ironic localism, deregulation and meaninglessness

While local government spent much of the last decade arguing for localism – by which was meant the empowerment of local government – the discourse of localism was deployed ironically by policymakers (Bennett and Orr, 2013) to distract from the policy of austerity. The legacy of this ironic localism can now be seen in the way in which the institutions, services and capacity of local government have become diminished with no corresponding empowerment. This is not to dispute that in some places austerity created a genuine sense of urgency, what Kotter would call an accelerator of change (Kotter, 2012), which led in some cases to valuable innovation and created the conditions to question traditional ways of working. But nor do we question the conclusion of the Conservative-led Local Government Association that the net result has been 'fragile services' that are 'no longer sustainable', and that councils have been left 'struggling to balance the books' (LGA, 2019).

One of the ironies involved in the recent austerity-as-localism is the way in which the abolition of the system of public performance reporting and external review was framed as a liberation of local government rather than a diminishment.

There is not space here to review the recent history of public audit and improvement. However, following Grace (2005), a significant point in the recent history of this debate is the 2001 Byatt and Lyons report on the role of 'external review', which stated that 'Future external review activity should recognise these accountabilities and be designed to support such leadership in effecting change' (Byatt and Lyons, 2001).

External review was being conceived and proposed as a resource to support leaders deliver change rather than as a retrospective audit of what went well or not. This repositioning of public services audit and inspection changed the traditional model, which had been linear with a one-way and simply retrospective relationship. The modern picture was far more connected, with two-way relationships between national government, local government and citizens (Grace, 2005).

As we shall see, this highly connected and networked form of governance, in which local government was understood to have relationships and responsibilities beyond its simple legal duties to auditors and beyond its democratic mandate from local voters, would became too heavy for the central–local relations to bear.

For while many saw accountability and external review as a necessary condition for local government's responsibility for strategic level priorities, regulation was seen as too burdensome and, more importantly, to impinge on local democratic virility.

In Chapter 9 of this volume, Dave Ayre sets out the evolution of the regulatory framework in England. As he argues, there was a glimmer of hope that the Best Value regime would be based more on collaboration than simple cost and competition considerations (Chapter 9).

In Scotland too, which had the power to develop a different legislative and regulatory framework for Best Value and community planning, ministers sought ideas on how to optimise the partnership between the new parliament and local authorities (Mair and Bennett, 1998). Some argued that *because* councils provide national priority services as a matter of statutory duty, and commit a low proportion of their resources to areas that are purely a matter of local discretion, this carried constitutional implications: 'Shared responsibility for these national services needs a partnership framework for planning and prioritisation. Indeed the ways in which these national programmes are run, and their consistency across Scotland, have clear implications for human rights' (Mair and Bennett, 2001).

Furthermore, given this context, it was argued what was needed was a much fuller framework of partnership between the Scottish Executive and local government that enshrined mutual recognition and shared responsibilities between the two levels of elected government. This fuller framework – which could be understood as a National Forum for Outcomes Delivery – involved mutual respect and recognition enshrined in a new partnership for governance. Concretely, it was proposed that councils recognise the rights of ministers to set national priorities that impact on local government, and ministers recognise that councillors are elected on a manifesto with commitments for local areas. Added to this was a protocol that developed how this mutual recognition and partnership should work in practice, including suggestions as to how subgroups could be focused on strategic themes.

A key argument was that strategic planning and budgeting should accommodate these partnerships – and promote mutual trust and understanding – avoiding the mundane conflict of indifference that had undermined many other previous efforts. The aim of the planning groups would be to put prioritised and costed three-year plans to the ministers and council leaders for consideration and decision. There would be disagreements and conflict around these initial plans, but the task would be to decide on a mutually agreed framework that would drive resource allocation and within which individual councils would develop their own detailed three-year plans.

Of course, the idea of a joint planning forum was not novel. There exist numerous central/local joint review and planning bodies, working groups etc. The novelty was suggesting in some detail how conflict could be reduced and how groups could be coordinated and focused through one joint planning forum centred on developing a three-year plan jointly agreed by ministers and council leadership as the basis for development. The proposal was that this might take the form of an outcome specified public service agreement (PSA) between the Executive and Scottish councils, but how detailed and prescriptive such a plan should be, and to what extent these could vary between councils, was to be a matter for negotiation. The minimum aim, however, was that it be stable and precise enough agreement of priorities, and performance expectations, including financial support for them, to allow councils stability for implementation and service development while respecting local circumstances.

If a PSA framework had been adopted, then it could have existed at different levels: a national framework agreement between local government collectively and the national government or detailed PSAs between individual councils and the Executive – or some combination of both to take account of local exceptions. This led to the idea that 'If PSAs were to be struck between individual councils and the Executive, then given the interrelated nature of councils and other local public agencies, developing the Community Plan as the focal point for local agreements would enable a joined up, programme approach. Detailed discussions will be necessary to establish at what level PSAs should be developed (collective or individual) between councils and the Executive' (Mair and Bennett, 2001).

An early evaluation of the impact of devolution in Scotland on local government found that devolution had not yet delivered the 'joining up' of public services that some had held out as a key aspiration (Bennett et al, 2002). Furthermore, the immediacy of the political landscape that devolution brought to Scotland meant that such issues could more easily be addressed and the possibility of partnership could be pursued. 'With the founding of the Parliament and the establishment of the Executive, there was now a stage upon which key actors could present their case. This stage was much closer to its audience and one where the actors might perhaps be more inclined to listen' (Bennett et al, 2002).

Despite this hope, the level of mistrust that continued to prevail between different levels of government in Scotland was a major countervailing force. 'While close interpersonal relations remained a key feature of the Scottish governance process, unlike the situation in England where the scale of local and national government makes personal relations less viable and useful, the institutionalising of mistrust between local and national government organisations continued in Scotland. Once again, much comment was generated on the need to build new processes and new links between the different levels of government in Scotland to overcome this situation. While personal contact will probably always be of significance in the "village" nature of Scotland's polity, progress was clearly needed to build institutional relations that mirrored some of the better aspects of interpersonal relations' (Bennett et al, 2002).

So while Community Plans did develop across Scotland, neither central or local government fully bought into a National Forum for Outcomes Delivery such as had been proposed. There was no national-level statement about how what central and local government priorities dovetailed towards agreed ends. More than ten years later, the Accounts Commission judged that implementation had not been successful, saying that there was a 'wider ambiguity both nationally and locally about the extent to which the focus of community planning should be on local needs or about delivering national priorities' (Accounts Commission, 2014). In other words, community planning existed in name at a local level but had no anchor in the political reality and no connection to the distribution of national resources. In early 2020, the Accounts Commission raised very similar criticisms of the new wave of City Deals (Accounts Commission, 2020).

In Scotland, local and central government continue to try to evolve a settlement on a mutually acceptable balance of freedom and accountability. Yet while there is a general acceptance of the principle of interdependence, there is no agreement about how to put this into practice. In England, the idea of partnership has been largely rejected by both sides, with central government reducing local government's resources in return for greater local 'discretion' over what local authorities now do.

Indeed, in retrospect we can see that neither central nor local government leaders were really ready for the implications of collaboration and partnership. National-level governance never trusted or respected local government sufficiently to accept it as an equal partner, and local government in England, after a short dalliance with strategic regulation, Comprehensive Performance Assessment and other forms of external review, chose localism and freedom over power-sharing and interdependency.

In England as in Scotland, then as now, what seemed to be required was for someone, in either central or local government, 'to make the first move to break the cycle of mistrust that in turn generates other barriers to improved central–local relations' (Bennett et al, 2002).

Some senior people in local government are beginning to regret the alacrity with which the sector swallowed what seemed to be the sweet success of their lobbying against external review. It appears to many that this new-found freedom has turned out to be empty. Local government has found itself isolated and irrelevant, with its voice silenced and its status reduced. To put it in existential terms, local government has found that being-in-and-for-itself is empty of meaning when compared with the significance of being-for-another. In more modern terms, local government has found that being reduced to statutory responsibilities is to exist as a delivery arm for government. This is a far cry from the integrationist ambitions of the place-shaping traditions (Lyons, 2007; Bichard, 2010) and ignores the importance of relationality to local leadership (Orr and Bennett, 2017).

Local government is familiar with the maxim that we measure what matters, but seemed blind to the logic that by abolishing measurement they were forsaking mattering. As Michael Lyons has argued, the Audit Commission's approach – while flawed and imperfect – 'encouraged more consistent comparisons between local authorities and put the spotlight on council management, showing that outstanding leadership made a difference and it wasn't just about putting in money. It also showed the importance of consistent achievement' (quoted in Burton, 2015). The practice and reporting of council performance was flawed, imperfect and gave licence for gaming, but it also provided opportunities for showing how local government mattered to the world and how individuals, teams and public service organisations could make a difference to the social conditions of their citizens.

On reflection, the effort that the government and its army of public audit, inspection and regulators made was at least a symbol of respect, an acknowledgement of the essential interdependence of local and central governance around key outcomes (Midwinter and Mair, 1987); that what local government did had meaning. Yes, the Audit Commission was high-handed. Yes, the inspectors could be cloth-eared to local needs. But however much the abolition of external review was framed as a compliment, it may have turned out to be no more than sarcastic flattery.

To put it another way, perhaps local government collectively did not sufficiently appreciate Isaiah Berlin's distinction between two concepts of freedom, negative and positive (Berlin, 1969). One interpretation might be that they grabbed at the chance of what Berlin calls negative freedom, which is the absence of (or freedom from) externalities without enough thought about what this might mean for positive freedom, the ability to (or the freedom to) act in the way one chooses. They chose localism over interdependence.

Recently, a number of significant figures in local government have begun to call for the reinvention of national system comparison and what we would see as an attempt at helping the sector towards a new national meaning. Rob Whiteman, the chief executive of the Chartered Institute of Public Finance and Accountancy, has proclaimed the 'failure of self-regulation'.

Donna Hall, until recently chief executive of Wigan Metropolitan Borough Council, made an explicit call to bring back the Audit Commission and a revised version of its Comprehensive Performance Assessment (CPA): 'Although the CPA process was much maligned by some colleagues at the time, I thought it was a useful whole-system approach which is not in place systematically across the UK now. Data could be compared across every council in the land through their relative performance overviews. This helped drive up aspirations and provide rich learning for everyone. ... We need something which rigorously challenges us and compares us collectively as providers of integrated, high quality, easy-to-access services, supportive employers in the locality, as civic leaders, community champions and authentic leaders of place' (Hall, 2018).

One way of understanding these interventions, and others like them, is alarm at the way in which local government has retreated from its historical position as the front line of defence against social evils. Local government has accepted a need to adapt to changing central government whims, but has never achieved strategic reforms that would have enhanced its constitutional position and protection. On the contrary, it welcomed with open arms the diminishments of localism and retrenchment.

While local government's resilience and ability to adapt to new administrative demands is a feature of its survival (Bennett and Orr, 2013; John, 2014), its embrace of ironic localism and freedom from external review have surely been false moves. Instead of finding new powers in their liberation, local government has become downgraded and isolated. UK governance is based on a series of interdependencies – involving localities, regions, central departments and agencies, not to speak of devolved national governments and supranational partnerships. This has been demonstrated once again by the UK response to COVID-19. National and local government, as well as public, private and voluntary sectors have worked together. Local government has performed exceptionally well shielding the vulnerable in their communities, working across boundaries with the NHS and others.

Yet these inter-relationships, these mutual dependencies also show that sovereignty is not complete in any of these domains, but is shared and based on complex and evolving partnerships. These partnerships can be contested and involve grey areas, but by seeking to become 'free' from central government, local government has become divorced from its partners in governance. Milan Kundera describes to us in *The Unbearable Lightness of Being*, 'The absolute absence of burden causes man to be lighter than air … his movements as free as they are insignificant.' Local authorities in England fought so long to shed their burdens that they ended up losing their responsibilities too. Regulation was a burden, for sure, but carrying that burden brought meaning. Councils were being measured because they were thought to matter. The central state depended on local government and recognised their mutual dependence – not least in the areas of public health and creating good social conditions. Over the last decade, deregulation, austerity and an unwillingness to accept the trade-offs of being a part of national governance has ushered in freedom but also dawning insignificance.

Dedicated to Colin Mair, 1952–2019

References

Accounts Commission (2014) 'Community planning: turning ambition into action', Edinburgh: Audit Scotland.

Accounts Commission (2020) 'Scotland's city region and growth deals', Edinburgh: Audit Scotland.

Allen, G. (2010) 'Recession and recovery', in Key Issues for the New Parliament 2010, House of Commons Library Research, London.

Amin-Smith, N. and Phillips, D. (2019) 'English council funding: what's happened and what's next?', London: Institute for Fiscal Studies.

Bennett, M., Fairley, J. and McAteer, M. (2002) 'Devolution in Scotland: the impact on local government', York: Joseph Rowntree Foundation.

Bennett, M. and Orr, K. (2013) 'Ironic Localism and a Critical History of English "Reform"', in G. Sansom and P. McKinlay (eds) *New Century Local Government: Commonwealth Perspectives*, London: Commonwealth Secretariat, pp 74–86.

Berlin, I. (1969) 'Two concepts of liberty', Berlin's inaugural lecture as Chichele Professor of Political and Social Theory at Oxford University. Available from: http://berlin.wolf.ox.ac.uk/published_works/tcl/tcl-a.pdf [Accessed 5 May 2020].

Bichard, M. (2010) 'Total place: a whole area approach to public services', London: HM Treasury.

Bonner, A. (ed) (2018) *Social Determinants of Health: An Interdisciplinary Perspective on Social Inequality and Wellbeing*, Bristol: Policy Press.

Bryant, J.H. and Rhodes, P. (2019) 'Public health', *Encyclopaedia Britannica*. Available from: https://www.britannica.com/topic/public-health/National-developments-in-the-18th-and-19th-centuries [Accessed 10 July 2019].

Burton, M. (2015) 'The sector "needs its own OBR" – interview with Sir Michael Lyons', *The MJ* (30 March). Available from: https://www.themj.co.uk/The-sector-needs-its--own-OBR/200160 [Accessed 10 July 2019].

Byatt, I. and Lyons, M. (2001) 'Role of external review in improving performance', Public Services Productivity Panel, HM Treasury.

Cattan, S., Conti, G., Farquharson, C. and Ginja, R. (2019) 'The health effects of Sure Start', London: Institute for Fiscal Studies.

Dahlgren, G. and Whitehead, M. (1991) *Policies and Strategies to Promote Social Equity in Health*, Stockholm: Institute for Futures Studies.

DfE (Department for Education) (2019) 'Characteristics of children in need in England, 2018–19', London: DfE. Available online at: https://www.gov.uk/government/statistics/characteristics-of-children-in-need- 2018-to-2019

Fielding, J.E. (1999) 'Public health in the twentieth century: advances and challenges', *Annual Review of Public Health*, 20(1): xiii–xxx.

Ford, M. (2018) 'Local government hits out at Dawes', *The MJ* (26 November). Available from: https://www.themj.co.uk/Local-government-hits-out-at-Dawes/212387 [Accessed 13 April 2020].

Gorsky, M., Lock, K. and Hogarth, S. (2014) 'Public health and English local government: historical perspectives on the impact of "returning home"', *Journal of Public Health*, 36(4) (1 December): 546–51.

Grace, C. (2005) 'Change and improvement in audit and inspection: a strategic approach for the twenty-first century', *Local Government Studies*, 31(5): 575–96.

Gray, S., Pilkington, P., Pencheon, D. and Jewell, T. (2006) 'Public health in the UK: success or failure?', *Journal of the Royal Society of Medicine*, 99(3): 107–11.

Hall, D. (2018) 'Let's bring back the audit commission', *The MJ* (28 March). Available from: https://www.themj.co.uk/Donna-Hall-Lets-bring-back-the-Audit-Commission/210548 [Accessed 10 July 2019].

Harris, J. (2009) '"Social evils" and "social problems" in Britain, 1904–2008', York: Joseph Rowntree Foundation.

John, P. (2014) 'The great survivor: the persistence and resilience of English local government', *Local Government Studies*, 40(5): 687–704.

Kelly, E., Lee, T., Sibieta, L. and Waters, T. (2018) 'Public spending on children in England: 2000 to 2020', London: Institute for Fiscal Studies, Children's Commissioner for England.

Kotter, J. (2012) 'Accelerate', *Harvard Business Review*. Available from: https://hbr.org/2012/11/accelerate [Accessed 13 April 2020].

Laming, H. (2009) 'The protection of children in England: a progress report by Lord Laming, 2009', HC 330, London: The Stationery Office.

LGA (Local Government Association) (2019) *Councils Can*, London: Local Government Association.

Longfield, A. (2018) 'Foreword', in 'Public spending on children in England: 2000 to 2020', pp 2–3, London: Institute for Fiscal Studies, Children's Commissioner for England.

Lyons, M. (2007) 'Lyons Inquiry, Final Report and Recommendations', London: HM Treasury.

Mair, C. and Bennett, M. (1998) Beyond DLOs: best value, competition and outsourcing in Scottish local government: report to Scottish ministers, Glasgow: Scottish Local Authorities Management Centre, University of Strathclyde.

Mair, C. and Bennett, M. (2001) Towards joint objectives: proposals for a future planning system in Scottish local government finance: report to Scottish ministers, Glasgow: Scottish Local Authorities Management Centre, University of Strathclyde.

Marmot, M. (2010a) 'Fair society, healthy lives', The Marmot Review, Institute of Health Equity. Available from: http://www.instituteofhealthequity.org/resources-reports/fair-society-healthy-lives-the-marmot-review [Accessed 8 April 2020].

Marmot, M. (2010b) 'Foreword', in F. Campbell (ed) *The Social Determinants of Health and the Role of Local Government*, London: Local Government Association, p 4.

Midwinter, A. and Mair C. (1987) *Rates Reform: Issues, Arguments & Evidence*, Edinburgh Mainstream.

Neville, J. (2012) 'Explaining local authority choices on public hospital provision in the 1930s: a public policy hypothesis', *Medical History*, 56(1): 48–71.

ONS (Office for National Statistics) (2003) 'Health statistics quarterly – no. 18', Summer. Twentieth Century Mortality Trends in England and Wales, London: Office for National Statistics.

ONS (Office for National Statistics) (2017) 'Causes of death over 100 years', London: Office for National Statistics.

Orr, K. and Bennett, M. (2017) 'Relational leadership, storytelling and narratives: practices of local government chief executives', *Public Administration Review*, 77(4): 515–27.

Rowlands, J. and Statham, J. (2009) 'Numbers of children looked after in England: a historical analysis', *Child and Family Social Work*, 14: 79–89.

Travers, T. (2018) 'Funding combined authorities and city regions' in British Academy (ed) *Governing England: Devolution and Funding*, pp 63–71, London: British Academy.

19

Devolution and the health of Scottish housing policy

Isobel Anderson

Introduction: housing in the Scottish parliament

Following the 1997 referendum, Scotland has had its own parliament since July 1999. The Scotland Act 1998, which established the parliament, specified those matters that would remain reserved powers of the United Kingdom (UK) Parliament, and devolved all remaining matters to the new Scottish Parliament. Housing, health, social care, education, most local authority services and civil law were fully devolved to the Scottish Parliament. The UK Parliament retained powers in the areas of employment, social security (including housing benefit) and migration, as well as on the common market for UK goods and services, consumer protection, and vehicle licensing. The UK's asymmetric model of devolution complicates comparison across its jurisdictions. The devolved powers of the Scottish Parliament are more substantial than those of the Welsh and Northern Ireland Assemblies, while Westminster retained authority over all matters for England (albeit with some devolution to the London Assembly and other combined authorities, such as Greater Manchester).

In 2019, the Scottish Parliament celebrated 20 years of operation and local authorities celebrated the 100th anniversary of the landmark Addison Act of 1919, which precipitated the expansion of council housing up to the 1980s. Just over half of the Scottish population lived in council or public housing by 1980, but the latter decades of the 20th century saw significant decline in the local authority landlord role across the UK, through sales to sitting tenants and lack of new investment (Stephens et al, 2019, p 111, Table 17b). Growth in the independent housing association (now registered social landlord) sector through stock transfers and new investment did not prevent the overall decline of the social rented sector continuing into the 21st century. Housing has, however, been a key area where the Scottish Parliament has delivered a distinct agenda from the rest of the UK, largely through local authorities and their partners.

Home and housing represent a key sphere in which local authorities can contribute to the health and wellbeing of their residents (Dahlgren and Whitehead, 1991), including the most marginalised groups in society. Scottish local authorities have strategic responsibility for assessing housing need and planning housing provision across all tenures, and all but six of Scotland's 32 local authorities remain council housing landlords. Prior to devolution, Scotland had some policy autonomy and Scots Law has long been distinct from the rest of the UK. Nonetheless, devolution represented a step change in the capacity of the Scottish policy community to shape its own destiny. The next two sections review key developments in housing policy under the devolved administrations led first by the Labour/Liberal Democrat coalition and then by the Scottish National Party. Implementation of housing policy remains heavily dependent on local authorities and their partners. The chapter then presents evidence from three examples of local housing as a social determinant of health in Scotland: the core benefits of moving from precarious to settled housing; meeting the housing needs of disabled people; and housing-led community regeneration. Conclusions are then drawn about the achievements of, and challenges for, housing and health in devolved Scotland.

The Labour/Liberal Democrat coalition (1999–2007)

The first two terms of the Scottish Parliament saw the electoral system of proportional representation deliver a Labour/Liberal Democrat Coalition government. UK New Labour politics were influential in some areas such as antisocial behaviour (Anderson, 2011), but the new Scottish Parliament also gave its members the opportunity to develop bespoke housing policy.

The first major housing policy review document in the post-1999 period was the 2000 White Paper *Housing: Better Homes for Scotland's Communities* (Scottish Executive, 2000). The policy ideas from this review fed into the Housing (Scotland) Act 2001, a wide-ranging Act that remains influential for housing practice in Scotland. It enhanced the local authority strategic housing role, including through reforms to the repair and improvement grants system for private housing, action on fuel poverty and an emphasis on promoting equal opportunities in housing. The Act abolished the non-departmental public body Scottish Homes, replacing it with Communities Scotland (itself subsequently abolished and replaced by the Scottish Housing Regulator), and introduced a single regulatory framework for registered social landlords (Housing Associations) and local authority landlords, facilitating important change in the social rented sector and local authority homelessness duties.

Social rented housing

The tenancy regime in Scotland changed through the introduction of Scottish Secure Tenancy for council and housing association tenants by the Housing (Scotland) Act 2001. Importantly, housing association and cooperative tenants transferred from 'assured tenancies', which had less security of tenure, to having the same rights as council tenants. Arguably, the 2001 Act underpinned the use of the umbrella term 'social' housing to embrace both local authority and housing association rented tenancies in Scotland. It introduced new responsibilities on landlords for tenant participation and enacted the first reforms to moderate the long-standing 'Right to Buy', which allowed social housing tenants to purchase their home at discount. The coalition restricted this right for new tenants in the social rented sector.

Legislative change was paralleled by the encouragement of local authorities to transfer their stock out of public ownership in order to take advantage of more favourable investment conditions through the New Housing Partnership initiative (Taylor, 2004; Kearns and Lawson, 2008; McKee, 2009). By the end of this period, only six local authorities had completed whole stock transfers. In some key areas (for example, Edinburgh City Council), tenants voted to remain as local authority tenants. Consequently, Scotland has not seen the degree of local authority stock transfer experienced in England although dwellings had been transferred from other public bodies, such as Scottish Homes and former New Towns (Taylor, 2004). Despite recognition of the importance of social rented housing, the sector declined as a proportion of overall housing stock from 32 per cent to 23 per cent during this period (Berry, 2019), and less new investment was achieved than had been anticipated. Notwithstanding the Scottish Parliament's 'creation' of a single social rented sector, council tenants themselves placed their faith in a continuing role for local authorities as housing providers, alongside the independent housing association sector.

Homelessness policy review

Perhaps of greatest significance in this period was the work of the Scottish Parliament's Homelessness Task Force (HTF). The key social determinants of homelessness lie in poverty and disadvantage, which contribute to housing exclusion, often exacerbated by adverse childhood and life experiences and exclusion from employment and health care (Bramley and Fitzpatrick, 2017). Since 1977, taking action on homelessness had been a significant responsibility of local authorities across the UK. Existing legislation placed a duty on local housing authorities to secure housing if a household was homeless according to the legal definition, was in a recognised 'priority need' group, had not become homeless intentionally and had a connection with the local authority where assistance was being sought (for example, through prior residence, family or work). This long-standing framework was selected for early review by the Scottish Parliament.

The HTF was set up in 1999 with wide housing sector representation and chaired by the Housing Minister. It commissioned research, heard evidence and spoke to homeless people in a variety of contexts, producing interim and final reports and recommendations (Homelessness Task Force, 2000, 2002) that had wide sector support and ready acceptance by government. Recommendations of the first report (Homelessness Task Force, 2000), which were incorporated into the Housing (Scotland) Act 2001, included the introduction of new local authority duties to produce a homelessness strategy (subsequently incorporated into local housing strategies), to ensure free homelessness advice services and to provide temporary accommodation to all homeless households while their applications are being assessed (typically for 28 days). Where there was a duty to secure long-term housing, this should result in a secure tenancy (subsequently amended in 2012, by the Scottish National Party (SNP) government to include a minimum 12-month short assured tenancy in the private rented sector) and the 2001 Act also introduced a provision for local authorities to refer homeless households for rehousing by registered social landlords (Section 5 referrals).

The final report (Homelessness Task Force, 2002) proposed a series of wide-ranging multi-agency measures to prevent homelessness and strengthen the legislative framework. Notably, the Homelessness etc. (Scotland) Act 2003 provided for the gradual abolition of the differential treatment of households according to whether they were considered to have 'priority need' or not, over a ten-year period. In effect, all homeless people would have equal priority, widely acknowledged as introducing a legal 'right to housing' (Anderson, 2012; Anderson and Serpa, 2013). Implementation of the 2003 Act was planned over a ten-year period with the abolition of the priority need distinction largely achieved by the target date of 31 December

2012 (Anderson and Serpa, 2013). The Coalition lost power before the end of the implementation phase, but the subsequent SNP government continued to implement the Act.

The rights-based approach to housing adopted by the Homelessness Task Force was widely seen as leading homelessness practice internationally (Anderson, 2012; Anderson and Serpa, 2013). While aspects of policy review could be characterised as rational policymaking (Simon, 1959; Hogwood and Gunn, 1984), implementation by local authorities was not without some conflict; for example, the increasing proportion of lettings to homeless households and increased time spent in temporary accommodation as the safety net widened (Anderson and Serpa, 2013). Although commitment to abolishing the test of priority need was sustained, local-level resistance to other proposals to abolish tests of intentionality and local connection meant that these recommendations were not fully implemented by the end of 2012 (Anderson, 2019).

Private housing sector review

The Labour/Liberal Democrat Coalition also began to review quality and conditions in private sector housing. Measures in the Housing (Scotland) Act 2006 included raising the Tolerable Standard for private housing stock and reforming local authority powers to deal with disrepair (UK Legislation, 2006). Changes to licensing of Houses in Multiple Occupation were introduced and the basic repair and maintenance requirement for private landlords (the Repairing Standard) was enhanced. The 2006 Act also introduced a Private Rented Housing Panel as an alternative to the main court system for housing disputes, and created a framework for the regulation of private tenancy deposits (subsequently introduced in 2011). More radical review and reform of privately rented housing would not be undertaken until prioritised by the subsequent SNP governments.

The Scottish National Party era (2007–20)

From 2007, Scotland saw greater political divergence from Westminster as the SNP achieved a minority government (2007–11) followed by a majority government (2011–16) and then a further minority administration from 2016, supported by the Green Party in Scotland (Aiton et al, 2016). During the same period, the 2010 UK elections saw a Conservative/Liberal Democrat government in power at Westminster, with a very different policy agenda to New

Labour – especially on welfare and public services. Following the 'No' vote in the September 2014 referendum on Scottish independence, Scotland remained part of the UK. The 2015 General Election saw a Conservative government with a slim majority, but with an unprecedented 56 SNP Scottish MPs at Westminster. When Britain voted to leave the European Union in 2016, Scotland voted firmly to remain. The subsequent 2017 Westminster election resulted in a minority Conservative government (and a reduced SNP presence at Westminster), culminating in a change of Conservative party leader and prime minister in the summer of 2019, with a decisive Conservative majority government returned in the ensuing December 2019 election. The Labour Party's representation in Scotland (in the Scottish, Westminster and European parliaments) had declined very significantly after 2007, and a similar trend became apparent in England in December 2019. By comparison, in the 2017 Scottish local government elections, none of the main political parties achieved overall control of any Scottish local authorities (BBC, 2019).

A key contextual change in the policy landscape for the incoming SNP government in 2007/8 was the impact of the general financial crisis, and ensuing austerity measures implemented by the Westminster government. The 2012 Welfare Reform Act applied across the whole of the UK, impacting negatively on the poorest groups in society (Beatty and Fothergill, 2018). The SNP government used its devolved powers to mitigate the clawback of housing benefit for notional under-occupation (the 'Bedroom Tax'), but a parallel freeze on council tax increases undoubtedly squeezed local authority service provision. That said, housing remained an important area for policy and for government investment (Anderson, 2019).

The 2007 consultation paper *Firm Foundations: The Future of Housing in Scotland* emphasised building more houses across all tenures with a target to increase new construction to 35,000 houses per annum by 2015 (Scottish Government, 2007, p 1). The ministerial statement also emphasised helping first-time buyers, prudential borrowing by local authorities to build homes to rent (Scottish Government, 2007, p 2) and ending the Right to Buy for new dwellings, with the aim of safeguarding new public housing for the benefit of current and future tenants. The public body Communities Scotland was to be abolished, with its investment and development functions incorporated into central government, and its regulation functions transferred to a new Scottish Housing Regulator.

Social rented housing

The Housing (Scotland) Act, 2010, addressed two key areas of housing policy: reform of the Right to Buy and the modernisation of housing regulation (UK Legislation, 2010). Regulatory reform resulted in 'lighter touch' regulation of registered social landlords and local authority housing and homelessness services, but with the parallel creation of a Scottish Social Housing Charter with performance targets. The reform of the Right to Buy legislation, to preserve the remaining social rented housing stock, is a key example of where Scottish housing policy diverged from England. The 2010 Act ended the Right to Buy for tenants moving into *new supply social housing* and for *new tenants* entering social housing. The Right to Buy was fully abolished in Scotland from 1 August 2016, through further review in the Housing (Scotland) Act 2014. The devolution period from 1999 to 2018 saw around 136,000 sales to tenants, but only 82,400 new social housing units constructed (Berry, 2019). Wales subsequently also abolished the Right to Buy, but it remained in place in England and Northern Ireland. The localism agenda of the Conservative/Liberal Democrat UK government, which introduced fixed term social tenancies, characterised as 'ambulance service housing' in England by Fitzpatrick and Pawson (2014), was never adopted in Scotland, and the proportion of households in social rented housing remained reasonably constant from 2007 until 2019 (Berry, 2019).

Homelessness and homelessness prevention

The SNP government largely continued implementation of the Homelessness etc. (Scotland) Act 2003, albeit with a parallel emphasis on homelessness prevention (Scottish Government, 2009; Christie, 2011). Homelessness prevention policy did not result in legislative change but was influential on the practice of local authorities, for example through the Housing Options approach (Scottish Government, 2016) of examining all available housing options for those seeking help from local authorities, including those at risk of homelessness. National policy development was seen to shift local outcomes without further legal change (Anderson and Serpa, 2013, p 31). The Housing (Scotland) Act 2010 introduced a duty to provide housing support for homeless households and important pre-eviction action requirements for social housing rent arrears cases, strengthening protection from eviction for Scottish social housing tenants.

Anderson and Serpa (2013) noted the impact of austerity on homelessness policy implementation. The post-2008 effects on mortgage finance, pressures in the home ownership and construction sectors, and constraints on budgets for welfare and investment in new social housing all contributed to increasing the pressure on local housing authorities as they sought to expand their homelessness services to include previously excluded groups. While Scotland retained a slightly larger social rented sector than the rest of the UK, a substantial decline in vacancies over the implementation period suggested the risk of losing social housing as an effective solution to homelessness should not be ignored. As Scotland passed the 2012/13 milestone, evidence indicated success in abolishing the priority need test, but continuing challenges in providing settled accommodation for homeless households (Anderson and Serpa, 2013, p 34; Mackie and Thomas, 2014).

By 2016, it was clear that homelessness policy in the devolved period had not ended street homelessness in Scotland or solved the most acute experiences of those with complex health and social care needs (Macías Balda, 2016). The Scottish Government's own analysis indicated that the ground to be gained from prevention was achieved relatively quickly, while the underlying causes of homelessness had changed little (Anderson et al, 2016). By 2017, the Scottish Government had constituted a new multi-agency Homelessness and Rough Sleeping Action Group, and the Convention of Scottish Local Authorities and Scottish Government (COSLA and Scottish Government, 2018) 'Ending Homelessness Together' action plan marked a renewed drive to tackle acute homelessness through rapid rehousing strategies and the Housing First approach, which provided intensive support in ordinary housing settings (Johnsen, 2013; Quilgars and Pleace, 2016; Anderson, 2019).

Private housing sector review

Though less directly relevant to the local authority role, the SNP government's review of private rented housing (Robertson and Young, 2018) had the potential to contribute significantly to improved wellbeing of tenants in this growing sector. The Private Housing (Tenancies) (Scotland) Act 2016 replaced assured and short assured tenancies in Scotland's private rented sector with a single Private Residential Tenancy, for all new tenancies from 1 December 2017 (UK Legislation, 2016). The new model provided considerably more security for tenants and also aimed to ensure appropriate safeguards for landlords, lenders and investors. The reform effectively ended 'no fault eviction' in Scotland's private rented sector – a proposal that was being debated in England during 2019.

Going local: housing interventions to enhance health and wellbeing

Despite the challenges of proving cause and effect, links to health benefits can be identified across the raft of policy changes on housing and homelessness since Devolution. Housing remains an important social determinant of health (Marmot, 2010) and a significant tool for local authorities to tackle health and wellbeing inequalities. Garnham and Rolfe (2019a) found a positive relationship between being well-housed and being well, while experiences such as homelessness or other housing problems had negative health effects. While poverty and inequality were also important contributing factors, evidence reviewed by Garnham and Rolfe (2019a) was reasonably clear that poor physical housing quality was bad for both physical and mental health (Marsh et al, 2000; WHO Europe, 2007; Fisk et al, 2010; Braubach et al, 2011; Thomson et al, 2013; Liddell and Guiney, 2015). This was also the case in relation to homelessness, particularly the most acute experiences such as rough sleeping (Anderson and Barclay, 2003; Muñoz et al, 2005; O'Connell, 2005; Wolf et al, 2016). Evidence was less clear on whether different tenures were better or worse for health, although insecurity of tenure appeared to negatively affect mental and physical health (Jelleyman and Spencer, 2008; Downing, 2016), and some research suggested that housing that feels like 'home' can generate psycho-social benefits (Kearns et al, 2000; Hiscock et al, 2001; Garnham and Rolfe, 2019a). This section presents research evidence of the contribution of Scottish local housing interventions to enhancing the health and wellbeing of marginalised groups: benefits of a secure tenancy, accessible housing for disabled people and housing-led community regeneration.

A sense of home: moving from precarious to settled housing

Garnham and Rolfe (2019a) examined the ways in which moving into settled housing impacted on the physical and mental health of less advantaged groups. The three-year study focused on housing provided through three 'social enterprises' (registered social landlord, private landlord and tenancy deposit scheme). Although no local authority landlord was included, the data was mainly collected within one local authority area, and the findings have applicability to the local authority sector in terms of identifying factors that help establish a sense of home for new tenants. The study tracked the experiences of more than 70 new tenants at three points over the first year in their new homes, and their self-rated health and wellbeing generally improved in all three housing organisations. Improvements were particularly notable when tenants had a positive relationship with their housing provider, their property was of high quality and their rating of their neighbourhood was positive (Garnham and Rolfe, 2019a, p 13). The fundamental affordability of rents remained important in sustaining settled housing, often supported by further financial help from the landlord, for example with welfare benefits, utilities and the management of any arrears. Positive landlord–tenant relationships can be supported by tenants being able to work with one key staff member who understands their individual situation (Garnham and Rolfe, 2019b). Ensuring high-quality repair and maintenance (especially when moving in) supports tenants in making their property feel like a home. Importantly, choice in the neighbourhood for new tenants helps them feel safe and develop a sense of belonging in their home and community.

The research demonstrated that strategic approaches to housing need to be centred on tenants' stability and security in their home, empowering and prioritising tenants to achieve sustainable tenancies (Garnham and Rolfe, 2019b). The potential contribution of housing as a social determinant of health should also be embedded in public health policy and practice, but the difference that quality housing makes in moving from precarity to a settled home is perhaps best expressed by a participant in the Garnham and Rolfe (2019a) study:

> I mean, it's mental to have your own place, and having somewhere to stay … But I mean, I've changed, eh, I've changed. Because likes of, when you come out of addictions, you know, and you're trying to get into recovery, having your own place is like, it's a vital part of your recovery, you know. So I've changed, with the way I look at the flat … I have more gratitude for it, you know. And I'm really quite lucky to have a flat like this, and I think of all the positive stuff. (p 35)

Accessible housing for disabled people

Local authorities and their partners also have a key role in providing accessible and adapted affordable housing to meet the needs of those with disabling impairments. Research conducted in three Scottish local authorities examined lettings practice for accessible and adapted social rented housing and tracked the experiences of 28 disabled home seekers and new tenants over a one-year period (Anderson et al, 2019a). Importantly, this study identified a key shift in local authority lettings practice towards a social (rather than medical) model of disability. However, there remained some distance between the needs and aspirations of disabled home seekers and the capacity of local authorities and their partners to meet those needs. The research revealed the extent to which disabled people's extended lived experience of inappropriate housing, while waiting for a more accessible home, caused considerable physical and mental harm, as in Tina's case (p 45):

> Tina stays in a 3-bedroom semi-detached house with her two sons, aged in their twenties, who have autism. They have lived in a private rental property for seven years. However, Tina requires wheelchair accessible accommodation and is struggling to use the stairlift currently installed. Her youngest son has experienced anti-social behaviour in the area and Tina feels that a social tenancy would provide greater security and stronger rights for any repairs to be carried out since their current private rented property has dampness, and other safety issues that require attention. As Tina explained:
>
>> I'd feel more secure in a Housing Association or Council house because you don't want the phone to go and our landlord wants his house back. And all of a sudden you become homeless and there's a rush to move. The anxiety of having perhaps 2 months to move, I'd feel more secure.

The process of applying for housing remained complex and confusing for applicants, and only two home seeker participants received offers of a suitable home to meet their needs during the tracking period (Anderson et al, 2019a, p 76). However, where local authorities were able to achieve creative solutions to resolving complex cases, the benefits to health and wellbeing could be transformative:

> A family staying in a private let, two-storey house had a child who had an assessed need for an adapted property.

The mum had been carrying the child up and down the stairs but as the child was getting older (9 years old) this was becoming more difficult. A solution was found when a two-bedroom bungalow was allocated to them with the agreement that the council would build an extension in order to make the property a three-bed home. The bungalow was already adapted with a wet floor shower.

> it is about knowing who is on the list and who is in the most need and then thinking how could we help …
> It is about thinking outside the box and we are reliant upon housing officers doing that. (Local Authority, quoted in Anderson et al, 2019a: 57).

Movers and tenants outlined the emotional and social benefits of moving to an adapted/accessible property. Among the Movers, Dougie was happy to be next door to a good friend who provided financial guardianship and social support. Sam declared that, 'I can do the dishes now' and was looking forward to cooking, moving unaided around the house − and enjoying rediscovering her relationship with her husband as stress reduced and he had fewer caring tasks. Jess was enjoying a sense of community since she is able to get out, meet neighbours and participate in local activities. (p 86)

The 'Match Me' study identified a number of ways in which local authorities could further improve lettings practice (Anderson et al, 2019a, pp 90–1). These included establishing co-production groups to involve disabled people in policy reviews; canvassing beyond their own housing registers where no immediate match emerges; and making better use of new technology to improve intelligence on stock and to enable remote viewings for applicants who are unable to visit in person. Local authorities should also consider widening needs assessment criteria for disabled applicants, for example by including access to a garden and neighbourhood features such as public transport links and access to a doctor and other services.

Housing led community regeneration

The health and wellbeing benefits of housing-led investment in poor neighbourhoods are well established and further demonstrated by evaluation of community transformation in the Broomhill area of Greenock, in Inverclyde (Anderson et al, 2019b). As Inverclyde Council had transferred its housing stock, the regeneration was led by River Clyde Homes Housing Association, in partnership with the local authority and the local tenants and residents association. Prior to regeneration, the area was perceived as blighted by deteriorated housing stock, high vacancy rates and a range of social issues, including crime, antisocial behaviour and drug/alcohol-related behaviours. A programme of more than £20 million of regeneration improvements was undertaken during 2014–18. Evaluation drew on analysis of available policy documents and outcome data, as well as qualitative discussion groups and interviews with around 40 staff, tenants and partner stakeholders.

The extensive programme of housing refurbishment brought all stock up to the Scottish Housing Quality Standard and Energy Efficiency Standard for Social Housing. Housing improvement underpinned a substantial and visible transformation of the neighbourhood, significantly enhancing the quality of living for residents and contributing to improved wellbeing and financial inclusion. While improved housing quality underpinned the Broomhill regeneration project, the broader aims for neighbourhood regeneration included more resident involvement, sustainable employment, improving health, reducing drug and alcohol misuse, and reducing crime and antisocial behaviour (River Clyde Homes, 2017).

By the end of the regeneration, the estate was virtually fully occupied, with clear demand for the refurbished homes. Evidence suggested regeneration had contributed significantly to revitalising community identity and a sense of belonging for residents. Feelings of wellbeing and safety were enhanced and there was a strong sense that crime and antisocial behaviour had reduced. Resident involvement was recognised as contributing significantly to the delivery of the regeneration. Participants identified a growing sense of pride in the neighbourhood and a feeling that local life was improving. One long-term resident summarised changing perceptions as:

> and of course, people used to say 'are you moving to Broomhill?' But now it's ... they say to me there's people trying to get into here now. (Resident, Anderson, et al, 2019b, p 32)

Conclusion

This chapter has presented key milestones that indicate where devolved Scottish housing policy has diverged from the rest of the UK in the post-devolution era, along with evidence of housing's positive contribution to health and wellbeing, which can be achieved at local authority level. While much has been achieved, many challenges remain, notably in relation to reserved Westminster powers such as social security, which impact significantly on the Scottish housing sector but could not be discussed in greater detail in this chapter.

The initial Labour/Liberal Democrat administration could be characterised as undertaking a 'blank sheet', rational policymaking approach (Simon, 1959; Hogwood and Gunn, 1984), but was also influenced by New Labour evidence-based policy (Nutley et al, 2007) and partnership working (Glendinning et al, 2002). Policymaking in the SNP-led period was more incremental (Lindblom, 1959) in relation to social rented housing and homelessness – but led the way on reform of private renting. The later period also saw more dissonance from Westminster, for example with the abolition of the Right to Buy and resistance to the 'bedroom tax'. Policymakers increasingly recognised housing as a social determinant of health and highlighted the critical links between health, housing and homelessness (Hetherington and Hamlet, 2015, 2018; Tweed, 2017), but particular challenges remain in relation to homelessness and health and the commissioning of specialist services to support those with complex needs (Parkes et al, 2019).

To an extent, housing policy outcomes may be explained by a degree of path dependency (Bengtsson and Ruonavaara, 2010; Anderson et al, 2016), even within the devolved framework. After the general financial crisis of 2007/8, national housing policy was found to demonstrate a degree of resilience (Anderson et al, 2016). Despite austerity measures, recorded homelessness in Scotland declined during 2010–15, at least partly explained by homelessness prevention activities (Anderson et al, 2016). However, the impact of prevention was already slowing by 2015, housebuilding was well below its 2007 peak and social housing completions fell by 44 per cent during 2010–14, increasing pressure within the housing system (Anderson et al, 2016). Berry (2019) has also reviewed 20 years of devolved housing policy in Scotland. The population had grown by 13 per cent and was ageing significantly. Owner occupation had remained proportionately stable while the private rented sector saw growth and the social rented sector had declined. House prices rose in the early 2000s, but the impact of the global financial crisis was that 'prices stalled rather than collapsed' (Berry, 2019), although sales volumes and new private housebuilding remained below the peaks of the early–mid-2000s. Berry acknowledged that investment had improved the condition of council and housing association housing, while private rented sector tenancy reform in Scotland represented a more radical change than in other UK countries. Despite these outcomes, Berry (2019, p 1), also observed that:

> During the first debate on homelessness in September 1999, the Minister talked about the government's ambition to end rough sleeping. Fast forward almost 20 years to the most recent debate on homelessness in November 2018. The Minister spoke of his plans to, yes you've guessed it, end rough sleeping.

Devolved housing in Scotland has provided important examples of innovatory approaches that have shaped health and wellbeing, often coordinated by local authorities in partnership with the third sector, community organisations and the private sector. New thinking on housing is still required. Housing must remain a top priority for promoting health and wellbeing, as well as being recognised as a human right. Housing policy needs to deliver secure, affordable housing for those in need, recognising the importance of home and community as well as housing quality. One hundred years after the Addison Act, which provided for council housing across the UK and 40 years after the introduction of the Right to Buy, which heralded decades of decline in social rented housing, local authorities remain the core agency for housing needs assessment, planning and coordination of policy delivery. The 2020s commenced with the shattering global COVID-19 pandemic, which had a highly uneven impact across age, race and social class groups (McKee et al, 2020). While media attention understandably focused on healthcare responses, frontline housing and homelessness services also reacted urgently to protect tenancies and communities, and to support roofless people in emergency accommodation. Documenting their contribution will be a future research priority. As they emerge from the COVID-19 crisis, the ensuing economic and social impact will demand further creative responses from local authorities. They will retain a crucial role in delivering the health benefits from sustainable homes and communities throughout the 21st century, albeit with different methods from those used in the 20th century.

References

Aiton, A., Burnside, R., Campbell, A., Edwards, T., Liddell, G., McIver, I. and McQuillen, A. (2016) *SPICe Briefing Election 2016*, 11 May, 16/34. Edinburgh: Scottish Parliament Information Centre (SPICe).

Anderson, I. (2011) 'Evidence, policy and guidance for practice: a critical reflection on the case of social housing landlords and antisocial behaviour in Scotland', *Evidence and Policy*, 7(1): 41–58.

Anderson I. (2012) 'Policies to Address Homelessness: Rights-Based Approaches', in S.J. Smith, M. Elsinga, L. Fox O'Mahony, Ong Seow Eng, S. Wachter and S. Fitzpatrick (eds), *International Encyclopedia of Housing and Home*, vol. 5, pp 249–54, Oxford: Elsevier.

Anderson, I. (2019) 'Delivering the right to housing? Why Scotland still needs an ending homelessness action plan', *European Journal of Homelessness*, 13(2): 131–59.

Anderson, I. and Barclay, A. (2003) 'Housing and health', in A. Watterson (ed) *Public Health in Practice*, pp 158–83, London: Palgrave.

Anderson, I., Dyb, E. and Finnerty, J. (2016) 'The "arc of prosperity" revisited: homelessness policy change in north western Europe', *Social Inclusion*, 4(4): 108–24.

Anderson, I. and Serpa, R. (2013) 'The right to settled accommodation for homeless people in Scotland: a triumph of rational policy making?', *European Journal of Homelessness*, 7(1): 13–39.

Anderson, I., Theakstone, D., Lawrence, J. and Pemble, C. (2019a) *Match Me: What Works for Adapted Social Housing Lettings? Action Research to Enhance Independent Living for Disabled People*. Edinburgh: Housing Options Scotland.

Anderson, I., Tokarczyk, T. and O'Shea, C. (2019b) *Transforming Broomhill: Community Regeneration Evaluation*, Home, Housing and Communities Research Programme, University of Stirling.

BBC (2019) 'Scotland local elections 2017' (8 July). Available from: https://www.bbc.co.uk/news/topics/c50znx8v8m4t/scotland-local-elections-2017 [Accessed February 2020].

Beatty, C. and Fothergill, S. (2018) 'Welfare reform in the UK 2010–16: expectations, outcomes and local impacts', *Social Policy and Administration*, 52(5): 950–68.

Bengtsson, B. and Ruonavaara, H. (2010) 'Introduction to a special issue on path dependence in housing', *Housing, Theory and Society*, 27(3): 193–203.

Berry, K. (2019) *Scotland's Changing Housing Landscape*, Edinburgh: SPICe (Scottish Parliament Information Centre). Available from: https://spice-spotlight.scot/2019/05/15/scotlands-changing-housing-landscape/ [Accessed February 2020].

Bramley, G. and Fitzpatrick, S. (2017) 'Homelessness in the UK: who is most at risk?', *Housing Studies*, 33(1): 96–116. Available from: https://doi.org/10.1080/02673037.2017.1344957 [Accessed February 2020].

Braubach, M., Jacobs, D. and Ormandy, D. (2011) *Environmental Burden of Disease Associated with Inadequate Housing*, Copenhagen: WHO Europe.

Christie, C. (2011) *Commission on the Future of Public Services*, Edinburgh: Public Services Commissioner.

COSLA (Convention of Scottish Local Authorities) and Scottish Government (2018) *Ending Homelessness Together – Action Plan*, Edinburgh: Scottish Government.

Dahlgren, G. and Whitehead, M. (1991) *Policies and Strategies to Promote Social Equity in Health*, Stockholm: Institute for Futures Studies.

Downing, J. (2016) 'The health effects of the foreclosure crisis and unaffordable housing: A systematic review and explanation of evidence', *Social Science and Medicine*, 162: 88–96.

Fisk, W., Eliseeva, E. and Mendell, M. (2010) 'Association of residential dampness and mold with respiratory tract infections and bronchitis: A meta-analysis', *Environmental Health: A Global Access Science Source* 9(1): article 72.

Fitzpatrick, S. and Pawson, H. (2014) 'Ending security of tenure for social renters: transitioning to "ambulance service" social housing?', *Housing Studies*, 29(5): 597–615.

Garnham, L. and Rolfe, S. (2019a) *Housing as a Social Determinant of Health: Evidence from the Housing through Social Enterprise Study.* University of Stirling and Glasgow Centre for Population Health. Available from: https://www.gcph.co.uk/assets/0000/7295/Housing_through_social_enterprise_WEB.pdf [Accessed February 2020].

Garnham, L. and Rolfe, S. (2019b) *Housing through Social Enterprise Recommendations.* University of Stirling and Glasgow Centre for Population Health. Available from: https://www.gcph.co.uk/assets/0000/7367/HTSE_recommendations.pdf [Accessed February 2020].

Glendinning, C., Powell, M. and Rummery, K. (eds) (2002) *Partnerships, New Labour and the Governance of Welfare*, Bristol: Policy Press.

Hetherington, K. and Hamlet, N. (2015) *Restoring the Public Health Response to Homelessness in Scotland*, Scottish Public Health Network.

Hetherington, K. and Hamlet, N. (2018) 'Health and homelessness', in A.B. Bonner (ed) *Social Determinants of Health: An Interdisciplinary Perspective on Social Inequality and Wellbeing*, pp 195–210, Bristol: Policy Press.

Hiscock, R., Kearns, A., MacIntyre, S. and Ellaway, A. (2001) 'Ontological security and psycho-social benefits from the home: qualitative evidence on issues of tenure', *Housing, Theory and Society*, 18(1–2): 50–66.

Hogwood, B. and Gunn, L. (1984) *Policy Analysis for the Real World*, Oxford: Oxford University Press.

Homelessness Task Force (2000) *Helping Homeless People: Legislative Proposals on Homelessness*. Edinburgh: Scottish Executive.

Homelessness Task Force (2002) *An Action Plan for Prevention and Effective Response*. Homelessness Task Force final report. Edinburgh: Scottish Executive.

Jelleyman, T. and Spencer, N. (2008) 'Residential mobility in childhood and health outcomes: a systematic review', *Journal of Epidemiology and Community Health*, 62(7): 584–92.

Johnsen, S. (2013) *Turning Point Scotland's Housing First Project Evaluation*. Final Report. School of the Built Environment, Heriot-Watt University.

Kearns, A., Hiscock, R., Ellaway, A. and Macintyre, S. (2000) '"Beyond four walls". The psycho-social benefits of home: evidence from west central Scotland', *Housing Studies*, 15(3): 387–410.

Kearns, A. and Lawson, L. (2008) 'Housing stock transfer in Glasgow – the first five years: a study of policy implementation', *Housing Studies*, 23(6): 857–78.

Liddell, C. and Guiney, C. (2015) 'Living in a cold and damp home: frameworks for understanding impacts on mental well-being', *Public Health*, 129(3): 191–9.

Lindblom, C. (1959) 'The science of muddling through', *Public Administration Review*, 19(2): 78–88.

Macías Balda, M. (2016) 'Complex needs or simplistic approaches? Homelessness services and people with complex needs in Edinburgh', *Social Inclusion*, 4(4): 28–38.

Mackie, P. and Thomas, I. (2014) *Single Homelessness in Scotland*, London: Crisis.

Marmot, M. (2010) 'Fair society, healthy lives', The Marmot Review, Institute of Health Equity. Available from: http://www.instituteofhealthequity.org/resources-reports/fair-society-healthy-lives-the-marmot-review [Accessed 8 April 2020].

Marsh, A., Gordon, D., Heslop, P. and Pantazis, C. (2000) 'Housing deprivation and health: a longitudinal analysis', *Housing Studies*, 15(3): 411–28.

McKee, K. (2009) 'Learning lessons from stock transfer: the challenges in delivering second stage transfer in Glasgow', *People, Place & Policy*, 3(1): 16–27.

McKee, K., Pearce, A. and Leahy, S. (2020) 'The unequal impact of Covid-19 on Black, Asian, Minority Ethnic and Refugee Communities', UK Collaborative Centre for Housing Evidence, Blog post, 6 May. Available from: https://housingevidence.ac.uk/the-unequal-impact-of-covid-19-on-black-asian-minority-ethnic-and-refugee-communities [Accessed 8 May 2020].

Muñoz, M., Crespo, M. and Perez-Santos, E. (2005) 'Homelessness effects on men's and women's health', *International Journal of Mental Health*, 34(2): 47–61.

Nutley, S., Walter, I. and Davies, H. (2007) *Using Evidence: How Research Can Inform Public Services*, Bristol: Policy Press.

O'Connell, J. (2005) *Premature Mortality in Homeless Populations: A Review of the Literature*, Nashville, TN: National Healthcare for the Homeless Council.

Parkes, T., Cuthill, F., Carver, H., Fotopoulou, M., Anderson, I., Wallace, J., Liddell, D., Budd, J., Johnsen, S., Doyle, E. and Burley, A. (2019) 'Homelessness, health and harm reduction', University of Stirling, Salvation Army Centre for Addiction Services and Research.

Quilgars, D. and Pleace, N. (2016) 'Housing first and social integration: a realistic aim?', *Social Inclusion*, 4(4): 5–15.

River Clyde Homes (2017) 'Getting it right for Broomhill governance group: aims and outcomes 2017–2020', River Clyde Homes.

Robertson, D. and Young, G. (2018) *An Evaluation of Rent Regulation Measures within Scotland's Private Rented Sector. A Report to Shelter Scotland*, Edinburgh: Shelter Scotland.

Scottish Executive (2000) *Housing: Better Homes for Scotland's Communities*, Edinburgh: Scottish Executive.

Scottish Government (2007) *Firm Foundations: The Future of Housing in Scotland*, Edinburgh: Scottish Government.

Scottish Government (2009) *Homelessness Prevention Guidance*, Edinburgh: Scottish Government.

Scottish Government (2016) *Guidance on Housing Options*, Edinburgh: Scottish Government. Available from: http://www.gov.scot/Resource/0049/00494940.pdf [Accessed February 2020].

Simon, H. (1959) 'Theories of decision-making in economics and behavioural science', *American Economic Review*, 49(3): 253–83.

Stephens, M., Perry, J., Wilcox, S., Williams, P. and Young, G. (eds) (2019) *UK Housing Review 2019*, Coventry: Chartered Institute of Housing.

Taylor, M. (2004) 'Policy emergence: learning lessons from stock transfer', in D. Sim (ed) *Housing and Public Policy in Post-Devolution Scotland*, Coventry: Chartered Institute of Housing, pp 126–47.

Thomson, H., Thomas, S., Sellstrom, E. and Petticrew, M. (2013) 'Housing improvements for health and associated socio-economic outcomes', *Cochrane Database of Systematic Reviews*, 2. Available from: https://www.ncbi.nlm.nih.gov/pubmed/23450585 [Accessed 14 April 2020].

Tweed, E. (2017) 'Foundations for well-being: reconnecting public health and housing. A practical guide to improving health and reducing inequalities', Scottish Public Health Network (ScotPHN).

UK Legislation (2006) Housing (Scotland) Act 2006. Available from: http://www.legislation.gov.uk/asp/2006/1/contents [Accessed February 2020].

UK Legislation (2010) Housing (Scotland) Act 2010. Available from: http://www.legislation.gov.uk/asp/2010/17/contents/enacted [Accessed February 2020].

UK Legislation (2016) Private Housing (Tenancies) (Scotland) Act 2016. Available from: http://www.legislation.gov.uk/asp/2016/19/contents/enacted [Accessed February 2020].

WHO (World Health Organization) Europe (2007) *Large Analysis and Review of European Housing and Health Status (LARES): Preliminary Overview*, Copenhagen: WHO Europe.

Wolf, J., Anderson, I., van den Dries, L. and Filipovic-Hrast, M. (2016) 'Homeless women and health', in P. Maycock and J. Bretherton (eds) *Women's Homelessness in Europe: A Reader*, London: Palgrave, pp 155–78.

20

Public health and local government in Wales: every policy a health policy – a collaborative agenda

Catherine Farrell, Jennifer Law and Steve Thomas

Introduction

This chapter focuses on public health in Wales and the context within which it is delivered. As a devolved service, health policy and the wider public policy legislative framework are the responsibility of the devolved Welsh Government tasked under the Government of Wales Act 2006 with developing and implementing policy, exercising executive functions and making subordinate legislation. Focusing on public health, part two of the chapter outlines the organisations involved and the context of the policy in Wales. It also explores the political drive for more collaboration between different organisations as a mechanism for the delivery of better services. Part three examines a unique piece of legislation in Wales, the Well-Being of Future Generations Act 2015 (WFG Act), and identifies how this may influence the work of local authorities and other organisations in relation to health and its social determinants. In part four, we draw on the available evidence on how this is working so far and focus on two key policy areas jointly driven by the Cymru Well Wales partnership – 'Adverse Childhood Experiences' (ACEs) and 'The first 1,000 days'. Finally, our conclusions indicate that regardless of where public health is located, the policy context in Wales is quite different, and the key issue is whether this will lead to improved public health outcomes for everyone in Wales.

Public health in Wales

The onset of devolution of health services across the United Kingdom (UK) has seen significant divergence through an asymmetric process where distinctive national characteristics of public services delivery have emerged (Bevan et al, 2014). Prior to this, as McClelland

(2002, p 325) states, the National Health Service (NHS) in Wales was perceived as 'forming an adjunct to the English health service'. Since 1999, legislative and policy frameworks have been viewed by the predominantly Welsh Labour-led devolved governments as a mechanism to assert political demarcation from Westminster. This was famously encapsulated in the term 'clear red water' set out in a speech delivered by the First Minister Rhodri Morgan in December 2002 (Morgan, 2017). While this philosophy was originally constructed in differentiating Welsh Labour from the marketisation strategies of New Labour in London, it grew in contextual importance. Osmond has argued that in the first decade of devolution it was the 'one really distinctive political philosophy [that] has really stuck in the public mind' (Osmond, 2010, p 1).

The Welsh NHS has consequently been conditioned by policies that firmly locate it in the orbit of a social democratic framework. Policies ending the quasi-market system in health, general practitioner (GP) fundholding, free prescriptions and eye tests, and the abolition of car park charges at hospitals were the visible manifestations of this. They were captured by the term 'progressive universalism', in essence a commitment to the breadth of universal services, but with additional provision for those most in need (Drakeford, 2007).

From the outset of devolution, there has been a strong emphasis on public health. Moon (2012) argues that the Welsh government pursued a public health agenda, rather than focusing on cutting waiting lists. Underpinning this, cross-sectoral partnerships and collaboration with local government have been regarded as the vehicle to tackle the determinants of ill health. In 2001, the National Assembly for Wales published 'Improving Health in Wales – A plan for the NHS with its Partners' (NAFW, 2001). In a long foreword to the document, Jane Hutt, the Minister for Health and Social Services, drew upon a concurrent review by the sociologist Professor Peter Townsend when she argued that health improvement and a reduction in health inequalities must determine strategy and resources (Townsend, 2002). In particular, this recognised Wales's industrial past, particularly within the South Wales valleys where the rate of long-term limiting illnesses is much higher than in many areas of the UK and linked to the decline of traditional industries in coal and steel (Michael, 2008). A seminal report from Derek Wanless that cogently addressed this point followed in 2003, arguing that 'a step-change in individuals' and communities' acceptance of responsibility for their health is needed' and recognising 'that securing better health cannot be accomplished by the state or by the health service, acting alone' (Wanless, 2003, p 61).

This explicit focus on public health, prevention and working in collaboration as the driver of Welsh health policy indicates a distinctiveness from England, and also heralded a sweeping reorganisation of delivery structures. As Greer (2016, p 19) contends:

> Welsh health policy was more radical, with an explicit effort to de-emphasize health care, particularly targets and shibboleths like waiting times, and refocus on intersectoral work for public health. It included a reorganization that produced 22 Local Health Boards coterminous with local government responsible for primary care and commissioning.

The creation of a single National Public Health Service (NPHS) in April 2003, which was hosted by an NHS trust, came about as a result of this reorganisation. Its ambitious vision to 'drive health improvement and wellbeing in Wales to that of the best in Europe' was to be achieved by seeking collaborative advantage through close working with local authorities and others to improve the health and wellbeing of the population (NPHS, 2004). However, the long-term focus of these 'localist' reforms soon hit political turbulence and expediency.

The abolition of the existing five strategic health authorities and the alignment with 22 councils was the core structural reform, but this was not only vigorously contested by Welsh opposition political parties but also within the secondary care sector. Problems of scale and the issue of critical mass of specialist services dominated this narrative (*Western Mail*, 2008). An increasingly acrimonious debate developed in Cardiff Bay and within Westminster, and Jane Hutt was replaced as a Minister in January 2005. In addition, escalating problems surrounding waiting list times, and delayed transfers of care meant that the 'localist' approach lasted barely five years. In 2009, a new Minister for Health and Social Care, Edwina Hart, called time on the reforms, with a new structure for the NHS being introduced, this time based on a unification of the planning and delivery functions of primary, secondary and tertiary care on a geographical basis in seven local health boards (LHBs) (Longley, 2013).

While the Health and Social Care Act 2012 led public health in England to move significant responsibility and resource to local government within a framework of local democratic accountability, this has not happened in Wales. A drawn out and failed process of local government reform in Wales during the 2010s effectively crowded out any discussion on additional powers for councils (WLGA, 2014). As a result, the 2009 health reorganisation effectively settled the issue of the location of public health in Wales, with solidification of a centrally based organisation responsible to the devolved Welsh Government. There were nevertheless local government-specific public health interventions, such as the GP exercise referral scheme, linked to local authority leisure facilities, and more latterly, the establishment of a National Autism Service, both within the Welsh Local Government Association (WLGA).

The NPHS evolved into Public Health Wales (PHW) as a separate trust with seven Directors of Public Health based in the LHBs. Each of these seven local health boards has a staff of public health experts who commission and deliver services in that area. In resource terms, this has meant that because of the relative protection of NHS funding in Wales, the public health function has not suffered the scale of cuts experienced by counterparts within English councils (Luchinskaya et al, 2017). The result has also seen a renewed focus on partnership working with local government through the establishment of public services boards (PSBs) across Wales, set within an innovative policy backdrop framed by the WFG Act. In Wales, these policies contribute to the 'health in all policies' approach, with health impact assessments mandatory as a result of the Public Health (Wales) Act 2017 and a focus on shared outcomes through the Public Health Outcomes Framework.

The WFG Act is the overarching legislative driver for public service change in Wales. As in the rest of the UK, public services in Wales have historically been delivered by a range of different organisations, each with their own responsibility for that particular area. Each service has its 'silos', whether these be professional groups, their own buildings, their own staff with different working conditions or separate funding streams, and a particular issue has been a lack of integration between each of these (Beecham, 2006). The need for more integrated joined-up working is a huge challenge, and this is not unique in Wales. The paradigm of 'new public governance' has highlighted the need for systems leadership where public sector alliances across organisational boundaries will create 'collaborative advantage' and by implication, deliver better outcomes for service users (Osborne, 2010). Despite a government agenda in Wales of collaboration in a range of different services, evidence up to the passing of the WFG Act suggests that there had not been sufficient collaboration across organisations in service planning or delivery (Williams, 2014). In this critical review of public services in Wales, while many examples of good practice are identified, the evidence indicates that organisations and services continue to operate within their own traditional areas and there is an unwillingness to let go of some responsibilities. This seems to confirm key research findings, which argue that 'collaborations are inherently paradoxical, characterised by tensions and contradictions, and that they are notoriously challenging to manage. Rather than yielding collaborative advantage, many end up in a state of inertia' (Vangan et al, 2017, p 7).

In relation to public health, partnership working is recognised as crucial. Taylor-Robinson et al (2012, p 1) argue that 'partnership working is widely advocated in order to implement strategies to influence the wider determinants of health and health inequalities, and thus secure population health improvement'. Partnership arrangements are frequently put forward in 'recognition that no single agency can possibly embrace all the elements that go to contribute to a policy problem or its solution' (Hunter et al, 2010). It has been argued that effective public health provision in the UK needs to be characterised by this type of strategic partnering, and this reflects the closer working between health organisations and local government over the last 15 years (Taylor-Robinson et al, 2012). The key finding from this study is that respondents were positive about this model of working and recognised that this approach is more likely to influence the health agenda and also impact on inequalities in health. In Wales, a cornerstone of the drive towards greater collaboration is the WFG Act, which sets this agenda within a legislative framework, and it is to this piece of legislation that the chapter now moves.

The Well-Being of Future Generations Act

The WFG Act has the potential to lead to significant changes in the way that local authorities and other organisations work, perhaps especially in complex and interconnected policy areas such as public health. It is an ambitious piece of legislation that seeks to introduce a new way of working in Wales – one that is based on the principle of sustainable development. This is defined as 'the process of improving the economic, social, environmental and cultural well-being of Wales by taking action, in accordance with the sustainable development principle, aimed at achieving the well-being goals' (Welsh Government, 2016, p 5). It states also that sustainable development means that public bodies 'must act in a manner which seeks to ensure that the needs of the present are met without compromising the ability of future generations to meet their own needs'. The Act came into force in 2016, and it is intended to lead to significant changes in the ways that organisations conceptualise, plan and deliver services. It applies to the Welsh Government, health boards, local authorities, fire and rescue authorities, and Natural Resources Wales, as well as to bodies such as the Sports Council and Public Health Wales. It has also been fully embraced by non-devolved services including the police as a core theme in preventative and collaborative work (FGCW, 2018a).

The Act encourages a wider responsibility for health beyond health boards and Public Health Wales. It does this partly through the introduction of a wellbeing duty on public organisations and a shared set of national wellbeing goals to which they must all seek to contribute. These shared wellbeing goals are a prosperous Wales, a resilient Wales, a healthier Wales, a more equal Wales, a Wales of cohesive communities, a Wales of vibrant culture and thriving Welsh language, and a globally responsible Wales. All public bodies must demonstrate how they can maximise their contribution to all seven goals by setting out objectives, publishing these and presenting their performance against them in an annual report. It also encourages a focus on understanding the wider social determinants of health as the guidance draws attention to the interconnected nature of the seven goals and the need for this to be recognised. For example, the objective of 'a more equal Wales' highlights the fact that organisations should be looking beyond aspects of equality such as race, gender and disability to incorporate issues such as socio-economic disadvantage.

Adhering to the broad principle of sustainable development, the WFG Act requires organisations to follow five ways of working. These are:

- Long term – the importance of balancing short-term needs with the need to safeguard the ability to also meet long-term needs;
- Prevention – how acting to prevent problems occurring or getting worse may help public bodies meet their objectives;
- Integration – considering how one organisation's wellbeing objectives may impact on each of the wellbeing goals or on the objectives of other public bodies;
- Collaboration – services and organisations acting in collaboration with each other;
- Involvement – the importance of involving people with an interest in achieving the wellbeing goals and ensuring that those people reflect the diversity of the area that the body serves.

Reflecting the need for greater collaboration and integration in public service delivery, the Act encourages this through the establishment of statutory PSBs, based largely on local authority boundaries, which are made up of the local authority, the health board, Natural Resources Wales and the fire and rescue service, plus other invited organisations including the police where this responsibility is not devolved. These boards are required to operate a system of local integrated planning by assessing the state of wellbeing in the local area, setting out objectives in a Local Well-Being Plan and taking all reasonable steps to meet those objectives. The key issue here is that there is now a statutory body in place to promote a collaborative, integrated, locally focused service agenda. Whilst these bodies are 'virtual', PSBs provide a new governance structure to enable a more joined-up and integrated way of working across different organisations to helping to resolve some of the key issues and problems in our society. Many of these focus on aspects of health and include issues within the wider health agenda, including loneliness, for example. Integration of public health issues in these boards is supported by the fact that the representative of the health board on the PSB is usually the Director of Public Health.

The WFG Act ensures accountability through a Future Generations Commissioner as well as the Auditor General for Wales. The commissioner acts as a guardian of the interests of future generations and provides support and guidance to public bodies in meeting their wellbeing objectives. She provides advice and challenge, conduct reviews and make recommendations to public bodies, which are obliged to respond publicly to these; and has outlined her expectations that the Act will encourage a new way of working, moving away from traditional 'silos' and short-term approaches (FGCW, 2017). There is a need for organisations to look for the root causes of problems, and to work jointly on solving these (FGCW, 2018b). The commissioner provides advice to the PSBs on their objectives, and many PSBs have focused on issues such as ACEs and alternative models for improving health and wellbeing, such as social prescribing, which the commissioner highlighted as some of her priorities in her term of office (FGCW, 2018c). There is also a role for the Auditor General for Wales in auditing the extent to which public bodies have acted in accordance with the sustainable development principle in setting their objectives and in meeting them.

Public Health Wales has argued that the WFG Act presents 'key opportunities to work differently across different sectors and with communities – to address the increasing health, social and economic challenges in a more effective and sustainable way' (Public Health Wales, 2016, p 3). Further, operating within the context of systems working, its focus is 'to improve the public's health, i.e. taking a whole systems approach which aligns public policies, financial flows and accountability with local public, private and third sector delivery and shared outcomes. A collaborative approach with an emphasis on prevention and public health will address the current and future health, social and economic challenges in Wales' (Public Health Wales, 2016, p 12). An additional component of the new ways of working is the 'sign up' of public and third sector organisations to the Academi Wales One Welsh Public Service values, which emphasise the need for all public bodies in Wales to put citizens first, work for the long term and work together; these values sit alongside the WFG Act wellbeing goals (Academi Wales, 2018). The idea is that if all organisations have these values central to their activity, it will lead to a more joined-up public service delivery for the citizens of Wales.

How well is it working? The evidence to date

A key driver for joined-up, collaborative and integrated public services in Wales has been put in place by the WFG Act and the wider context of the One Welsh Public Service values framework. This section of the chapter now moves on to present some of the evidence that shows the impact of this new way of working on public health. As the legislation only took effect in 2016, with the first wellbeing assessments put in place in April 2017, it is still quite early to consider the impact of this new policy environment. However, an examination of these wellbeing assessments put forward by the PSBs shows that many focused on health within the wider context. For example, 'by the time Torfaen children reach reception class in school, factors associated with where they live are already affecting their weight, health and well-being' (FGCW, 2017, p 11). All of the assessments highlight obesity as a key issue, and the need to promote both healthier eating and solutions that are not medically based, such as exercise and local activities, including clubs. For example, the Cardiff assessment indicates that 'food poverty means not being able to afford or access food for a healthy diet. It is not just about quantity, it is also about having physical access to shops that sell healthy foods and the social issues which affect which foods are eaten' (FGCW, 2017, p 6). One of the conclusions of this review was that while these first assessments were valuable, 'further work should be undertaken to provide a deeper understanding of people's lived experiences through gathering and using far more of the information that partner organisations hold about people's wellbeing as well as making use of the "day-to-day intelligence" that is gathered on the ground in communities by a range of services' (FGCW, 2017, p 50).

In 2018, the Auditor General for Wales undertook a review of the ways in which public bodies had responded to the WFG Act. Overall, this report indicates that the vast majority of respondents indicated that the Act provided an 'opportunity' to their organisation rather than a 'distraction' in terms of their service. Furthermore, many intended to use the legislation to 'transform' services in ways, including 'we will use the Act to help us address some of the major challenges facing our organisation' (WAO, 2018, p 14). The conclusion of the review indicates that 'it will take time for public bodies to fully apply the principles of the Act. The Wales Audit Office welcomes honest self-reflection on progress … Over the medium to long term, the WAO will expect public bodies to be able to demonstrate how the Act is shaping what they do' (WAO, 2018, p 25).

An early assessment of the wellbeing objective setting and reporting by public bodies indicates that many individual public bodies are also including health and health-related objectives in their wellbeing plans: '99 objectives set by 38 public bodies relate to health, social care, social prescribing, safeguarding and ageing well' (FGCW, 2018d). However, it also suggests that there is some way to go before the policy works effectively; in the first year of operation, 'few have shown how they have considered if their services currently contribute to the seven national well-being goals' (FGCW, 2018c, p 15). The commissioner has also stated that there is a need to dig deeper to gain a richer understanding of the wider social, economic, cultural and environmental factors that contribute to wellbeing. To date, there is limited evidence to date on the impact of the WFG Act on public health and outcomes for the people of Wales. This evidence base will grow over the coming years as the Act beds in and studies emerge of its impact. The Act itself provides the framework for new ways of working to be developed and a governance structure for services and organisations to come together.

In addition to the evidence given here, there are other initiatives that have been driven by joint work between the Welsh Local Government Association and Public Health Wales through their establishment of Cymru Well Wales. This is described as a 'movement of motivated organisations that are committed to working together today to secure better health for the people of Wales tomorrow'. It seeks to take a 'whole system approach' and has three initial priorities: 'Adverse Childhood Experiences', 'The first 1,000 days' and 'Employability'. This section presents details of the first two of these priorities.

Vignette 1: Adverse Childhood Experiences

ACEs are regarded as traumatic experiences in childhood that are remembered and have an impact on future life. These include neglect, abuse, family breakdown and exposure to domestic violence or living in a household where there are problems of substance misuse and incarceration. This issue has been publicised by Cymru Well Wales, which has published research on ACEs and the impact that they have, as well as strategies to build resilience to these events in order to raise awareness and momentum for action. A number of PSBs and other partnerships are now starting to try and jointly address these issues, and this has been further supported through additional funding of £6.87 million that was won by a partnership of police commissioners in Wales, the four chief constables, Public Health Wales and a range of other organisations from the statutory and voluntary sectors from the Home Office transformation fund. This will focus on both root cause prevention and intervention. In a recent review of one local authority's focus on ACEs, which has the objective to 'work with partners to ensure that we target support to those children at risk of adverse childhood experience in the first 1,000 days of their lives', the Auditor General found that while there are many strengths in what the authority is doing, there are also some areas for improvement. These are: 'the Council needs to collect data so it can: – understand the issues in sufficient detail; – establish what success looks like (based on outcomes); and – know how it is going to measure outcomes'. In addition 'the Council needs to consider how it will evaluate the impact of working with families in a more collaborative way in the short, medium and long term' (WAO, 2019, p 6). While these findings indicate the complexities involved in working together to undermine adverse childhood experiences and capturing the outcomes of these activities, this focus on ACEs means that the joined-up approach to resolving this particular challenge may be successful.

Vignette 2: The first 1,000 days

This collaborative activity focuses on the first 1,000 days of a child's life and seeks to share knowledge and best practice on improving existing service between a range of agencies. The aim is to encourage all services to recognise this timeframe as a priority and to commit to make systems change for reasons associated with the improvement of future health, wellbeing and deep health inequalities that originate from this period of life. The background to this joint initiative is that 'there is often a great deal of activity around the first 1,000 days in any local area but the connections and links between services is very limited. They do not function as a collective system' (Public Health Wales, 2017). In terms of the impact of this joint initiative, there is evidence of a changing service focus. In a recent Public Health Wales report, it is highlighted that 'participation by local partnerships in the First 1,000 Days programme has increased, and 11 of the 19 Public Services Boards in Wales are now actively engaged in the programme. In addition, eight of the 11 are pathfinders in Welsh Government's Early Years Integration Programme, and the First 1,000 Days programme is working closely with the Welsh Government to develop the focus on the first 1,000 days within their Early Years Integration programme' (Public Health Wales, 2019).

Clearly, then, in terms of public health, and public services more generally, the WFG Act is central to the development of collaborative services, and a key part of this is the work of the PSBs. Shifting from existing patterns of service provision to a systems approach will be important. As highlighted by one PSB, 'although there is no new money to support different ways of working, we recognise that in working together and involving our communities, we can be more efficient, provide more focused services, share our assets and have a much bigger impact locally. We will develop radical and innovative ways of working, creating the momentum needed to improve the wellbeing of all in this area' (Cwm Taf, 2018). These examples and evidence highlight that while much rests on PSBs in the planning, commissioning and delivery of new activities, there is no additional money for their activities either from the Welsh government or from each of their component organisations. However, both individual organisations and PSBs clearly recognise the role that they play in terms of health in Wales and share high-level outcomes such as 'a healthier Wales'. Initiatives such as those driven by the Cymru Wales Well partnership initiated by the WLGA and PHW have had success in identifying areas of work such as the first 1,000 days and ACEs, which have been picked up by many organisations. This sense of a shared responsibility for health is enhanced by the need for statutory bodies to do health impact assessments and the general approach in Wales of 'every policy a health policy'.

In relation to local authorities and public health, while authorities are a statutory member of the PSB and effectively administer these bodies, responsibility for public health in Wales rests formally with the NHS. In this sense, local authorities in Wales as democratic bodies have not gained the control of public health that their counterparts in

England have secured. This mirrors a much wider tension in terms of central–local relations in Wales, where it has been argued that

> when it comes to functions, local government has pushed for additional functional areas like public health, elements of primary care and health scrutiny, but all have been effectively ruled out without a debate. Indeed, there is clear evidence of councils losing functions to non-elected bodies. Meanwhile, the local accountability and democratic oversight arrangements in the existing system of centrally appointed Local Health Boards are almost non-existent. (Thomas, 2018, p 4)

Although the issue of where public health should be located is an important one, recent approaches to complex policy areas suggest that it is more important to consider building effective systems. Randle and Anderson (2017) suggest that in order to work effectively, these systems need factors such as a focus on place-based strategies and plans, place-based outcomes, collaborative governance and leading systems rather than organisations. In relation to public health in Wales, the building blocks for effective systems are in place. These include the WFG Act with its focus on outcomes, shared responsibilities, area-based assessments and plans, but also existing relationships and the ability in a small nation to bring relevant individuals and organisations together (Rabey, 2015). The One Welsh Public Service values should also be central to this agenda and shared governance arrangements through the PSBs. At this stage, however, it is too early to say if the presence of these enabling factors will lead to real change in the health of the Welsh population or if organisations will simply be stuck in collaborative inertia.

Conclusion

Health and its wider determinants are of crucial importance in Wales. Life expectancy in Wales is still lower than the average for England, and it has clear health inequalities, as do other parts of the UK. Wales has chosen to deal with these issues in ways that are different to other countries, both in terms of structures and policies, where public health is formally provided through the health service (both the central agency of PHW and directors of public health in local health boards), rather than through local government. The Welsh government has also encouraged a partnership approach with local government as well as other agencies through the PSBs, and has sought to widen responsibility for this policy area; it takes a 'health in all policies approach' with a duty on public organisations to undertake health impact assessments. The WFG Act provides a shared set of national wellbeing goals for all organisations to contribute to, which includes 'a healthier Wales', as well as statutory partnership bodies that must undertake a local wellbeing assessment and plan. Do these differences in structure and policy approaches really matter? Previous research has indicated that health policy divergence in the UK did not lead to matching divergence of performance (Bevan et al, 2014). Early signs in relation to recent policies such as the WFG Act indicate that it has the potential to enable systems change, as the framework for collaborative and joined-up public services are in place to deliver improved public health. It is too early to identify whether this is happening. However, even if it does act in this way, given the number of factors that may contribute to ultimate changes in a population's health, it will be difficult to isolate any one influence on this much desired outcome.

References

Academi Wales (2018) 'One Welsh public service'. Available from: https://academiwales.gov.wales/pages/one-welsh-public-service [Accessed 23 April 2019].

Beecham, J. (2006) *Making the Connections – Delivering Beyond Boundaries, Transforming Public Services in Wales*, Cardiff: Welsh Assembly Government.

Bevan, G., Karanikolos, M., Exley, J., Nolte, E., Connolly, S., and Mays, N. (2014) 'The impacts of asymmetric devolution on health care in the four countries of the UK – research report', Health Foundation and The Nuffield Trust.

Cwm Taf (2018) 'Creating the Cwm Taf we want'. Available from: http://www.ourcwmtaf.wales/SharedFiles/Download.aspx?pageid=286&mid=613&fileid=210. [Accessed 13 April 2020].

Drakeford, M. (2007) 'Social justice in a devolved Wales', *Benefits*, 15(2): 171–8.

FGCW (2017) 'Well-being in Wales: planning today for a better tomorrow – learning from well-being assessments'. Available from: [https://futuregenerations.wales/wpcontent/uploads/2017/07/FGCW_Well-being_in_Wales Planning_today_for_a_better_tomorrow_2017_edit_27082017.pdf1 (Accessed 10 March 2019].

FGCW (2018a) 'Putting ACEs front and centre with the Wellbeing and Future Generations Act'. Available from: http://futuregenerations.wales/news/acesdecember-putting-aces-front-and-centre-with-the-well-being-of-future-generations-act/ [Accessed 12 March 2019].

FGCW (2018b) 'Future generation frameworks for projects'. Available from: https://futuregenerations.wales/wp-content/uploads/2018/11/FGCW-Framework.pdf [Accessed 12 March 2019].

FGCW (2018c) 'The people's platform'. Available from: http://futuregenerations.wales/news/the-peoples-platform/ [Accessed 10 March 2019].

FGCW (2018d) 'Well-being in Wales: the journey so far'. Available from: https://futuregenerations.wales/wp-content/uploads/2018/11/FGCW-1-year-Report-_English.pdf [Accessed 10 March 2019].

Greer, S. (2016) 'Devolution and health in the UK: policy and its lessons since 1998', *British Medical Bulletin*, 118: 17–25.

Hunter, D.J., Perkins, N., Bambra, C., Marks, L. and Hopkins, T. (2010) 'Partnership working and the implications for governance: issues affecting public health partnerships'. Final report. NIHR Service Delivery and Organisation programme.

Longley, M. (2013) 'Wales', in C. Ham, D. Heenan, M. Longley and D. Steel (eds) *Integrated Care in Northern Ireland, Scotland and Wales: Lessons for England*, London: The King's Fund.

Luchinskaya, D., Ogle, J. and Trickey, M. (2017) 'A delicate balance? Health and social care spending in Wales'. Wales Public Services 2025. Available from: http://www.walespublicservices2025.org.uk/files/2017/03/Wales-health-and-social-care-final_amended_04-2017.pdf [Accessed 9 March 2019].

McClelland, S. (2002) 'Health policy in Wales – distinctive or derivative?', *Social Policy and Society*, 1: 325–33.

Michael, P. (2008) 'Public health in Wales (1800–2000) A brief history', Welsh Assembly Government. Paper commissioned by the Chief Medical Officer for Wales to mark the Faculty of Public Health Conference held in Cardiff on 3–5 June . Available from: http://www.wales.nhs.uk/documents/090203historypublichealthen[1].pdf [Accessed 9 March 2019].

Moon, D. (2012) 'Rhetoric and policy learning: on Rhodri Morgan's "clear red water" and "made in Wales" health policies', *Public Policy and Administration*, 28(3): 306–23.

Morgan, R. (2017) *Rhodri: A Political Life in Wales and Westminster*, Cardiff: Cwasg Prifysgol Cymru/University of Wales Press.

NAFW (National Assembly for Wales) (2001) 'Improving health in Wales – A plan for the NHS with its partners', Crown Copyright. Available from: http://www.wales.nhs.uk/publications/NHSStrategydoc.pdf [Accessed 28 March 2019].

NPHS (National Public Health Service Wales) (2004) 'NPHS report on 2003/04', Cardiff: NPHS. Available from: http://www.wales. nhs.uk/sitesplus/documents/888/EXTNPHS0304.pdf [Accessed 30 March 2019].

Osborne, S. (2010) *The New Public Governance – Emerging Perspectives on the Theory and Practice of Public Governance*, London: Routledge.

Osmond, J. (2010) 'Making the "red water" really clear', *Institute for Welsh Affairs* (10 July). Available from: https://www.iwa.wales/ click/2010/07/making-the-%E2%80%98red-water%E2%80%99- really-clear/ [Accessed 9 March 2019].

Public Health Wales (2016) *Making a Difference: Investing in Sustainable Health and Well-being for the People of Wales*, Executive Summary, Cardiff: Public Health Wales.

Public Health Wales (2017) 'Y 1,000 diwrnod cyntaf | First 1,000 Days FTD 24 Ymateb gan: Iechyd Cyhoeddus Cymru, Response from: Public Health Wales', *CYPE*, 5-29-17 – Paper 2. Available from: http://www.senedd.assembly.wales/documents/s67718/CYPE5- 29-17%20-%20Paper%202%20-%20Public%20Health%20Wales%20 -%20Response%20to%20First%201000%20days%20consultation.pdf [Accessed 21 January 2020].

Public Health Wales (2019) 'Working to Achieve a Healthier Future for Wales, Annual Report 18-19'. Available from: https://phw.nhs. wales/files/annual-reports/working-to-achieve-a-healthier-future- for-wales-annual-report-2018-19/ [Accessed 21 January 2020].

Rabey, T. (2015) 'Connection, coherence and capacity: policy making in smaller countries', Public Policy Institute for Wales. Available from: https://sites.cardiff.ac.uk/ppiw/files/2015/10/Connection- coherence-and-capacity_-Policy-making-in-small-countries-final- report-FINAL.pdf [Accessed 15 March 2019].

Randle, A. and Anderson, H. (2017) 'Building collaborative places: infrastructure for system change', Collaborate in association with Lankelly Chase. Available from: http://wordpress.collaboratei.com/ wp-content/uploads/Building-Collaborative-Places_Digital-Report- Pages-2.pdf [Accessed 20 March 2019].

Taylor-Robinson, D.C., Lloyd-Williams, F., Orton, L., Moonan, M. and O'Flaherty, M. (2012) 'Barriers to partnership working in public health: a qualitative study'. *PLOS ONE*, 7(1): e29536. Available from: https://doi.org/10.1371/journal.pone.0029536 [Accessed 18 May 2020].

Thomas, S. (2018) 'Welsh government and Welsh local government – "is this town big enough for the both of us"?' Valedictory Lecture to The Morgan Academy, Swansea. Available from: https://www.swansea.ac.uk/media/Valedictory-Speech-1.pdf [Accessed 21 January 2020].

Townsend, P. (2002) 'Inequalities in health: the Welsh dimension 2002–2005', Welsh Assembly Government. Available from: http://www.healthcarealliances.co.uk/public/documents/Townsend%20final%20report%200512.pdf [accessed 30 March 2019].

Vangan, S., Potter, K. and Jacklin-Jarvis, C. (2017) 'Collaboration and the governance of public services delivery', paper prepared for the Symposium on the Policy and Reform Trajectory of Public Services in the UK and Japan, 8–9 November. Open University Online. Available from: http://oro.open.ac.uk/51742/3/Collaboration%20and%20the%20governance%20of%20public%20services%20delivery%20Vangen%20et%20al%20%281%29.pdf [Accessed 15 May 2020].

WAO (Wales Audit Office) (2018) *Reflecting on Year One: How Have Public Bodies Responded to the Well-Being of Future Generations Act 2015?*, Cardiff: WAO.

WAO (Wales Audit Office) (2019) 'Well-being of future generations: an examination of the step "we will work with partners to ensure that we target support to those children at risk of adverse childhood experiences in the first 1,000 days of their lives"', Neath Port Talbot County Borough Council, audit year: 2018–19. Available from: https://www.audit.wales/system/files/publications/neath_port_talbot_wfg_adverse_childhood_experiences_english.pdf [Accessed 21 January 2020].

Wanless, D. (2003) 'The review of health and social care in Wales', report of the project team, Welsh Assembly Government. Available from: http://www.wales.nhs.uk/documents/wanless-review-e.pdf [Accessed 25 March 2019].

Welsh Government (2016) 'Shared purpose: shared future'. Statutory guidance on the Well-being of Future Generations Act, 2015.

Western Mail (2008). 'NHS managers calling for more change' (30 June).

Williams, P. (2014) *Commission on Public Service Governance and Delivery*, Cardiff: Welsh Government.

WLGA (Welsh Local Government Association) (2014) *In Defence of Localism: Elected Government in Wales and the Impact of Austerity*, Cardiff: WLGA. Available from: https://www.wlga.wales/SharedFiles/Download.aspx?pageid=62&mid=665&fileid=1218 [Accessed 15 March 2019].

21

Steadying the swinging pendulum – how might we accommodate competing approaches to public service delivery?

Nigel Ball

Introduction

As we have seen throughout this book, discourse around the social determinants of health is skewed towards the parts of the population whose adverse social circumstances harm their health the most. Local authorities are much closer to the complexities of service delivery than central government departments, and thus have an instrumental role to play in efforts to support these groups. As we have seen, they do not play this role alone – it is shared with other local delivery agencies, such as Sustainability and Transformation Partnerships in the National Health Service (NHS), as well as private providers and local community groups. There has always been much debate around what role each of these actors should play, and how they might interact with one another so as to create masterful theatre rather than a depressing farce. This question continues to be the focus of much policymaking, experimentation and debate. In this chapter, I will briefly take stock of the current state of thinking, before explaining my own recent attempt to make sense of the cocktail of approaches via the West London Zone for Children and Young People, a cross-sector delivery partnership. I go on to explore some of the intersecting themes across other efforts, drawing on research from the Government Outcomes Lab (where I now work). Finally, I explore the drivers behind the changes in approach that we are starting to see, and suggest some questions that we still need to answer if we are to truly make progress.

What is the problem?

Some of our most difficult work as public servants is serving those parts of the population whose lifestyle or circumstances cause them to interact with multiple aspects of the public services. This means we do not just meet them as they make use of health services, but perhaps housing, social care, employment support, criminal justice or any of a myriad of services that might have an influence on what we term the 'social determinants of health'.

However we choose to characterise this group, there are always people in society who need, and tend to receive, greater levels of support from society at large. In the modern era, we can trace attempts to meet this need on a universal basis to the Tudor poor laws. These had an ignominious provenance as an attempt to protect landowners when labour shortages after the Black Death pushed up prices in the mid-14th century. But by the time the Elizabethan Poor Law was enacted 250 years later in 1601, alms for the poor were funded through taxation.

On the surface, it is not so difficult to make the case for helping people out in hard times – whether they fall into them, are born into them or seem never to escape them. There are both economic and moral imperatives to do so. For this reason, the issues are ever present in the political discourse of the day.

The economic imperatives are well rehearsed. Some people in society exert a greater demand on universal public services than the wider population – for example, they might make more use of the NHS. There are people in society who make life harder for others, victimising them through crime or violence, which creates the need for public policing, courts and rehabilitation. Others need constant care, because they are very young, very old or incapacitated for some reason, which keeps their carers from adding value elsewhere in the economy. In each case, helping these people more effectively in the short term has a good chance of either saving money or raising productivity in the long term. It also tends to make life better for the people themselves – which is where the moral imperative comes in.

Accompanying this long-established political imperative is a wide canon of social reforms intended to achieve the politically desired change. Despite this seemingly endless stream of reform, many who have careers in the public sector are able to recognise some repeating themes. Just as teenaged trouser legs swing from baggy to skinny and the prevailing male chin from smooth to bristled, trends in public service delivery also seem to oscillate between a limited array of approaches. And a little like sartorial fashions, every new (or returning) idea seems to divide opinion into true believers and to-the-death sceptics.

We are at such an inflection point once again. An emerging discourse is turning us away from the marketisation trend in public services over the last few decades, which has seen public services attempting to simultaneously engage with and ape the private sector. Alongside this, recent attempts to apply the scientific experimental method that has worked wonders for testing medicines to social programmes are starting to raise eyebrows. This is despite the government recently opening its eighth What Works centre to 'bring that same transformative approach [from medicine] to other public sector professions.' (Gould, 2018).

Instead, conversation in local areas increasingly revolves around system change and place-based working. But these ideas might not be as novel as some suppose. Neither should we forget that the prior swing towards market-based and evidence-led approaches felt right to many at the time, and to others still does. Many would have agreed · that the post-welfare state public sector came to feel monolithic and lumbering, and decision-making seemed to be based on political or bureaucratic idiosyncrasies rather than facts. Is it that in addressing these issues we have created new ones? Or do our new ideas just never live up to their early promise? Are we really locked inside the public services grandfather clock, tied forever to its eternally swinging pendulum, or is there a way to genuinely move forward? How should a die-hard pragmatist, like me, cut through the noise and decide what approach to take next?

What I tried

Many attempts at reform are born of frustration. In my own case, after a short stint as a teacher in a cut-off corner of Salford, I went into the charity/VCSE sector – initially abroad and then at home. I quickly discovered that the inspiring and energetic desire to help others that typifies the sector was often being undermined by misaligned incentives. This manifested in two ways. First, the personal agency of the people we tried to help was under-utilised – things were 'done for' them more than 'done with' them. Secondly, the potential for organisations to work together to clear the barriers for those people to exercise their agency was under-explored. This led me on a search for a way to fund the work of charitable organisations that better aligned with what mattered for the people they helped, and better enabled them to collaborate with one another. That search led me to join an effort to set up an 'operating system' for the social sector that relied on a more constructive set of incentives, which became the West London Zone for Children and Young People. Put simply, we set out to:

1. understand the unique needs of people in a particular place;
2. get charities to pull in the same direction towards an agreed set of shared outcomes that would meet those unique needs;
3. realign the financial incentives for the charities around those shared outcomes.

Achieving these three deceptively simple steps turned out to be much harder than I expected. It required us to combine a set of existing innovations in radically new ways. But the lessons we learnt are an instructive example of a broader change in practice that we are witnessing up and down the country.

Understanding the unique needs of a particular place

The chosen place was 3 square miles straddling parts of four London boroughs around the Harrow Road. Following many years of research and relationship-building prior to my arrival, our motivating problem was that in this poor part of West London, one in five children were at risk of negative outcomes in adulthood. We concluded that this was 'due to a lack of effective identification of need and a lack of connectivity between professionals and agencies (in the public and social sectors)' (West London Zone, 2016).

Unearthing statistics on 3 square miles of West London that covered part of four boroughs, but the whole of none of them, was hard: most data is collected and shared at borough level. Nor did it help us much. It gave very little insight into the needs of young people in the area beyond high-level (and sadly unsurprising) insights into educational attainment and poverty. But we couldn't fix poverty, and we needed to know why the poor educational outcomes were occurring. What saved us was a remarkable piece of research that the then-named Dartington Social Research Unit (DSRU) had done in Scotland, which surveyed every single child in five local authorities via their school on a wide range of risk factors, including wellbeing, family relationships and drug use (DSRU, 2016). We could not have repeated the feat in England because unlike in Scotland, few schools were still under direct local authority control. But even if we could have, that alone would still not have been enough – we needed to know *which* children were most at risk, not just aggregated patterns of risk. No existing dataset helped – the local authorities knew who was in contact with statutory social care services and early help but couldn't breach privacy and tell us – and besides, our target cohort was wider. We wanted to reach children before their circumstances led them to those services. So we borrowed DSRU's survey, adapted it for our area and went to local schools one by one, asking them to run it with all their children – with the added benefit to them of a set of insights useful to their own decision-making. By combining this quantitative data with qualitative insights from school staff members and local early help teams, we worked out which children we ought to be working with.

This unique mix of rich quantitative and qualitative data, and the computer system sitting behind it, had the added benefit that it enabled us to track progress over time. By repeating the survey and collecting data from schools at least annually, we were able to maintain a relentless focus on outcomes throughout delivery. Importantly, it also set up a long-term relationship between our organisation and local schools, which turned out to be integral to the model.

Getting charities to pull in the same direction towards an agreed set of shared goals that would meet those unique needs

West London is fortunate, and not representative of much of the country, in that it has a rich ecology of local charities. Our starting point in leading a collaboration between them drew from the five principles of collective impact, a much-vaunted collaborative framework imported from the United States (Kania and Kramer, 2011). Our effort as leaders of the collaboration was to be separately incorporated into an independent 'backbone organisation', the existence of which is one of the principles. The other four are a common agenda, shared measurement systems, mutually reinforcing activities and continuous communication. When we first started to sit down with the massed charities of inner West London, we were both surprised and caught out. What surprised us was the level of appetite from the charities for such an initiative – it seemed that most charity leaders, at least in this example, acutely recognised the same shortcomings in the sector as we did, and welcomed an effort to work in a new way.

What caught us out was that we supposed that enacting the collective impact principles alone would be enough: if West London Zone, independent backbone organisation, could get everyone more coordinated, our problem would be solved, we said. But we had underestimated the effect of the current fragmentation on the children and young people we aimed to work with. How would we collectively engage them? How would we collectively maintain their engagement? And how would we collectively liaise with schools and councils to ensure that the joined-up nature of the work extended as far as possible across those realms as well?

These questions led us to adopt a link worker model. After identifying a cohort as described previously, it was up to the link worker to approach the child and family, and sit down with them to jointly work out a package of support from the partnership of charities that suited their strengths and needs. This enabled a personalised form of support that aligned with a broader framework of cross-cutting outcomes that all partners had bought into. Through the link workers, we had a way of balancing the outcomes important to society with those important to the young person. We could also talk to them as much about what they had as what they lacked. Based in the child's school, the link worker would build a relationship over time to ensure continued engagement with the support. We recruited link workers from within the local community as much as possible.

As well as this child-facing role, the link workers would also face outwards to the 'system'. They were a common denominator for both the child and the other adult facilitators across the different types of charitable support provided, and they acted as a single point of liaison for the sector with other professionals in schools and local authorities. It was important that the link workers were operating from within the social sector, which seemed to make it easier to build relationships of trust with children and their families. All this helped to ensure that a link worker did not become 'yet another professional'.

Realign the financial incentives for the charities around those goals

We didn't expect the collaboration to succeed if financial incentives still pulled charities towards different sets of goals, encouraged them to compete and did not allow a narrative to emerge of the whole being greater than the sum of its parts. It was essential to work out how resources flowed around the young people we had identified, how these might be used more efficiently and how success might collectively be demonstrated for the sake of those committing in cash and in kind. For this part, we turned for inspiration towards social impact bonds (SIBs).

The first SIB was famously pioneered in Peterborough prison. In a similar model to ours, a set of charities offering rehabilitation to ex-offenders were coordinated through the One Service. The work of the One Service and its partner charities was financed by investors who only got their money back if offending was reduced relative to a national comparison cohort (Disley et al, 2015). While it was fiendishly complex to set up, we believed that a similar mechanism might help us too to align the flow of money with the end goals collectively desired. By focusing on end outcomes rather than pre-specified activities, we believed it might also unlock the flexibility needed to be truly responsive to the strengths and needs of the children we aimed to help.

The work of West London Zone and its partner charities was ultimately paid for from four sources: local authorities, local schools, local (and sometimes national) individual philanthropists and grant-making bodies, and the National Lottery Community Fund. Each paid on the basis that the collectively agreed outcomes would be achieved – since some of this funding was paid in arrears, a 'social investment' deal of repayable finance plugged the gap. Only because we had a way of arriving at a collective view of need and of delivering joined-up support did these partners agree to provide funding. Schools in particular regarded the support to be good value for money. The required funding, it seemed, existed in the system – but was not used in a joined-up manner. The benefits of this financing model are summed in the charity's recent Collective Impact in Practice report: 'We cannot give up on any child, no matter how challenging the work. We can provide more support than any of these parties could afford on their own. We are not reliant on one source of funding alone' (West London Zone, 2018).

Others who are trying it

West London Zone continues to thrive and is starting to show promising signs of impact. But what is the relevance of a voluntary sector initiative to local authorities? In many ways, it is aligned with the broader shift in thinking that is occurring. Elements of what we were doing in West London are being repeated up and down the country as part of a broader shift to more collaborative approaches. At the Government Outcomes Lab at Oxford University's Blavatnik School of Government, where I now work, we did some work to try to learn more about this shift – both to give more examples of how it works and to identify common themes. This culminated in the 2019 report, 'Are We Rallying Together? Collaborative Approaches to Public Service Reform' (Blundell et al, 2019).

The report looked at ten areas of the country that reported they were working in collaborative ways, and among these identified four different modes of collaboration. West London Zone is an example of a 'systems connector', better aligning and leveraging existing resources to respond to a specified challenge.

A second type was 'agents of change'. Like system connectors, these operate independently from outside a system, but rather than aligning resources, they agitate change by flagging up blockages or weaknesses in the system to its actors, with a particular focus on improving existing front-line practice. For example, in Ignite Coventry, agents worked with a housing provider to reduce the incidence of failed tenancies by changing the way staff interact with clients.

A third type was 'collaborative markets'. These seek to change the prevailing orthodoxy in a locality from one where competition is seen to provide best value, to one where collaboration does. System incentives are realigned to promote joint working. In Plymouth, an 'alliance contract' has been used to procure services from the local provider market jointly. This means there is a single contract between a purchaser and partner organisations with a collective goal, interdependent responsibilities and shared risks and rewards.

The fourth category is 'collaborative councils': 'programmes of change which span the responsibilities of local government' (Blundell et al, 2019). In these:

> collaboration is a mechanism through which the local authority attempts to reform their own way of working and the way residents, central and local government departments, schools, local business and charitable entities, all work together. Collaborative councils see their role as leaders of their wider community and all its constituent parts. Rather than leaders of their own organisation, they see themselves as 'leaders of place'. (Blundell et al, 2019)

Our report looked at how Wigan, Wirral and Oldham were enacting changes in this spirit. But we have come across similar thinking up and down the country: Staffordshire, Essex, Barking and Dagenham, Camden, Sutton, the Greater Manchester Combined Authority, and no doubt many other places, are starting to think in this way.

Across all these different modes of collaboration, we observed some common approaches to leadership, culture, infrastructure and community that enabled the approaches to be ingrained.

Leadership shifted from being about decision-making exerted through traditional hierarchies to the facilitation of relationships. This type of 'collaborative' leadership is quite well understood in the literature. We saw stewards, who listen to partners and create a shared understanding of the issue; mediators, who negotiate differences of opinion and nurture the building of trust; and catalysts, who identify opportunities for new approaches and help mobilise partners to pursue them (Ansell and Gash, 2008).

Culture had to change. Giving front-line staff more decision-making power and freedom to operate came with risks for those staff as well as their managers and organisation leaders. It represented a major change of working culture. Communicating and accepting a shared imperative to work in a different way early on was essential.

Infrastructure had to be put in place. New ways of capturing data and sharing information were needed. Co-location was sometimes identified as a major facilitator, but was not always essential, nor enough on its own. Many sites used new types of meetings to improve communication and relationships between teams, and some provided access to shared digital or computer systems.

Communities were always involved, though in varied ways. Sometimes community members were used as innovators, coming up with ideas that one public sector leader claimed bureaucrats would never think of. Sometimes assets such as libraries and swimming pools were transferred to the community to run – though this came with risks in terms of competencies and maintaining equality of access. Many places tried to change the conversation with citizens from 'what can we do for you?' to 'what can we help you do for yourselves?'

The work we observed was genuinely inspiring, but it left many questions unanswered.

One was about how information was used. There was an overwhelming consensus that ensuring healthy flows of information was invaluable for the sake of learning and decision-making. But despite this consensus on the purpose of sharing information, the type of information captured varied widely. Some places relied on indicators of 'system health', such as staff turnover, absences and sicknesses. Others defined a 'theory of change' and measured outcomes against it. Some relied on individual stories of success and failure, gathered at the front line. And some made promises to the community and tracked the progress being made towards them.

However, a further, deeper, question was raised through the work about how accountability should work. True collaboration rests on equal relationships between partners, underpinned by an empowered and entrusted workforce. So who is in charge? Who sets the level of ambition, measures success and is answerable if things go wrong? Not everyone agreed that there was a role for the information they collected beyond learning – for example, using it to account for the success of their collaborative endeavour.

Answering this question will be critical if the current move towards more collaborative approaches continues to accelerate. At the moment, much store is set by the intuition of those leading these approaches that the status quo is manifestly failing and working together is the only way to cope. When we asked the places in the Rallying Together research why they were working in these new ways, the responses sounded more like articulations of the end goals or perceived effects, rather than the driving forces: a desire to share responsibility, to use the voluntary sector more, to increase impact and value, and to make the public sector a better place to work (Blundell et al, 2019). But is this a genuine step forward to more effective practice or simply a pendulum swing back to a less equitable and accountable system of public service delivery? Are we inadvertently designing a 21st-century version of Victorian patronage, with idiosyncratic decision-making on resource allocation and weak public accountability?

Why this, now?

It is imperative that we make sure that the new approaches we are seeing do not repeat the mistakes of the past. We should seek to maintain the benefits of what came before, and address the shortcomings. To do this, it is worth exploring the social, economic and political drivers of the trend. If we can explain what makes the pendulum swing, perhaps we can do a better job of steadying it. There are multiple possible explanations for the current shift in thinking, which intersect.

Cash-starved councils

One popular explanation says that of course local authorities have turned to their communities for help delivering vital services. Post-austerity, they are starved of cash: councils spent almost 25 per cent less per person in 2017/18 than in 2009/10 (Phillips, 2019), so they look for resources from elsewhere (including non-financial ones). Donna Hall, until recently the Chief Executive of Wigan (seen as a vanguard of the new approach), admits: 'We were honest with residents about the challenge we faced and, with humility, asked for their help in delivering services...' (Hall quoted in Lent and Studdert, 2019).

This explanation suggests citizens will one way or another step into the gap left by the rolling-back of the state – by donating money and time voluntarily. If this is indeed the driver, then citizens will need to adjust to a fundamental shift in the terms of engagement between citizen and state. Donna Hall says that in Wigan they aimed for 'the building of a very different relationship with our residents, their networks and communities' (Hall quoted in Lent and Studdert, 2019).

No longer are we passive recipients of universal public services that we have the right to. Now, citizens and public servants are mutually dependent because each holds mutually important resources (a perspective which has a theoretical underpinning known as 'resource dependence theory'; Pfeffer and Salancik, 1978).

This may not be quite as bad as it sounds – and nor is it completely new. In his book *The Future of Capitalism*, Paul Collier (2018) explores the sense of reciprocal obligations that was essential to the founding of the welfare state. The post-war social contract unlocked the level of taxation that enabled universal public services. While 'rampant individualism' has eroded this in the decades since, Collier believes it must return. 'People enter into reciprocal commitments, the essence of community', which 'can be restored and enhanced by policies that rebalance power' (Collier, 2018, p 19).

Volunteering can help to do this because it can have benefits beyond free labour. Claire Bonham examines this in detail in the predecessor to this book: 'There is evidence to suggest that more diverse, heterogeneous groups have higher levels of trust and cohesion, and thus the work that volunteers do is capable of transforming society through building inclusive communities' (Bonham, 2018, p 131). And Andy Haldane, Chief Economist at the Bank of England, has argued that we should be ready for an almost-doubling of volunteering resource in the coming decades owing to, among other things, the large-scale automation of jobs (Haldane, 2019).

Rising demand

Augmenting the issue of falling budgets, of course, is rising demand – itself an explanation for the shift in thinking. At the simplest level, there is an increase in the overall amount of demand on services, which is most often attributed to natural demographic change, such as an ageing population. But there is another element to the demand increase: needs are becoming more acute owing to increases in poverty. This is probably at least partly attributable to deliberate political decisions, including the introduction of universal credit.

The Institute for Fiscal Studies has shown that reforms to the tax and benefit system since 2010 have reduced incomes for the poorest tenth of households by 10 per cent, compared with less than 1 per cent for the general population (*Economist*, 2018). But there is also an increasingly recognised issue of in-work poverty: figures released by the government in 2019 show that '69 per cent of all children in low income households were in working families' (Department for Work and Pensions, 2019).

Why should an increase in the severity of need drive towards more collaboration? Perhaps because those with severe needs are often (perhaps euphemistically) regarded as 'complex'. But are the people complex or is it the system serving them? Nigel Hewett observed in chapter 19 of the predecessor to this book that 'We often dismiss groups as "hard to reach"; [perhaps] the services, and not the patients, are "hard to reach"' (Hewett, 2018, p 265).

Certainly, our top-down and siloed system of public service delivery seems to have serious limitations. It no longer makes sense to think of education, health, social care and criminal justice in isolation when so many members of the population have interconnected issues that cannot be portioned off in this way. Paul Collier argues that 'dedicated professionals on the front line are trapped in a compartmentalised hierarchy designed for control' (Collier, 2018, p 158). There is a recognition that staff and services within and outside the public sector need to work together to become more preventative and reduce 'failure demand' (when a problem is not solved first time round, and a person bounces around the system from one service to another).

Increased system complexity

Rising demand is exposing the complexity of our public services system, which could be driving the move to collaborate. But it could also be argued that the increasing complexity itself is driving the change, independently of other factors.

A quick examination of the history of public services systems can help us understand where this complexity might have come from. In a recent report, Adam Lent and Jessica Studdert of the New Local Government Network (Lent and Studdert, 2019) delineate four distinct approaches or 'paradigms' over the last century or so. First was the pre-war Victorian 'civic paradigm', which largely relied on charities and patronage to care for those who couldn't afford to care for themselves. Then came the universal welfare state, free for all, administered from the top by bureaucrats. When it was felt this was too big to be efficient, inspiration was taken from market-based approaches, and a purchaser–provider split was imposed on much of the public sector. They propose that the recent change represents a fourth, emerging paradigm, which they call the community paradigm.

A paradigm shift narrative is compelling, but the reality is that the shift is more incremental. In our Rallying Together research, we identified that the move to privatise in the 1980s led to the increased use of third parties to deliver public services. The change in thinking supposed that market forces applied to public service would drive up efficiency and quality. It also vastly increased the number of independent actors involved in the delivery of services, and led to an increasingly dense web of contractual relationships. As an example of the scale of the change, the amount of public spending on voluntary organisations in the UK grew to £15.3 billion in 2014/15 (House of Commons, 2017).

But attempts to deal with this complexity are not brand new. In fact, they could be said to have their root in the emergence of 'commissioning' as a concept. In a 2018 paper, Gary Sturgess acknowledges that commissioning is a contested term, sometimes used to refer to procurement and sometimes strategic planning. But despite the association with outsourcing, he says 'it is widely argued that the concept applies as much to publicly-delivered public services' (Sturgess, 2018, p 156). As far back as 1995, the UK Department of Health defined commissioning as 'a strategic activity of assessing needs, resources and current services, and developing a strategy of how to make the best use of available resources to meet needs' (Sturgess, 2018, p 157). Importantly, the verb 'to commission' implies a delegation of power and authority to complete a task – to set a broad goals and parameters but let the person doing the work figure out how to achieve them – as you might if you commissioned a painting or a building. Indeed, this was why the word was chosen for the application of this concept in public services. Though its meaning has meandered, the idea of devolving decision-making authority sounds remarkably aligned to the new collaborative approaches.

Similarly, the idea that local authorities should take a holistic view of all the resources in their community, not just those that they themselves control, is not new. Sturgess traces it back to a 1984 speech by UK Health Secretary Norman Fowler, and mentions a response a few years later to an Audit Commission report that criticised 'fragmentation and poor coordination between health and social care authorities' – which proposes in response that local authorities act as enablers, rather than deliverers, within their local communities (Sturgess, 2018, p 157).

Sturgess then walks his reader through 30 years of attempts to join up services and delegate decision-making power. He concludes thus: 'None of these attempts at joined-up commissioning has yet proved to be an outstanding success, which demonstrates how difficult it is in a modern society to integrate the diversity of complex human services, based on different policy paradigms, staffed by professionals with different backgrounds, and delivered by agencies reporting to different governments and ministers with competing priorities' (Sturgess, 2018, p 163).

Political drivers

From time to time, these bureaucratic dilemmas find their way into political discourse. Some of the rhetoric being used around the current shift in thinking has popped up in political narratives, which could also be a driver of the change. But the party-political ownership of the ideas is ambiguous and contested. In 2009, before becoming prime minister, David Cameron famously stated that 'our alternative to big government is the big society'. In the Hugo Young lecture that year, he set out a vision that contains many of the elements we recognise in the practice we are seeing ten years on: the state

> must help families, individuals, charities and communities come together to solve problems. [...] The first step must be a new focus on empowering and enabling individuals, families and communities to take control of their lives [...] we can give people power over the services they use. (Cameron, 2009)

Surprisingly, though, the ideas must be untainted by this association, because some of the most active proponents of the approach are in Labour councils. Most of the ten places that the Rallying Together research looked at were Labour-run local authorities (Blundell et al, 2019). Other active proponents are part of the Cooperative Councils Innovation Network, which was started in 2013 by Steve Reed, who was Lambeth Council Chief Executive before he changed jobs to become Croydon North's member of parliament (Bibby, 2013). The network now represents 6.6 million citizens and holds an annual directly managed budget of £8.75 billion (Co-operative Councils Innovation Network, 2019a). Though it claims to be non-party political, a quick glance at the 'associate member' page belies this, peppered as it is with local Labour Party logos (Co-operative Councils Innovation Network,

2019b). The network promotes 'councils working in equal partnership with local people to shape and strengthen communities; replacing traditional models of top down governance and service delivery with local leadership [and] genuine co-operation' (Co-operative Councils Innovation Network, 2019c). This is despite the shift in Labour party thinking under Corbyn towards a very different model that looks much more like the top-down 'statism' of old (Labour Party, 2019).

While the ideas may pop up across the political spectrum, it is difficult to argue that there has been no party political driver to the change we are seeing, or that the ideas are yet to be picked up politically.

Citizen demands

A fifth and final explanation attributes the shift to broader social changes, seemingly happening at a faster pace than ever before. The feelings of alienation and anti-establishment sentiment expressed in the Brexit vote manifest at the level of public service delivery too. Many citizens seem to have lost confidence that the government is working in their own interests, and feel they have lost control of the agenda. Alongside this, ever-increasing individualism in the consumer domain is extending to a similar expectation for personalised public services, in direct contrast to the one-size-fits-all universalism promoted in earlier decades. Social media are giving people new opportunities to influence their lives and those of people around them. Is the emerging new practice an attempt by the public sector to adapt to these new expectations? If we do not, might we find ourselves increasingly out of step with the public mood and hamstrung by endless criticism, demotivating our already overstretched workforce?

One way this broader societal shift is showing up in the social sector and local public agencies is in the buzzwords of 'lived experience', 'expert by experience' and 'user voice'. These signify a genuine and laudable attempt to include traditionally marginalised groups in decision-making and to change prevailing power structures that are perceived to exclude their perspective. It stems from a legitimate desire by those who hold power to restore trust in public institutions and give greater control to those whom they aim to help. But we should take care not to return to a time when the voice of one person was taken to be representative of a whole community, or even the whole of society (unless the community or society at large has endorsed them in that role – by electing them, for example). Gen Maitland-Hudson describes the risk eloquently: 'When we each define our own truth, then expertise is necessarily of diminished importance.

The idea of objectivity, the view from outside, loses a great deal of its force. Statistical abstraction, after all, never tells *my* story' (Maitland-Hudson, 2018).

Clearly, there is a need to respond to the urge citizens are expressing to have more say over services that affect them. But we probably need highly informed people with a good understanding not just of individual stories, but also of patterns and trends of data, to make decisions that ensure quality and fairness – to decide the right array of sophisticated health services to meet complex needs, for example. Gen Maitland-Hudson again: 'Social justice, and the common good, rely on the fair distribution of finite resources in necessarily imperfect ways' (Maitland-Hudson, 2018).

Conclusion: where do we go from here?

I started this chapter by cautioning us against being too captivated by old ideas dressed up in snazzy new clothes. I tried to show through my own attempts, and that of others, that the practical work of addressing the social determinants of health locally is messy and incremental, not heroic and revolutionary. But despite this, there are clear drivers behind a genuine change in approach.

So how do we make sure that the current inflection point in public service delivery does not repeat the mistakes of the past? Clearly, there are powerful forces driving people to think about systems holistically and find ways to join up services, collaborate and devolve power to front-line workers and the community. There are bold, and diverse, attempts to put these principles into practice. But we must also beware of making services vulnerable to the very weaknesses that previous rounds of reforms were an attempt to correct.

This means we must meet the challenge of working hand in hand across public services and with citizens themselves to solve collectively defined problems in a place. But we must not do so at the expense of quality and accountability. The risks are real: at worst, the active creation of a postcode lottery, large-scale capture of services by interest groups and easy routes to fraud. Addressing these risks in the new approach will be critical if local authorities want Whitehall to clear the barriers to working in more joined-up ways locally. Ongoing regulation, target-setting and red tape from national government make it harder for localities to put these new ideas into practice. Yet there are many reasons why central government policymakers could yet fail to be convinced. Some will think the ideas have already been tried. Others will consider them too risky as the implementation cannot be controlled from the centre. Still others will dismiss them until they see hard evidence that the approach will produce better outcomes, efficiency or productivity. Setting the ideas in the context of what has come before, and showing how they build on that, is one way of tying the conversation locally to the discourse centrally.

As we face this challenge, we should perhaps recall the economist Marianna Mazzucato's rallying cry to government: 'the state is not just a spender but an investor and risk taker' (Mazzucato, 2018, p 263). We need to be bold, but we need to be pragmatic. Recognising that reform moves in cycles, we should look backwards to look forwards. Understanding where we have come from, and why things are changing, will enable us to slow the swing of the pendulum from one disappointment to another, and ensure we genuinely move forward.

References

Ansell, C. and Gash, A. (2008) 'Collaborative governance in theory and practice', *Journal of Public Administration Research and Theory*, 18(4): 543–71.

Bibby, A. (2013) 'Co-operative councils: the future for local authorities?' Available from: https://www.theguardian.com/social-enterprise-network/2013/mar/22/co-operative-councils-local-authorities [Accessed 31 July 2019].

Blundell, J., Rosenbach, F., Hameed, T. and FitzGerald, C. (2019) 'Are we rallying together? Collaboration and public sector reform', Government Outcomes Lab, University of Oxford, Blavatnik School of Government.

Bonham, C. (2018) 'Building an inclusive community through social capital: the role of volunteering in reaching those on the edge of community', in A. Bonner (ed) *The Social Determinants of Health: An Interdisciplinary Approach to Social Inequality and Wellbeing*, pp 121–34, Bristol: Policy Press.

Cameron, D. (2009) 'The big society', speech given at Hugo Young Lecture, Kings Place (10 November). Available from: https://conservative-speeches.sayit.mysociety.org/speech/601246 [Accessed 31 July 2019].

Co-operative Councils Innovation Network (2019a) 'Our members'. Available from: https://www.councils.coop/about-us/our-members [Accessed 31 July 2019].

Co-operative Councils Innovation Network (2019b) 'Our associate members'. Available from: https://www.councils.coop/about-us/our-associate-members/ [Accessed 31 July 2019].

Co-operative Councils Innovation Network (2019c) 'A network of UK local authorities who are driving global municipal co-operative policy'. Available from: https://www.councils.coop/wp-content/uploads/2019/07/Introducing-the-CCIN.pdf [Accessed 31 July 2019].

Collier, P. (2018) *The Future of Capitalism*, London: Allen Lane.

Department for Work and Pensions (2019) 'Households below average income: an analysis of the UK income distribution: 1994/95–2017/18'. Available from: https://assets.publishing.service.gov.uk/government/uploads/system/uploads/attachment_data/file/789997/households-below-average-income-1994-1995-2017-2018.pdf [Accessed 31 July 2019].

Disley, E., Giacomantonio, C., Kruithof, K. and Sim, M. (2015) 'The payment by results social impact bond pilot at HMP Peterborough: final process evaluation report', RAND Europe as part of Ministry of Justice Analytical Series.

DSRU (Dartington Social Research Unit) (2016) *Transforming Children's Services: Using the Best Evidence to Get it Right for Every Child*, Dartington: DSRU.

Economist (2018) 'Keep the benefits: if universal credit is to succeed, the government must act now'. Available from: https://www.economist.com/britain/2018/10/27/if-universal-credit-is-to-succeed-the-government-must-act-now [Accessed 31 July 2019].

Gould, J. (2018) 'The What Works Network: Five Years On', What Works Network. Available from: https://assets.publishing.service.gov.uk/government/uploads/system/uploads/attachment_data/file/677478/6.4154_What_works_report_Final.pdf [Accessed 11 May 2020]

Haldane, A. (2019) 'The third sector and the fourth industrial revolution', speech given to Pro Bono Economics Annual Lecture, The Royal Society, London (22 May).

Hewett, N. (2018) 'What works to improve the health of the multiply excluded?', in A. Bonner (ed) *The Social Determinants of Health: an Interdisciplinary Approach to Social Inequality and Wellbeing*, pp 265–78, Bristol: Policy Press.

House of Commons (2017) 'House of commons briefing paper no SN05428 charities and the voluntary sector: statistics'. Available from: https://researchbriefings.parliament.uk/ResearchBriefing/Summary/SN05428 [Accessed 31 July 2019].

Kania, J. and Kramer, M. (2011) 'Collective impact', Stanford Social Innovation Review. Available from: http://www.ssireview.org/articles/entry/collective_impact [Accessed 31 July 2019].

Labour Party (2019) 'Democratising local public services: a plan for twenty-first-century insourcing'. Available from: https://labour.org.uk/wp-content/uploads/2019/07/Democratising-Local-Public-Services.pdf [Accessed 31 July 2019].

Lent, A. and Studdert, J. (2019) 'The community paradigm: why public services need radical change and how it can be achieved', London: New Local Government Network. Available from: http://www.nlgn.org.uk/public/wp-content/uploads/The-Community-Paradigm_FINAL.pdf [Accessed 15 May 2020].

Maitland-Hudson, G. (2018) 'It's not me, it's you: why we need objectivity to develop the social economy'. Available from: https://medium.com/@genmh_80488/its-not-me-it-s-you-why-we-need-objectivity-to-develop-the-social-economy-1372daa24803 [Accessed 31 July 2019].

Mazzucato, M. (2018) *The Value of Everything: Making and Taking in the Global Economy*, London: Allen Lane.

Pfeffer, J. and Salancik, G.R. (1978) *The External Control of Organizations: A Resource Dependence Perspective*, New York: Harper & Row.

Phillips, D. (2019) 'Local government finance: chop and change', Institute for Fiscal Studies. Available from: https://www.ifs.org.uk/uploads/a/Presentation/2019-01-16%20%20(David%20Phillips)_1547666389.pdf [Accessed 31 July 2019].

Sturgess, G. (2018) 'Public service commissioning: origins, influences, and characteristics', *Policy Design and Practice*, 1(3): 155–68.

West London Zone (2016) 'Summary of the West London Zone pilot implementation study', West London Zone. Available from: https://www.westlondonzone.org/collective-impact-report-and-annual-accounts [Accessed 31 July 2019]

West London Zone (2018) 'Collective impact in practice', West London Zone. Available from: https://www.westlondonzone.org/collective-impact-report-and-annual-accounts [Accessed 31 July 2019].

Conclusion

Adrian Bonner

The five parts of this book build on ideas developed in the previous volume in the Social Determinants of Health series (Bonner, 2018), which focused on the issues related to health and wellbeing of individuals at the edge of the community.

Throughout the book, various lenses through which local authorities link with central government and with their communities are viewed from the perspectives of health and social care, local authority institutions, social policy and business/management research, the third sector, the private sector and the legal profession. Each of these approaches to understanding the needs of people and enabling them in their local communities has developed over many years.

As noted in Part I, the prolonged attempt to integrate health and social care and to recognise 'health' in all services provided by local councils is reviewed. An emerging approach in these multi-agency strategies is to encourage relationships between people and their communities. A report by Nesta (Wood et al, 2016) highlighted improved outcomes for individuals by person- and community-centred approaches to health and wellbeing, with respect to mental and physical health and wellbeing, National Health Service sustainability and wider social outcomes.

Although public health in the United Kingdom has mainly focused on non-communicable disease in response to modern epidemics of obesity, alcohol-related diseases and the politics of health care, communicative diseases can still have major health, social and economic impacts, as demonstrated by the COVID-19 pandemic, which is rapidly being transmitted across the globe (McKie, 2020). The challenge facing national governments is not restricted to practical issues related to limited diagnostic tools, no vaccines, or treatment, but also includes considerable financial threats to national and global economies. In March 2020, there was a significant drop in investments in world stock markets, on the same scale as the financial crisis of 2008 (Anon, 2020). On 7 May, the Bank of England warned of a historic recession with 3 million Americans filing for jobless claims in the preceding week, a 25% fall in the UK GDP in the January–March quarter, and a possible 14% shrinkage of the UK's GDP in 2020 (Weaden, 2020). On 5 May, despite information indicating that hospital deaths were declining from a daily peak of 800 deaths in English Hospitals on 8 April 2020 (LSHTM, 2020), there were major concerns about the rising numbers of deaths in care homes (Health Foundation, 2020).

In order to develop interrelationships and interdependencies across the various domains within a social determinants of health rainbow model (Dahlgren and Whitehead, 1991) (see Figure 2.1), there needs to be a good understanding and respect for each of these contributions to the health and wellbeing of people and their communities. The primary aims of this book have been to:

- Provide an accessible, interdisciplinary approach to support collaboration across the public, private and third sectors.
- Promote *social determinants of health* perspective in community organising.
- Give an insight into culture change in the management and commissioning of services in the community.
- Explore innovative responses to the challenges being addressed by local authorities provided by elected members, council officers, academic commentators, health and social care policymakers and service managers.

The cultural changes leading to the development of the welfare state and contemporary system transformations are reviewed in Chapters 9 and 18. Innovative approaches that involve shared responsibilities between statutory, third sector, community organisations and the private sector are suggested in Chapters 10, 16 and 17; these approaches demonstrate multisectoral collaborations that are needed to address the highly complex problems, reviewed in the previous volume (Bonner, 2018). These 'wicked issues' (Rittel and Webber, 1973), referred to in Chapters 4, 5, 7 and 13, identify 'a social or cultural problem that is difficult or impossible to solve due to; incomplete or contradictory knowledge, the number of people and opinions involved, the large economic burden, and the interconnected nature of these problems with other problems' (Kolko, 2012).

Poverty, for example, is linked with education, nutrition and the economic status of the family. Policymakers often struggle with these issues. Sometimes an issue is too big and cumbersome and is written off. This is a situation likely to be experienced by local authorities as they juggle with decreasing budgets and seemingly unsolvable issues related to inequality. However, understanding the nature of a specific issue and using an appropriate strategic framework, for example the 'rainbow' model of social determinants of health, can lead to design and planning that can mitigate against the negative consequences of single factor interventions. Complex or 'wicked issues' may be approached from multiple, sometimes competing perspectives and may have multiple possible solutions (Conklin, 2005). In the case of COVID-19 there is an increasing awareness of the impact of this 'wicked' issue on another; climate change (Figueres and Zycher, 2020).

Local authorities are increasingly innovative in calling on resources, including non-financial ones, from elsewhere. In Chapter 8 we read that Wigan Metropolitan Borough Council '[is being] … honest with residents about the challenge we faced and, with humility, asked for their help in delivering services'. Chapter 8 provides examples of how citizens filled the gap left by the rolling back of the state – by donating money and time voluntarily. The emergence of the 'local authority of citizens' is noted by Chasteauneuf in Chapter 16.

Developing collaborations between public, private and the third sector is important in procurement and commissioning processes, a key theme of Part III. This is particularly important in the provision of housing and the support of people across the lifespan (see Chapters 12 and 20). The case for building relationships and partnering is made in Part III, but the apparent shifting of a welfare state to an 'enabling' state presents the challenge of fostering a cultural change to a new relationship between citizens, communities and the state (The Carnegie Trust, 2018). An enabling state clearly requires a fair society and healthy lives (Marmot, 2010).

As noted many times in this book, decreasing funding from central government and increasing demands on their statutory services have resulted in a ten-year period of austerity in which health and social inequalities have widened, as reported in the Marmot Review (Marmot et al, 2020). The anticipated socio-economic impact of the COVID-19 pandemic could exacerbate the financial constraints on councils with ever greater threats to the health and wellbeing of individuals and communities.

In the ten year period of austerity preceding the COVID-19 crisis, many local authorities have radically reduced their social and health services for children and families (Chapter 11) and young people (Chapter 15), concentrating solely on those with the most acute need, those whom they have a legal obligation to support. Bennett, in Chapter 18, suggests that local government has 'retreated from its historical position as the front line of defence against social evils'. There remain major concerns about local authorities' ability to support their communities in the post-COVID-19 period. 'The COVID-19 crisis of 2020 has shown the capacity of local government to mobilise anew around public health issues but its fundamental fiscal and constitutional weaknesses show that a new settlement is needed more than ever' (Bennett, Chapter 18).

Although there are large numbers of reports and reviews aimed at local commissioning policies and practices, there is very little evidence to support the interrelated and interdependent approaches utilising a social determinants of health model that specifically addresses 'wicked issues'. Current issues such as COVID-19, climate emergency, housing and homelessness, and social care highlight the need for a social determinants of health approach to these 'wicked issues'.

The rationale and development of the Centre for Partnering is supported by chapters in this book, provided by authors based in universities involved in these formative discussions and a primary theme in this volume. This will hopefully contribute to this relational approach embracing the public–private and third sectors

References

Anon (2020) 'Coronavirus: global shares suffer worst week since financial crisis', BBC News (28 February). Available from: https://www.bbc.co.uk/news/business-51639654 [Accessed 13 April 2020].

Bonner, A.B. (ed) (2018) *Social Determinants of Health: An Interdisciplinary Perspective on Social Inequality and Wellbeing*, Bristol: Policy Press.

Carnegie Trust (2018) 'Places of kindness with Carnegie UK Trust'. Network of Wellbeing. Available from: http://networkofwellbeing.org [Accessed 13 April 2020].

Conklin, J. (2005) Wicked problems and social complexity', Cognexus Institute. Available from: https://cognexus.org/wpf/wickedproblems.pdf [Accessed 15 May 2020].

Dahlgren, G. and Whitehead, M. (1991) *Policies and Strategies to Promote Social Equity in Health*, Stockholm: Institute for Futures Studies.

Figueres C. and B. Zycher (2020) 'Can we tackle both climate change and Covid-19 recovery?', *Financial Times*, 7 May. Available from: https://www.ft.com/content/9e832c8a-8961-11ea-a109-483c62d17528 [Accessed 15 May 2020].

Health Foundation (2020) 'Care homes have seen the biggest increase in deaths since the start of the outbreak', COVID-19 chart series, The Health Foundation, 5 May. Available from: https://www.health.org.uk/news-and-comment/charts-and-infographics/deaths-from-any-cause-in-care-homes-have-increased [Accessed 15 May 2020].

Kolko, J. (2012) 'Wicked problems: problems worth solving', *Stanford Innovation Review*, 6 March. Available from: https://ssir.org/books/excerpts/entry/wicked_problems_problems_worth_solving [Accessed 15 May 2020].

LSHTM (London School of Hygiene and Tropical Medicine) (2020) 'Peak in COVID-19 deaths occurring in English hospital passed on 8 April', blog post, 27 April. Available from: https://www.lshtm.ac.uk/newsevents/news/2020/peak-covid-19-deaths-occurring-english-hospitals-passed-8-april [Accessed 20 April 2020].

McKie, R. (2020) 'Coronavirus. The huge unknowns'. Available from: https://www.theguardian.com/world/2020/feb/15/coronavirus-the-huge-unknows-by-robin-mckie [Accessed 13 April 2020].

Marmot, M. (2010) 'Fair society, healthy lives', The Marmot Review, Institute of Health Equity. Available from: http://www.instituteofhealthequity.org/resources-reports/fair-society-healthy-lives-the-marmot-review [Accessed 8 April 2020].

Marmot, M., Allen, J., Boyce, T., Goldblatt, P. and Morrison, J. (2020) 'Health equity in England: the Marmot review 10 years on'. London: Institute of Health Equity. Available from: http://www.instituteofhealthequity.org/resources-reports/marmot-review-10-years-on/the-marmot-review-10-years-on-full-report.pdf [Accessed 10 April 2020].

Rittel, W.J. and Webber, M.M. (1973) 'Dilemmas in a general theory of planning', *Policy Sciences*, 4(2): 155–69.

Weaden, G. (2020) 'Bank of England warns UK faces historic recession; US jobless claims hit 3.1 m-business live', *The Guardian*, 7 May. Available from: https://www.theguardian.com/business/live/2020/may/07/bank-of-england-interest-rates-covid-19-downturn-us-job-losses-business-live. [Accessed 15 May 2020].

Wood, S., Finnis, A., Khanand, H. and Ejbye, J. (2016) 'Realising the value: ten key actions to put people and communities at the heart of health and wellbeing'. Available from: https://www.health.org.uk/sites/default/files/RtVRealisingTheValue10KeyActions.pdf [Accessed 13 April 2020].

Appendix:
COVID-19 timeline

31 December 2019   A cluster of cases of pneumonia reported by the Wuhan Municipal Health Commission in China

4 January 2020   First recorded case of COVID-19 outside China, in Thailand

28 January 2020   The UK Foreign and Commonwealth Office updates its travel advisory, advising against all but essential travel to mainland China

31 January 2020   First recorded case of COVID-19 in the UK

2 March 2020   The government holds a COBRA (Civil Contingencies Committee) meeting to discuss its preparations and response to the virus, as the number of UK cases jumps to 36

3 March 2020   The government publishes its action plan for dealing with COVID-19. This includes scenarios ranging from a milder pandemic to a severe prolonged pandemic and warns that a fifth of the national workforce could be absent from work during the peak

5 March 2020   First death in the UK confirmed
Chief Medical Officer Chris Whitty, announces that the UK is moving to the second stage of dealing with COVID-19, from the 'containment' to the 'delay' phase

9 March 2020   FTSE 100 plunges again by over 10%, its biggest drop since 1987, with other markets around the world being similarly affected by the ongoing economic turmoil
UK Chief Medical Officers raise the risk to the UK from moderate to high
The UK advises people to work from home if possible and to avoid visiting public places
Public Health England stops performing contact tracing, as widespread infections overwhelm capacity

15 March 2020	Health Secretary Matt Hancock says that every UK resident over the age of 70 will be told 'within the coming weeks' to self-isolate for 'a very long time' to shield them from COVID-19
16 March 2020	Prime Minister Boris Johnson advises everyone in the UK against 'non-essential' travel and contact with others, to work from home if possible, and to avoid visiting social venues such as pubs, clubs or theatres. He urges pregnant women, people over the age of 70 and those with certain health conditions to consider the advice 'particularly important', and says they will be asked to self-isolate within days. The Department for Digital, Culture, Media & Sport states 'it is advised that large gatherings should not take place'
17 March 2020	Chancellor of the Exchequer Rishi Sunak announces that £330 billion will be made available in loan guarantees for businesses affected by the virus The Foreign and Commonwealth Office advises against all non-essential international travel due to the pandemic and the border restrictions put in place by many countries in response The UK government provides a £3.2 million emergency support package to help rough sleepers into accommodation
18 March 2020	The government announces that all schools in the country will shut from the afternoon of Friday, 20 March, except for those looking after the children of key workers and vulnerable children
19 March 2020	In an emergency move, the Bank of England cuts interest rates again, from 0.25% to just 0.1%, the lowest rate in the Bank's 325-year history The government announces £1.6 billion to help local authorities with the cost of adult social care and support for the homeless, and £1.3 billion to the NHS and social care so that up to 15,000 people to be discharged from hospital

20 March 2020	Sunak announces that the government will pay 80% of wages for employees not working, up to £2,500 a month, as part of 'unprecedented' measures to protect people's jobs Johnson orders all cafes, pubs and restaurants to close from the evening of 20 March, except to provide take-away food. All the UK's nightclubs, theatres, cinemas, gyms and leisure centres are told to close 'as soon as they reasonably can'
22 March 2020	Johnson warns that 'tougher measures' may be introduced if people do not follow government advice on social distancing
23 March 2020	In a televised address, Johnson announces a UK-wide partial lockdown to contain the spread of the virus. The British public is instructed to stay at home, except for certain 'very limited purposes' – shopping for basic necessities; for 'one form of exercise a day'; for any medical needs; and to travel to and from work when 'absolutely necessary'. The restrictions to come into force on 26 March
24 March 2020	Health Secretary Matt Hancock announces the government will open a temporary hospital, the NHS Nightingale Hospital at ExCel Centre in London, to add extra critical care capacity
26 March 2020	The Health Protection (Coronavirus, Restrictions) (England) Regulations 2020 (SI 350) (the 'Lockdown Regulations') come into effect, significantly extending the range of businesses that are required by law to close with immediate effect, including all retail businesses not on an approved list. These regulations also include significant restrictions on freedom of movement: 'no person may leave the place where they are living without reasonable excuse' The government announces that some self-employed people will be paid 80% of profits, up to £2,500 a month, to help them cope during the economic crisis

27 March 2020	Johnson and Hancock both test positive for COVID-19
3 April 2020	NHS Nightingale Hospital London opens at ExCel Centre in East London, employing NHS staff and military personnel, with 500 beds and potential capacity for 4,000. It is the first of several such facilities planned across the UK
4 April 2020	Keir Starmer is elected as the leader of the Labour Party
6 April 2020	Johnson is taken into intensive care at St Thomas' Hospital. It is announced that First Secretary of State Dominic Raab will deputise for him
16 April 2020	Raab announces a three-week extension to the nationwide lockdown measures as the number of confirmed COVID-19 cases in the UK surpasses 100,000
17 April 2020	Sunak extends the subsidised wage scheme for furloughed workers for another month, to the end of June
18 April 2020	Care England, the UK's largest care homes representative body, estimates that as many as 7,500 care home residents may have died because of COVID-19, compared to the official figure of 1,400 released a few days earlier Communities Secretary Robert Jenrick announces a further £1.6 billion in support for local authorities, on top of the £1.6 billion given on 19 March Jenrick says that the virus appears to be having a 'disproportionate impact' on the Black, Asian and minority ethnic (BAME) communities
23 April 2020	The first human trials of a COVID-19 vaccine in Europe begin in Oxford
27 April 2020	The government announces that the families of NHS and care workers who die because of COVID-19 will be entitled to a payment of £60,000

2 May 2020	Jenrick announces £76 million of funding to help vulnerable people, including children, victims of domestic violence and modern slavery, who may be 'trapped in a nightmare' during the lockdown restrictions
5 May 2020	The number of recorded deaths rises by 693 to 29,427, giving the UK the highest number of COVID-19 related deaths in Europe
7 May 2020	The Bank of England warns that the economy is on course to shrink by 14% in 2020 because of the impact of COVID-19, pushing the UK into its deepest recession on record
10 May 2020	The UK government updates its coronavirus message from 'stay at home, protect the NHS, save lives' to 'stay alert, control the virus, save lives'
13 May 2020	The Health Protection (Coronavirus, Restrictions) (England) (Amendment No.2) Regulations 2020 (SI 500) come into effect, allowing the re-opening of garden centres, sports courts and recycling centres. In addition to outdoor exercise, open-air recreation is also permitted with no more than one member of another household

Figure A.1: The Route Plan to opening UK society and the economy

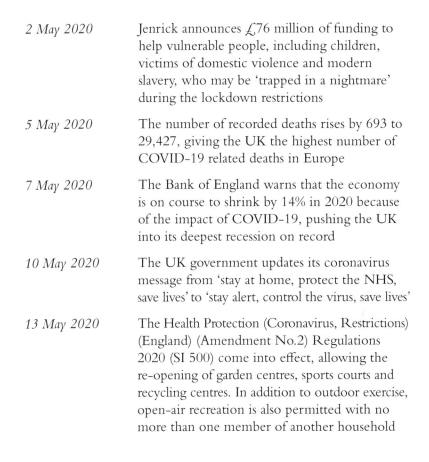

Note: R = [replication value] 0.5–0.9 on 10 May 2010.
Source: Bienkov and Colson, 2020

29 May 2020	Sunak announces that the Coronavirus Job Retention Scheme will cease at the end of October. Before then, employers must pay National Insurance and pension contributions from August, then 10% of pay from September, increasing to 20% in October. Self-employed people whose work has been affected by the outbreak will receive a 'second and final' government grant in August
1 June 2020	The Health Protection (Coronavirus, Restrictions) (England) (Amendment No.3) Regulations 2020 (SI 558) come into effect. Car and caravan showrooms, outdoor sports amenities and outdoor non-food markets may reopen. The prohibitions on leaving home are replaced by a prohibition on staying overnight away from home, with certain specific exceptions. Gatherings of people from more than one household are limited to six people outdoors and are prohibited entirely indoors, with exceptions including education. There are further exemptions for elite athletes
6 June 2020	Anti-racism demonstrations are held in cities across the UK; attendees are reported to be in the thousands
8 June 2020	Rules requiring travellers arriving into the UK to quarantine for 14 days come into force
9 June 2020	Business Secretary Alok Sharma confirms that all non-essential retailers in England can reopen from Monday, 15 June providing they follow safety guidelines. However, pubs, bars, restaurants and hairdressers must wait until 4 July 'at the earliest' to reopen. Johnson announces that zoos and safari parks will also reopen on 15 June
11 June 2020	Figures from the Office for National Statistics indicate those under the age of 30 have been hardest hit by a fall in income during the COVID-19 outbreak

12 June 2020	Office for National Statistics figures indicate deprived areas have been hit twice as hard by the COVID-19 pandemic when compared to more affluent areas. The impact has also been greater in urban areas compared to rural areas, with London experiencing the highest number of deaths per 100,000 inhabitants
13 June 2020 and 15 June 2020	The Health Protection (Coronavirus, Restrictions) (England) (Amendment No.4) Regulations 2020 (SI 588) come into effect
18 June 2020	The Bank of England announces plans to inject an extra £100 billion into the UK economy to help fight the downturn precipitated by the pandemic
19 June 2020	The UK's COVID-19 Alert Level is lowered from Level 4 (severe risk, high transmission) to Level 3 (substantial risk, general circulation). Figures from the Treasury show that UK debt stands at £1.95 trillion, making it larger than the economy for the first time in 50 years
29 June 2020	Following a spike in COVID-19 cases in Leicester, Hancock announces the reintroduction of stricter lockdown measures for the city, including the closure of non-essential retailers from the following day, and the closure of schools from 2 July
6 July 2020	The UK government announces grants and loans of £1.57 billion to support theatres, galleries, museums and other cultural venues affected by the COVID-19 outbreak. As concerns about increasing unemployment grow, the UK government announces a £111 million scheme to help firms in England provide an extra 30,000 trainee places, and £21 million to fund similar schemes in Scotland, Wales and Northern Ireland

8 July 2020	Sunak unveils a £30 billion spending package aimed at mitigating the economic impact of the pandemic, including a temporary reduction in VAT for the hospitality sector, a scheme to pay firms £1,000 for each employee brought back from furlough, a scheme to get young people into employment, and a temporary rise in the stamp duty threshold
9 July 2020	The Institute of Fiscal Studies warns that taxes will have to rise to pay off the support measures put in place by the government
11 July 2020 and 13 July 2020	The Health Protection (Coronavirus, Restrictions) (No 2) (England) (Amendment) Regulations 2020 come into effect, allowing outdoor swimming pools and water parks, nail bars and salons, tanning booths and salons, spas and beauty salons, massage parlours, tattoo parlours, and body and skin piercing services to re-open
15 July 2020	Johnson confirms an independent inquiry will be held into the handling of the pandemic, but says it would not be right to devote 'huge amounts of official time' to an inquiry while the pandemic is ongoing. A temporary cut in VAT worth £4 billion comes into force until 12 January 2021 as a means of helping the food and hospitality industries
17 July 2020	Johnson announces a further easing of lockdown restrictions for England, with plans for a 'significant return to normality' by Christmas. The new rules allow people to use public transport for non-essential journeys with immediate effect, give employers more discretion over their work places from 1 August, and give local authorities the power to enforce local shutdowns from 18 July
18 July 2020	Local authorities in England get new powers to close shops and outdoor public spaces, and to cancel events in order to control COVID-19.

21 July 2020	Sunak announces that 900,000 public sector workers, including doctors and teachers, will get an above-inflation pay rise of 3.1% in acknowledgement of the important role they have played during the pandemic
23 July 2020	A report published by the House of Commons Public Accounts Committee criticises the UK government for its 'astonishing' failure to plan for the economic impact of the COVID-19 pandemic
24 July 2020	Face coverings become compulsory in shops and most other enclosed public places in England
25 July 2020	Public Health England warns that being obese and overweight puts people at greater risk of severe illness or death as a result of COVID-19
19 August 2020	The Prime Minister announced that Public Health England would be abolished and replaced by the National Institute for Health Protection

Further reading

Anon (2020) 'Coronavirus: global shares suffer worst week since financial crisis', BBC News, 28 February. Available from: https://www.bbc.co.uk/news/business-51639654 [Accessed 13 April 2020].

Figueres, C., and Zycher, B. (2020) 'Can we tackle both climate change and Covid-19 recovery?', *Financial Times*, 7 May. Available from: https://www.ft.com/content/9e832c8a-8961-11ea-a109-483c62d17528 [accessed 28 July 2020].

Health Foundation (2020a) 'Care homes have seen the biggest increase in deaths since the start of the outbreak', COVID-19 chart series. The Health Foundation, 5 May. Available from: https://www.health.org.uk/news-and-comment/charts-and-infographics/deaths-from-any-cause-in-care-homes-have-increased [accessed 28 July 2020].

Health Foundation (2020b) 'COVID-19 policy tracker: A timeline of national policy and health system responses to COVID-19 in England', 4 July. Available from: https://www.health.org.uk/news-and-comment/charts-and-infographics/covid-19-policy-tracker [accessed 28 July 2020].

HMG (Her Majesty's Government) (2020) 'Guidance and Support', COVID-19 guidance updates. Available from: https://www.gov.uk/guidance/coronavirus-covid-19-information-for-the-public [accessed 28 July 2020].

McKie, R. (2020) 'Coronavirus: the Huge Unknowns', *The Guardian*, 15 February. Available from: https://www.theguardian.com/world/2020/feb/15/coronavirus-the-huge-unknows-by-robin-mckie [Accessed 13 April 2020].

References

Bienkov, A. and Colson, T. (2020) 'Boris Johnson has revealed his "road map" for ending the UK coronavirus lockdown', *Business Insider*, 11 May. Available from: https://www.businessinsider.com/boris-johnson-road-map-to-ending-the-uk-coronavirus-lockdown-2020-5?r=US&IR= [accessed 28 July 2020].

Index

Note: Page numbers for figures and tables appear in italics.